Handbook of Occupational and Environmental Medicine

Handbook of Occupational and Environmental Medicine

Edited by Kirk Anderson

AMERICAN
MEDICAL PUBLISHERS
www.americanmedicalpublishers.com

American Medical Publishers,
41 Flatbush Avenue,
1st Floor, New York,
NY 11217, USA

Visit us on the World Wide Web at:
www.americanmedicalpublishers.com

ISBN: 978-1-63927-449-9

Cataloging-in-Publication Data

Handbook of occupational and environmental medicine / edited by Kirk Anderson.
p. cm.
Includes bibliographical references and index.
ISBN 978-1-63927-449-9
1. Medicine, Industrial. 2. Environmental health. 3. Occupational diseases.
4. Occupational therapists. I. Anderson, Kirk.
RC963.3 .O33 2022
616.980 3--dc23

Table of Contents

Preface

Occupational medicine is a branch of medicine that deals with the maintenance of health in the workplace. It includes the prevention and treatment of diseases and injuries. It is dynamic in the field of occupational health and safety and aims to prevent diseases and promote wellness among workers. Environmental medicine, on the other hand, is an interdisciplinary field that involves the discipline of medicine, chemistry, environmental science, etc. Environmental medicine is concerned with the prevention of food-borne and water-borne infections. Some of the factors involved in causing environmental diseases are physical, chemical, biological and social factors. The scope of this domain comprises of the interaction between human health and the environment and the role the environment plays in causing and mediating diseases. This book studies, analyzes and upholds the pillars of occupational and environmental medicine and its utmost significance in modern times. It presents researches and studies performed by experts across the globe. Students, researchers, experts and all associated with these domains will benefit alike from this book.

The information shared in this book is based on empirical researches made by veterans in this field of study. The elaborative information provided in this book will help the readers further their scope of knowledge leading to advancements in this field.

Finally, I would like to thank my fellow researchers who gave constructive feedback and my family members who supported me at every step of my research.

Editor

1

Pulmonary injury associated with spray of a water-based nano-sized waterproofing product

Paul T. J. Scheepers[1*], Lucie Masen-Poos[2], Frits G. B. G. J. van Rooy[3], Arné Oerlemans[1], Eline van Daalen[1,6], Robbert Cremers[1,7], Hera Lichtenbeld[4], Bonne Biesma[2], Jorid B. Sørli[5], Ismo K. Koponen[5], Søren Thor Larsen[5], Peder Wolkoff[5] and Asger W. Nørgaard[5]

Abstract

Background: In most reported cases of lung trauma with water proofing products, volatile organic compounds (VOC) have a prominent role. Here we report on a case involving ten workers exposed to a sprayed product containing nanoparticles in a water solution with only a few percent VOC.

Case presentation: Ten workers suffered from respiratory symptoms following spray impregnation of hardwood furniture using a waterproofing product that contained positively charged fluorinated acrylate copolymer solid cores with a median diameter of 70 nm (1.3 w%) in aqueous suspension with 3.3 w% VOC and 0.3 w% quaternary ammonium. The worker who applied one liter of the product in a wood workshop, using an air mix spray gun, did not report any health complaints. Another worker, who entered the workshop 3 h later and had rolled and smoked two cigarettes, was hospitalized with severe chemical pneumonitis. A chest X-ray (CXR) showed bilateral infiltrative impairment in the lower lobe regions. On the next day a second CXR showed increased patchiness marking in all fields. A high-resolution Computer Tomography (CT)-scan demonstrated extensive bilateral areas of ground-glass opacities predominantly in the lower regions of the upper lobes, the right middle lobe and the apical regions of the lower lobes, compatible with severe chemical pneumonitis. On the following morning, nine workers in an adjacent workplace in the same building, experienced dry cough, chest tightness and substernal pain upon physical exercise. Reconstruction of the spray application in a climate chamber confirmed trimethyl silanol, glycol ethers and fluoroalkenes in the gas phase. Immediately after the spray application, aerosols were observed at a maximum concentration of 6.3×10^4 cm^{-3}. Mass concentrations were 0.095 and 10 mg/m^3 in the size ranges 5.6-560 nm and 0.22-30 µm, respectively, decreasing to less than 10 $\mu g/m^3$ in both size ranges after 15 h.

Conclusion: The hospitalized worker had smoked cigarettes contaminated with fluoropolymers which is a plausible explanation for the lung trauma. Respiratory symptoms in the nine workers may be caused by inhalation of particles that became airborne by resuspension from surfaces when workers entered the adjacent workplace the next day. A contribution from VOC appears less likely because measurements and modelling showed that concentrations in the mg/m^3 range could have occurred only if the building was assumed to be completely airtight.

Keywords: Chemical pneumonitis, Exposure reconstruction, Inhalation injury, Occupational accident, Waterproofing

* Correspondence: paul.scheepers@radboudumc.nl
[1]Research Lab Molecular Epidemiology, Radboud Institute for Health Sciences, Radboudumc, PO Box 9101, 6500 HB Nijmegen, The Netherlands
Full list of author information is available at the end of the article

Background

Waterproofing products are used to coat textile fabric, leather or solid surfaces to ensure water and dirt resistance. These products usually contain three key components: a water repellent (active compound), a solvent and a propellant (if the product is canned). The water repellent is generally a mixture of siloxanes or acrylate polymers – both with fluorocarbon or hydrofluorcarbon chains. In products marketed before 2000, the solvent used to be an aliphatic hydrocarbon and sometimes chlorinated or cyclic hydrocarbons were used [1–3]. Nowadays, aqueous mixtures of glycols and glycolethers are often used as solvents [4, 5]. Propellants are usually C_3-C_4-alkanes or CO_2 (Additional file 1: Figure S2).

Over the past 20 years, different health effects from the use of waterproofing agents have been described in approximately 20 reports involving exposure of over 200 individuals. The first report is from 1983 and described a case in the US of a consumer who used a 1,1,1-trichloroethane-based product [1]. Other reports describe cases with a variety of products, containing trimethylpentane solvent and paraffins [6], ethyl acetate and n-heptane [3] and petroleum hydrocarbons [7]. Most case-reports did not describe the product composition [2, 8–12]. Overall, these cases report mostly local effects on the airways and dyspnea with dry cough as the common denominator. However, tachypnea, tachycardia and mild cyanosis was also reported [6, 7, 10, 13, 14]. Only a few cases reported a slight increase of body temperature and only one study reported neurotoxic signs [5]. There is wide consensus that the use of propellants such as propane and butane isomers does not represent a hazard [2, 15]. In most case reports, the active fluorinated compounds were implicated as the agents responsible for the acute pulmonary response [2, 3, 7, 14, 16]. Only the first reported case of an intoxication [1] suggested the organic solvent 1,1,1-trichloroethane as the primary cause of the pulmonary complaints. More recent reports suggest involvement of an organic solvent to explain some of the specific local and systemic effects [5]. A change of isopropanol to heptane as a solvent was implicated as a probable cause of acute respiratory symptoms in a Swiss incident, but in this case the type of fluorocarbon resin used was also changed, along with the solvent [4]. In an incident in a supermarket alkylsiloxanes and C_9-C_{13} alkanes were involved [17]. Recently, two studies associated the airway toxicity of a perfluorinated silane with the number of hydroxyl groups in addition to the properties of the used solvent [18, 19].

Most of the aforementioned reports suggest that health complaints arise from inhalation of spray aerosols. Some studies suggest that the particle size and number characteristics of inhaled sprays could play a role in the acute pulmonary toxicity [2, 5, 20, 21]. Waterproofing agents that interact with the thin film of liquid covering the alveoli implicate lung surfactant deterioration as the cause of the respiratory problems [6, 17, 19–28]. Some authors have also made reference to "polymer fume fever", that has been observed after inhalation of pyrolysis products of e.g., polytetrafluoroethylene (Teflon) [2, 6, 29]. Two case reports described the use of waterproofing product in conjunction with smoking [11, 12].

In this study we describe the results from two reconstructions of the spraying process of wood coating with the purpose of identifying the potential causative agents.

Case presentation

Product application

The incident occurred in an occupational setting and relates to a self-employed carpenter (person A). Co-exposures involved his wife (person B) and a hired mechanic (person C). At 17.00 h on the day of the incident, a carpenter (person A, a non-smoking male of 47 y) treated two tabletops (approximate surface area of 2 m^2) with a waterproofing product (cf Table 1 for information on the composition). The spray application was performed in a wood workshop for the production of hardwood furniture with a volume of ca. 2.600 m^3 (h x l x w = 4 × 32.5 × 20 m) without mechanical ventilation (Additional file 1: Figure S1). One liter of the product was sprayed undiluted at a distance of approximately 0.5 m from the surface over a period of 4 min using an air mix spray gun (Eminex type E31 EHT M 01 with a 1.80 mm nozzle diameter, Eminent, Oss, NL) at a pressure of 2 bar. No gloves or respiratory protection was used. No other chemicals than the waterproofing product were used. During spraying, person A did not report any smell. Around 18:15 person B, the wife of the carpenter (non-smoker, 43 y) arrived and spent approximately 15 min in the workshop (see Additional file 1: Table S1 for a complete timeline). Both person A and person B reported not to have seen any mist or noticed

Table 1 Formulation of the waterproofing product as reported by the producer

Component	CAS[a]	Fraction (w%)
Water	7732-18-5	95.3
Fluoroalkyl ethyl acrylate co-polymer	–	1.3
Propylene glycol	504-63-2	1.3
Alcohols, C12-C14-secondary, ethoxylated	84133-50-6	1.3
Dipropylene glycol monomethyl ether	34590-94-8	0.3
Polyethylene glycol trimethylnonyl ether	84133-50-6	0.3
Quaternary ammonium compounds, bis(hydrogenated tallow alkyl)dimethyl chlorides	61789-80-8	0.3
Polyether (not specified)	–	0.1

[a]Chemical identification corresponding to CAS number reported in ChemIndex list of synonyms http://ccinfoweb.ccohs.ca/chemindex/search.html)

any unusual smell nor did they experience any health problems. At 19:45, person C, a mechanic (male, smoker of 5-20 cigarettes/day, 40 years of age) arrived to do some repair work. He spent about 10 min in the room where the tables had been sprayed. He also did not notice any spray mist or smell and was not wearing any skin or respiratory protection. Around 20:30 he spent another 15 min in the workshop repairing a milling machine. He did not have direct contact with the treated table tops. He picked up and used a vernier caliper that was lying around (at least) 10 m from the treated tabletops. During his work he did not wear gloves. He did not remember if his hands were somehow contaminated when returning to the office. Around 22:00 he rolled two cigarettes. He did not notice any strange smell or taste when smoking these cigarettes outside. At 23:15 he experienced serious dyspnea and asphyxiation (perceived as if 'drowning') and reported to the emergency room of the local hospital.

Secondary exposure

In the same building, next to the wood workshop, a mail sorting and distribution centre was located. This workshop (h x l x w = 4 × 30 × 20 m) had also no forced ventilation. There was an open air (space) connection near the roof of 0.1 m over a distance of about 20 m in a brick wall between the wood workshop and the mail sorting and distribution centre (see Additional file 1: Figure S1). The first worker who entered the building at 7:45 on the day after the application of the waterproofing spray, did not observe any mist or unusual smell. But around 8:30 he started to cough and by 10:00 another eight workers reported a painful and persistent dry cough. Some of them also reported chest tightness and sub-sternal chest pain upon physical exercise. Neither the employer nor the workers had been informed about the incident that had occurred in the wood workshop on the day before. On the morning of the second day after the incident the workers still suffered from cough; however, anamnesis and physical examination of four workers by an occupational physician did not reveal any abnormalities of respiratory function. During the following days the workers did not feel well, reporting fatigue and weakness. After a week all workers had fully recovered and had returned to their work. The outdoor weather conditions on the day of the incident and the day of the second exposure are presented in Additional file 1: Table S2.

Physical examination

Person C had no history of respiratory disease or pre-existing sensitivity, asthma or allergy. Upon arrival in the emergency room at 23:30 he suffered from dyspnea, cough and produced clear sputum. He felt cold, reported impaired vision, his hands were shaking and he also reported a tingling sensation in his extremities. Blood pressure was 125/61 mmHg and his pulse rate was 105/min. His body temperature was 39.0 °C that normalized within 6 h. Blood saturation was 93% on a non-rebreathing oxygen mask (15 L/min) and decreased to 60% rapidly without respiratory support. Heart sounds were normal and airway examination by stethoscope indicated vesicular respiratory sound on both sides. Analysis of a venous blood sample showed a leukocytosis (19.1·109/L) and an elevated C-reactive protein content (CRP, 57 mg/L), rising to a maximum of 112 mg/L on the third day of hospital admission. A chest X-ray (CXR) was taken at 2:00 in the night of admission (not presented). A high resolution computed tomography (HRCT) thorax (Fig. 1) indicated extensive bilateral areas of ground-glass opacities and predominantly in the lower regions of the upper lobes, the right middle lobe and the apical regions of the lower lobes. There were no signs of honeycombing. An aspiration pneumonitis as most probable course was suggested by the radiologist.

No antibiotics were given as, from the start, a pneumonitis due to chemical exposure was found to be the most likely diagnosis. During his stay at the emergency unit and afterwards at the pulmonology ward the Netherlands poison centre (NVIC) was contacted several times. Treatment was started and prednisolone was tapered after consultation of the poison centre. Person C was treated with oxygen, Salbutamol (2.5 mg) and

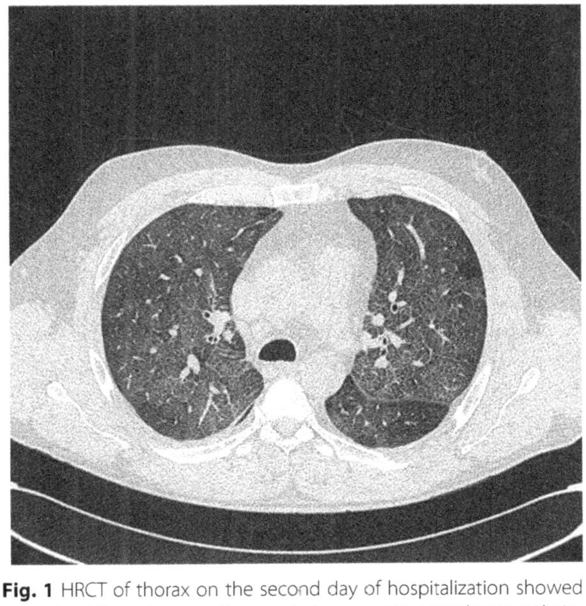

Fig. 1 HRCT of thorax on the second day of hospitalization showed extensive bilateral areas of ground-glass opacities predominantly in the lower regions of the upper lobes, the right middle lobe and the apical regions of the lower lobes, compatible with severe chemical pneumonitis

Atrovent (500 μg) by inhalation and received 50 mg of prednisone i.v. four times a day. The patient remained hypoxic with desaturation upon physical exercise, for a week. Recovery was slow, but oxygen supply could gradually be reduced. The patient was dismissed from the hospital five days after the incident and then followed-up in the outpatient clinic for another three weeks. Lung function showed a minimal obstruction: FVC 3.99 L (91% predicted), FEV1 2.89 L (80% predicted). FEV1/FVC 73.3 (92% predicted), and TLCO 7.56 mmol/min/kPa (74% predicted). Treatment with prednisone was gradually reduced and terminated within two weeks at the outpatient clinic. Two weeks after admission the patient did not report any airway complaints. The blood oxygen saturation was 96% without oxygen supplement and the CXR appeared normalized (not presented).

Methods

Chemicals

2-(2-Butoxyethoxy) ethyl acetate, decamethyl tetrasiloxane, di(propylene glycol) methyl ether (mixture of isomers), 2-ethylhexyl acrylate, hexamethyl disiloxane, methanol, 2-(2-methoxypropoxy)-1-propanol, 1H,1H,2H-perfluoro-1-decene, 1H,1H,2H,2H-perfluorodecyl acrylate, 1H,1H,2H,2H-perfluoro-1-octanol, toluene, trimethyl silanol were obtained from Sigma Aldrich (Brøndby, Denmark). 1H,1H,2H-perfluoro-1-tetradecene was obtained from Synquest Laboratories, Alachua, FL. All chemicals were of the highest available purity (98-99.9%).

Waterproofing product

The label of the product indicated it was water-based. According to the user's instructions it would make wooden surfaces water and dirt resistant and explain how it should be applied. The product was advertised for surface treatment of hardwood furniture (for both indoor and outdoor use). The label did not contain symbols referring to any health or environmental hazards, but the product contained the following phrases (translated from Dutch/French): 'Keep out of range of children; prevent direct contact with skin and eyes; use only in a well-ventilated area; store in closed bottle; do not induce vomiting if swallowed and consult a physician and show the package and label; we do not accept liability in the case of wrong use; attention: store frost-free'. The label did not provide further information about the composition, e.g. fluorinated compounds or nanoparticles. The manufacturer provided information about the formulation of the product to the authors (Table 1). On the label, instructions were given to rub the product on the surface using a cloth. However, in this case the product was sprayed by use of a spray gun.

Analysis of the product showed presence of nano-sized spheres with a median diameter of ca. 72 nm, with strong hydrophobic properties and with a slight positive charge (zeta potential of +31.3 mV, see Additional file 1: Figure S2-S5). These particles formed a stable suspension in water with a negligible tendency to form clusters. The particles were chemically characterized as water-free solid organic silica cores, with a soft shell consisting of tri-block-copolymers containing perfluoroalkyl acrylate, in addition to polyethylene oxide and polypropylene oxide, and presumably end-capped with ethylene oxide.

Reconstruction of spray incident

In order to obtain information about the emission of volatile organic compounds (VOC) and aerosols during and after application of the product, spray tests were carried out under different test conditions in two different test chambers (Experiments 1 and 2). Experiment 1 was carried out at 6-fold the concentration of the incident; Experiment 2 at 46-fold higher concentration for the evaluation of larger particles and collection of particle samples for further analysis (not presented here). In both experiments, the spray gun (Eminex type E31 EHT M 01, Eminent, Oss, NL) was equipped with similar nozzles and operated at the same spray pressure (2.0 Bar) as the one originally used in the wood workshop on the day of the incident.

Experiment 1

In this experiment, 47 g of product was sprayed in a uniform layer on a 0.6 m^2 untreated plywood surface placed inside a climate steel chamber (h x l x w = 2.29 × 3.46 × 2.56 m) with an ante-chamber (2.72 m^3) as inner entrance. The experiment was carried at a ventilation, temperature and relative humidity of 0.08 ± 0.03 h^{-1}, 22 ± 2 °C and 45 ± 5%, respectively. Immediately after the start of the experiment, three mixing fans were turned on for 60 s in order to ensure a homogeneous distribution of aerosols and VOC. The fans were placed in three corners on the floor and at 5 cm from the chamber wall. VOC were sampled through a 10 mm stainless steel sampling manifold placed at a height of 1.0 m from the floor and ca. 1.2 m from the spray position; air was sampled at 5 cm from the inner chamber wall. During the first 5 h, samples were taken in duplicate at 10-30 min intervals, starting the first sampling event 1 min after the spray application was initiated. Additional samples were taken after 23 and 25.5 h, following the start of the spray application, respectively. The time of sampling is given as the midpoint between start and end of each sampling period. VOC data are reported as mean of duplicates, corrected for chamber background air and rounded to the nearest integer. VOC were sampled on clean Tenax TA (60-80 mesh) adsorbent tubes (200 mg) with a sampling time of 10 min at 100 mL/min, using calibrated pumps (Gillian Gilair 5, Sensidyne, US). The

Tenax TA tubes were analyzed on a Perkin Elmer Turbo Matrix 350 thermal desorber (TD) coupled to a Bruker SCION TQ GC-MS system (Bruker Daltonics, Bremen, DE). Tube desorption was carried out at 275 °C for 20 min and the low and high temperatures of the cryo trap were −20 °C and 280 °C, respectively. Separation was performed on a 30 m GC column with 0.25 mm internal diameter and 0.25 μm film thickness (type VF-5MS, Agilent Technologies, Santa Clara, US). The oven program was as follows: 50 °C for 4 min, ramp 1: 4 °C/min to 120 °C, ramp 2: 50 °C/min to 250 °C, hold for 2 min. Helium was used as carrier gas at an inlet pressure of 0.97 bar (1.5 mL/min). The mass spectrometer was operated in SIM/scan mode using either electron ionization or chemical ionization with methane (5.0) as ionization gas. Argon of ultrahigh purity (99.999%) was used for collision induced dissociation (CID) experiments. Valves, transfer lines and ion source were kept at 270 °C. Six-point calibration was applied (r^2 > 0.99) using authentic standards in methanol. Identification of observed VOC was based on retention time and mass spectra of authentic standards, when applicable, in addition to library search [29], chemical ionization and CID.

Number size distribution measurements were conducted using a TSI Model 3091 Fast Mobility Particle Sizer (TSI, Shoreview, NM). The instrument was operated at 1-s time resolution in a measurement range of 5.6-560 nm. An optical particle spectrometer Grimm 1.109 (Grimm Aerosoltechnik, Ainring, Germany) was used to measure the number size distribution from 0.25 to 32 μm at 6 s time resolution (count distribution mode). Total number concentration was integrated from the number size distribution. Spherical SOA particles with a density of 1.0 g/ml was assumed for mass calculations. In addition, a density of 2.6 g/ml was used for comparison of mass results with experiment 2 measurements where an environmental mode was used (in the environmental mode a default density of 2.6 g/ml was also used to calculate mass concentration).

Experiment 2

In this experiment, ca. 0.7 l of the product was sprayed 'mid air' inside a 40 m^3 paint booth (h x l x w = 4.0 × 4.0 × 2.5 m) during a period of 10 min. During the last 2 min of spraying, the spray booth was turned off to allow the particles to remain in the booth and to describe the time-resolved post-spraying changes in particle size. Aerosol mass size distribution spectra in the size range from 0.25 to 32 μm were measured using a Grimm 1.109 operating at a time resolution of 6 min. The instrument was set to occupational mode (PM-10, PM-2.5, PM-1.0 in μg/m^3). A nephelometer (type IV Hazdust, Environmental Devices, Plaistow, NH, USA), equipped with a cyclone pre-seperator, was used for collection of the thoracic fraction (equivalent to PM-10) at a 10-s time resolution.

Filter samples were collected twice; the first period of 0-50 min after the start of application and a second period of 1-16 h after application. Inhalable dust was collected using an IOM sampler and a calibrated personal air sampling pump (A.P. Buck, Orlando, Florida, USA) at 2.0 L/min. A similar set-up was used to collect respirable particles by a Cassella cyclone (Cassella Measurement, Bedford, UK) at 1.9 L/min. Thoracic dust and respirable dust fractions were collected using PM-10 and PM-2.5 Harvard impactors, respectively, at 10.0 L/min. The filter samples were collected 2.0 m from the spray application at height of 1.2 m from the floor. All filters used were Teflon membrane filters (Sartorius, Göttingen, Germany).

Modelling

A two compartment model was constructed using Simulink/MatLab. This model was used to estimate the time pattern of VOC in the wood workshop and the mail sorting and distribution centre.

The air concentrations of VOC were modelled using the measurement data from experiment 1. The modelling was carried out by use of the data from total glycol ether which was by far the most abundant of measured VOCs. The initial concentration of the glycol ethers at the start of the spray application in the wood workshop was calculated to be 46 mg/m^3, using a standard spray scenario of the exposure model ConsExpo 5.0 (www.rivm.nl/en/Topics/C/ConsExpo). The inter-compartment flow (Qi) in the open air connection with the dimensions of 20 × 0.1 m (2.0 m^2) was estimated to be 7200 m^3/h for an air speed of 1 m/s (1 m/s × 2.0 m^2 = 2 m^3/s = 7200 m^3/h). We then estimated the concentration in the wood workshop over time by adopting an algorithm used by Vernez et al. [30]:

$$C_1 = \int \frac{1}{V_1} (Qi*C_2 - Qi*C_1 - Q*C_1) \quad (1)$$

where C_1 is the concentration in the wood workshop (initial concentration 46 mg/m^3),

C_2 is the concentration in the mail sorting centre (initial concentration 0 mg/m^3),

V_1 is the volume of the wood workshop (2600 m^3),

Q is the air exchange rate with outdoor air (0.08 h^{-1}, 1.0 h^{-1} and 2.5 h^{-1}),

Q_i is the inter-compartment flow (7200 m^3/h).

A second equation was used to calculate the concentrations over time in the mail sorting centre:

$$C_2 = \int \frac{1}{V_2} (Qi*C_1 - Qi*C_2 - Q*C_2) \quad (2)$$

where C_1 is the concentration in the wood workshop (initial concentration 46 mg/m^3),

V_2 is the volume of the mail sorting centre (2400 m^3),

C_2, Q and Qi are the same as in eq. (1).

The initial concentration in the mail sorting centre was assumed to be zero. As the complaints of the mail workers started at 8:00 am the next morning, we calculated the concentration at 15 h after the start of the spray event. We modelled three different air exchange rates. The first value of 0.08 h^{-1} is the air exchange rate of the measuring chamber and corresponds to a more or less airtight building. The other two values represent more realistic values to describe the type of naturally ventilated industrial building that is usually not very air tight, a low estimate of 1.0 h^{-1}, corresponding to a low natural ventilation in a situation with low wind speed and closed doors and a high value of 2.5 h^{-1} to a moderately ventilated building with doors opened and at moderate wind velocity conditions. The real situation was probably in the range between these two conditions.

Results

The concentration time-pattern following the spray application was followed in two separate experiments. Experiment 1 describes the results of a small-scale reconstruction in a measuring room, using only a small amount of product and focuses on submicron particles and VOC. Experiment 2 describes the use of a larger volume of the product in a spray booth. In this experiment the thoracic and respirable fractions were measured by optical instruments and filter sampling. The results of both experiments will be discussed below.

Experiment 1

Use of the wood impregnation product resulted in an instant release of VOC, mainly trimethyl silanol, glycol ethers, fluoroalkyl compounds and a siloxane (see Table 2 and Figs 2 and 3). Trimethyl silanol, the glycol ethers and the siloxane reached maximum concentrations of 1.6 mg/m^3, 1.6 mg/m^3 and 0.4 mg/m^3, respectively, within the first ca. 15 min after the spray event (Fig. 3a). Hereafter, the compounds decayed to concentrations of 9 µg/m^3, 80 µg/m^3 and 10 µg/m^3, respectively, after 23 h. The concentration of the fluoroalkyl compounds (Fig. 3a and b) were dominated by 1H,1H,2H-perfluoro tetradecene and peaked between 1 and 1.7 h after the spray event. After a plateau, lasting about 1 h, all fluoroalkyl compounds decayed from a total maximum concentration of 0.6 to 0.03 mg/m^3, after 23 h.

Figure 4a shows the number and mass concentration-time pattern for particles below 560 nm. An increase in the total number concentrations from 5.0 to 63 × 10^3 cm^{-3} was observed immediately after the spray event. During the next 3 min, the particle number concentration about halved, followed by a slower decay, presumably due to wall losses and ventilation. The concentration returned to the initial background in 10 h after spraying.

The mass concentration increased from 5 to 95 µg/m^3 during the first 2 min after the spray application, followed by a sharp decrease to 57 µg/m^3 after 4 min. This was followed by a decay due to chamber ventilation, resulting in a concentration corresponding to the pre-experiment value of ca. 2 µg/m^3, after ca. 24 h. The mass concentration did not decrease as fast as the number concentration during the first 1 h. Figure 4b presents

Table 2 Compounds identified in the gas phase after use of the wood impregnation product in Scenario 1. C_{max} and T_{max} are the maximum concentration and time of the maximum concentration, respectively

Peak	T_r (min)	Compound	CAS	Max conc. (µg/m^3)	Max conc. (µg/m^3 per g product)	T_{max} (min)	Boiling point (°C)	Vapor pressure (mbar)
1	1.7	Trimethyl silanol	1066-40-6	1582	33.7	5	99	21.0[c]
2	2.0	1H,1H,2H-perfluoro-1-decene	21652-58-4	31	0.7	16	146	8.5[d,e]
3	2.2	Hexamethyl disiloxane	107-46-0	392	8.3	16	100	56[d]
4	3.1	1H,1H,2H-perfluoro-1-dodecene[a]	30389-25-4	83[b]	1.8	60	202	1.3[d,e]
5	5.8	1H,1H,2H-perfluoro-1-tetradecene	67103-05-3	363	7.7	71	253	0.3[d,e]
6	8.0	1H,1H,2H,2H-perfluoro-1-octanol	647-42-7	97	2.1	16	90	0.5[d,e]
7	9.7	1H,1H,2H-perfluoro-1-hexadecene[a]	–	68[b]	1.4	102	–	–
8-10	10.6-11.3	Di(propylene glycol) methyl ether, mixture of isomers	34590-94-8	1581	33.7	5	203	0.13[d,e]
11	11.7	2-(2-methoxypropoxy)-1-propanol	13588-28-8	2	<0.1	5	190	0.67[d]
12	12.8	Decamethyltetrasiloxane	141-62-8	18	0.4	49	235[e]	0.13[d,e]
13	14.5	1H,1H,2H,2H-perfluorodecyl acrylate	27905-45-9	7	0.1	5	268	0.13[d,e]
14	19.5	2-ethylhexyl acrylate	103-11-7	8	0.2	16	233	0.13[d,e]
15	22	2-(2-butoxyethoxy)ethyl acetate	124-17-4	135	2.9	5	232[e]	0.13[d,e]

[a]) No standard; [b]) 1H,1H,2H-Perfluoro-1-decene equivalents; [c]) at 20 °C; [d]) at 25 °C; [e]) predicted values ACD/labs

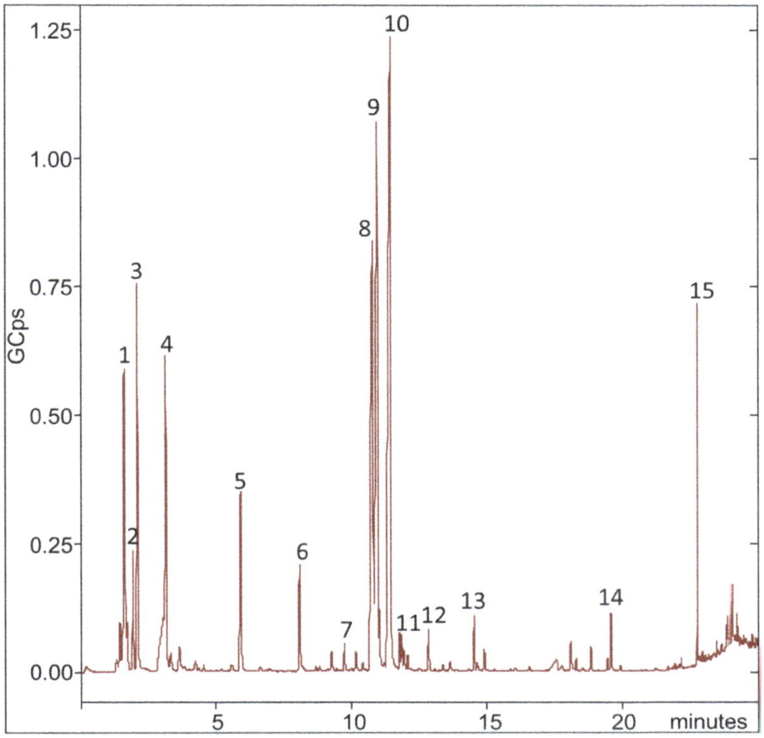

Fig. 2 Total ion chromatogram (TIC) showing VOCs emitted to the gas phase 5 min after spraying 47 g of the product on a 0.6 m^2 untreated wooden surface in Experiment 1 (see Table 2)

the evolution of the number size distribution over 24 h with 1 min time resolution. The initial particle number size mode shows a peak around 100 nm that appears relatively stable during the entire 24 h measurement period.

Experiment 2

The mass concentration profiles of aerosols are shown for PM-10, PM-2.5 and PM-1.0 in Fig. 5. When turning on the ventilation of the booth, the particle concentration dropped sharply and increased again when the spraying started. After shutting down the ventilation system at 16:25, the concentration of PM-10 peaked 16 min after spraying started at about 100 mg/m^3 at 16:36; this was confirmed by the Hazdust measurement (inset in Fig. 5). The particle concentration gradually decreased due to the room ventilation of the building until this system was automatically shut off at 19:00 h. This time point matches the delay of ~2.5 h after the spray application when worker C was first exposed. At this time point the concentrations of PM-10, PM-2.5 and PM-1.0 were 32, 26 and 14 μg/m^3, respectively. Over the period between 20:00 h and 1:00 h the three aforementioned PM fractions had very similar time-weighted average concentrations of 10, 9 and 8 μg/m^3, respectively. The concentrations of PM-10, PM-2.5 and PM-1.0 stabilized at 12, 8 and 4 μg/m^3, respectively. After the room ventilation was turned on at 7:00 the concentrations of all aforementioned particle fractions decreased rapidly to about 3 μg/m^3 at 8:00 h.

The particle mass size distributions shown in Fig. 6a and b suggest that the particles produced during spraying are of the thoracic size fraction. Due to settling of coarse particles the relative contribution of respirable particles and specifically submicron particles increased over a time frame of 5 h. In the first period after the spray application there is a considerable contribution from particles with a size of about 0.5 μm but they are lost due to evaporation or agglomeration.

The particle concentrations were also measured by filter sampling (results not presented) and show that the time-weighted average concentrations of inhalable, thoracic and respirable dust were high during the first 50 min after the start of the spraying. Over the post-exposure period the concentrations were much lower and approached levels, which corresponded to levels often observed as a normal background for a workplace in a production environment.

Modelled vapour concentrations

In Fig. 7 three scenarios are presented with three different air exchange rates. The concentration time pattern

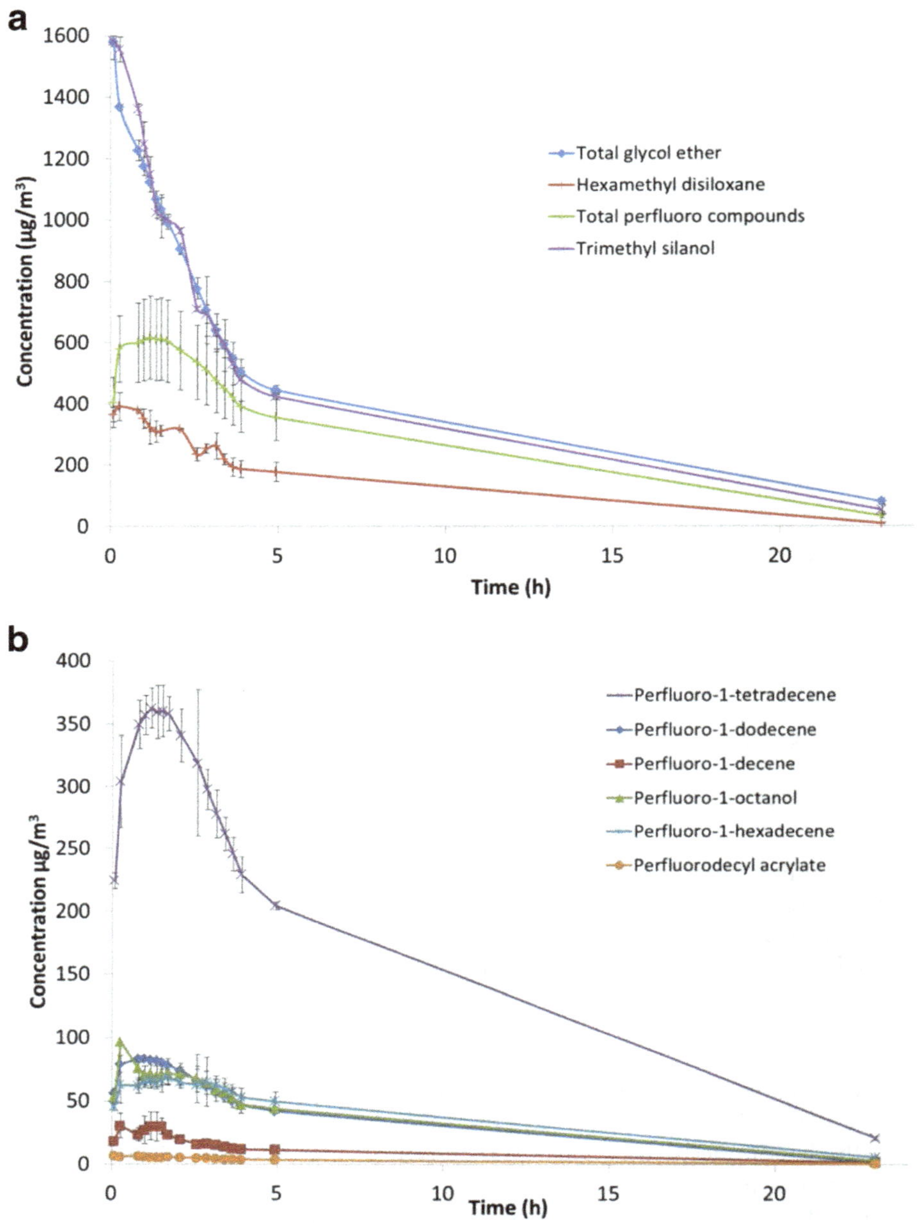

Fig. 3 Time-concentration profiles of trimethyl silanol (peak 1) total glycol ether (peaks 8-10), total fluoro compounds (peaks 2, 4-7 and 13) and hexamethyl disiloxane (peak 3) (**a**); time-concentration profiles of fluoro compounds (**b**)

concentration for the most abundant VOC was modelled in the wood workshop and in the mail sorting and distribution centre. In the wood workshop the concentration decreased lognormally. In the mail sorting centre the concentration increased rapidly until a peak is reached within 1-2 h. Then the concentration decreased in a similar way as in the wood workshop. The assumption of the air exchange rate has a profound influence on the concentration in the mail sorting room 15 h following application of the product in the wood workshop. At this time point we estimate a concentration of 7.2, 7.3 × 10^{-6} and 1.2 × 10^{-16} mg/m^3, corresponding to a respective assumed air exchange rate of 0.08, 1.0 and 2.5 h^{-1}.

Discussion and conclusion

In a recent review of health effects from exposure to waterproofing products (Hays and Spiller, 2014) [31] it is suggested that new formulations of fluropolymer sprays lead to formation of smaller particles. It is suggested that this is in line with the general understanding that ultrafine particles with a low water solubility have toxic properties [31–33]. Hays and Spiller [31] argued

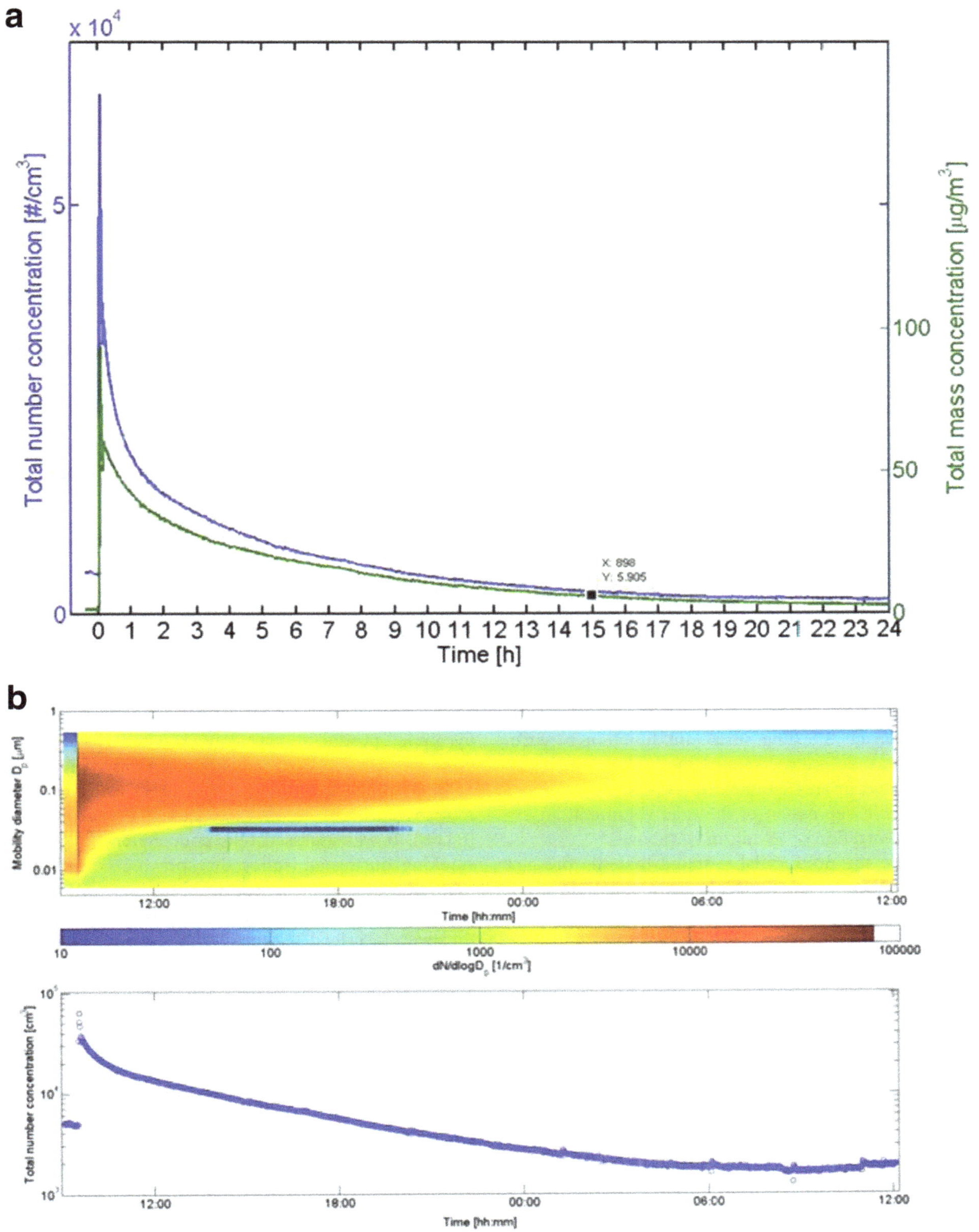

Fig. 4 **a** Total number and mass concentration (density 1) calculated from the FMPS measurements in Scenario 1; $t = C$ refers to the start of spraying. **b** Particle number size distribution and particle number concentration as the function of time

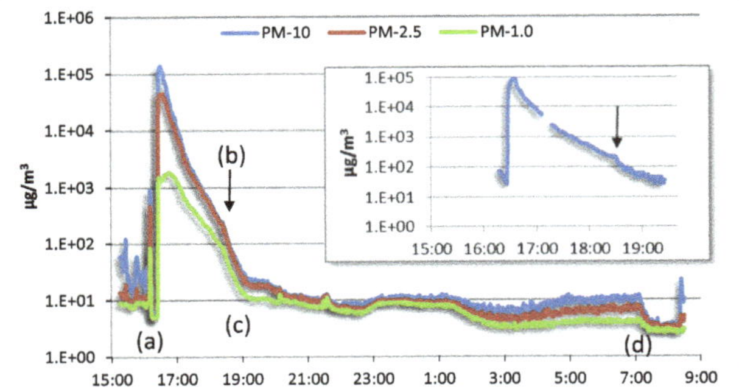

Fig. 5 Concentration of three particle fractions in µg/m^3 on a timescale representing local clock time during experiment 2. The inset shows the simultaneous registration of the concentration of the thoracic fraction (PM-10). (**a**) Paint booth ventilation turned on at 15:50 h; (**b**) increased ventilation due to a thunderstorm past over Nijmegen between 18:30 and 19:00 h causing a sudden decrease in dust concentration (see inset); (**c**) The ventilation system was shut off at 19:00. (**d**) The ventilation system is turned on at 07:00 h the next morning

that the increasing particle size of some fluoropolymer fumes was associated with a reduction in toxicity. A smaller particle size will also allow the product to reach deep into the lungs, to the alveoli and respiratory bronchioles that are covered by a thin liquid film of lung surfactant [34, 35]. The product used in the wood workshop has previously been tested in an assay assessing lung surfactant function in vitro and in a mouse bioassay. The breathing pattern of mice exposed to the product was monitored (referred to as "Wood impregnation" in Sørli et al. [17]. The waterproofing product was found to damage the lung surfactant function in vitro. Furthermore, it severely damaged the lungs of mice exposed to "wood impregnation". This was seen as a rapid and irreversible depression of the tidal volume at an exposure concentration of 39 mg/m^3 or above.

In our case the product label stated that the product should be rubbed on the surface using a cloth. However, the product label did not contain an explicit warning not to spray the product. The spraying of the product in the wood workshop left the applicant (person A) and his wife (person B) unaffected but caused a serious chemical-induced pneumonia in a mechanic (person C) who entered the workshop ca. 2-3 h later. On the next day (ca. 15 h after spraying) another nine workers in an adjacent room of the building suffered from mild airway symptoms. The prevailing wind direction supported the assumption of transfer of vapours and airborne particles by infiltration from the wood workshop into the mail sorting centre through a 2.0 m^2 open air connection in the wall. No exposures other than the use of the waterproofing product could be identified to explain the observed health complaints. The labor inspector found no chemicals in the wood workshop and the fire brigade did only detect organic vapours at low levels using a photoionization detector. A psychogenic mechanism in the occurrence of health complaints in the nine mail workers could be ruled out because the employer and the workers of the mail sorting area were unaware of the occupational accident that had occurred in the wood workshop the previous day.

Remarkably, the exposure of persons A-C showed an almost dichotomous response; person C was severely affected by a 30 min exposure with a latency of 2-3 h following the moment of spray application. This is in contrast to the unaffected persons A and B. Aside from the different exposure times, person C was an active smoker, as opposed to persons A and B. The response of the smoker is in accordance with some previously reported cases. For instance, a 25-yrs. old woman developed severe dyspnae, cough and slight fever 5 h after having used a waterproofing spray [8]. Following the spraying, she had smoked a cigarette with spray-contaminated fingers. The thermal degradation products were suggested to cause the severe hypoxemia and leukocytosis that was observed in the clinical examination. CXR and CT showed diffuse infiltration in both lungs and patchy alveolar infiltration. In another case, seven out of 13 workers reported symptoms of cough, fever, chills, aching and weakness after the application of a fluorocarbon polymer. Four of the seven workers reported shortness of breath. Those with symptoms, considered to be polymer fume fever, were all smokers, whereas most of the nonsmokers were without symptoms. The authors considered exposure to pyrolysis products via contaminated cigarettes to cause the symptoms [36]. In a third case, workers developed polymer fume fever after using a mold-release spray containing a polytetrafluoroethylene (PTFE). It was assessed that poor general hygiene and smoking during and after the spraying contributed to the symptoms [37]. A previously healthy 21-year old man who was machining PTFE, presented symptoms that were ascribed to polymer fume fever. The symptoms occurred suddenly while smoking a cigarette 2 h after leaving his workplace. The cigarette was from a pack that had been open and was lying next to his work station [38].

In experiments conducted in 1962 by DuPont, cigarettes were spiked with PTFE in doses ranging from 0.05 to 0.4 mg. Forty volunteers participated in the experiment. It was shown that smoking a cigarette spiked with 0.4 mg of PTFE induced polymer fume fever in 9 out of 10 subjects [39]. In a recent review of the literature, Hays and Spiller [31] conclude that specific precautions such as dermal protection and frequent hand washing is recommended to avoid the formation of pyrolysis products to be formed as a results of poor personal hygiene related to tobacco smoking.

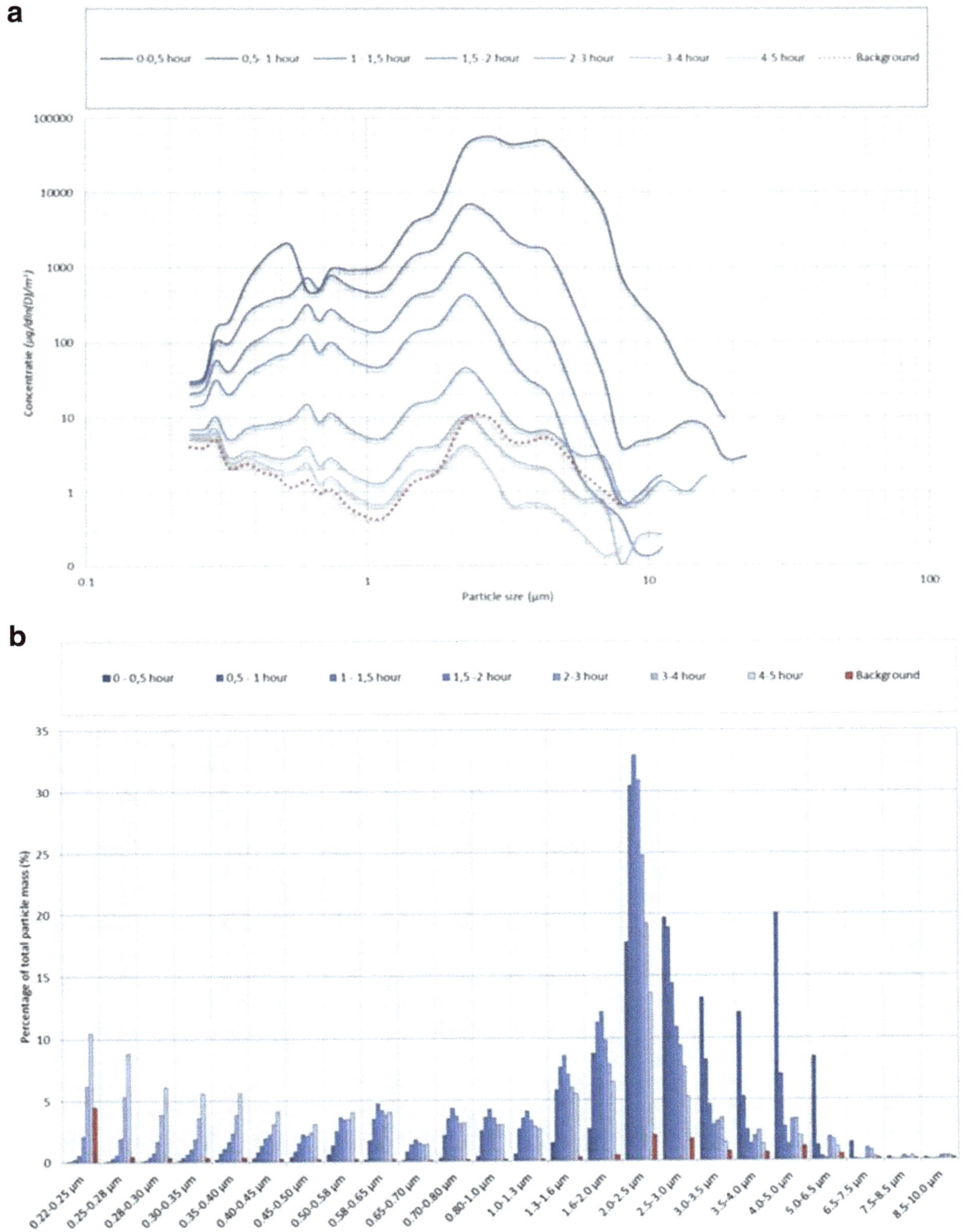

Fig. 6 (See legend on next page.)

(See figure on previous page.)
Fig. 6 Optical particle size distributions (experiment 2). **a** Particle mass size distribution at time intervals of 30 min. This distribution was recorded in the spray booth during 30 min prior to the start of the spray application (red dotted curve). **b** Relative change of the contribution of each channel to the total measured mass concentration with a time interval of 30 min. The relative contribution of the background to each channel is presented for reference (red bars)

Person C did not wear gloves when performing the repairs in the wood workshop where the waterproofing product had been sprayed. Although person C did not notice any contamination on tools or surfaces and declared not to have been in direct contact with the treated table top, we suggest that it is likely that his hands became contaminated with the waterproofing product due to handling of tools and touching of machinery. We suggest that during the break, person C rolled cigarettes with contaminated fingers. When smoking these cigarettes perfluorinated contamination in the cigarettes became pyrolized, followed by inhalation during smoking. It is a fair assumption that surfaces in the workplace had been covered with the product from a wide deposition in the work environment. This assumption is supported by the rapid decrease of the contribution of particles with a mass median aerodynamic diameter (MMAD) of 2.5 to 6.5 μm in the first half h after the application (Fig. 6b). The soiling of surfaces with the product is likely enhanced by the positive charge of the perfluorinated nanospheres in the product.

A similar case of secondary exposure involved eleven workers with severe dyspnea [17]. These workers had been exposed following an open air discharge of pyrolysis products from fluorocarbon monomers at a distance of 35 m between 20:00 and 0:00. Perfluoroisobutylene, hydrogen fluoride, hexafluoropropylene, tetrafluoroethylene, chlorotrifluoroethylene were detected in the sub mg/m^3 range, 22 h after the release. Five workers were diagnosed with an acute respiratory distress syndrome

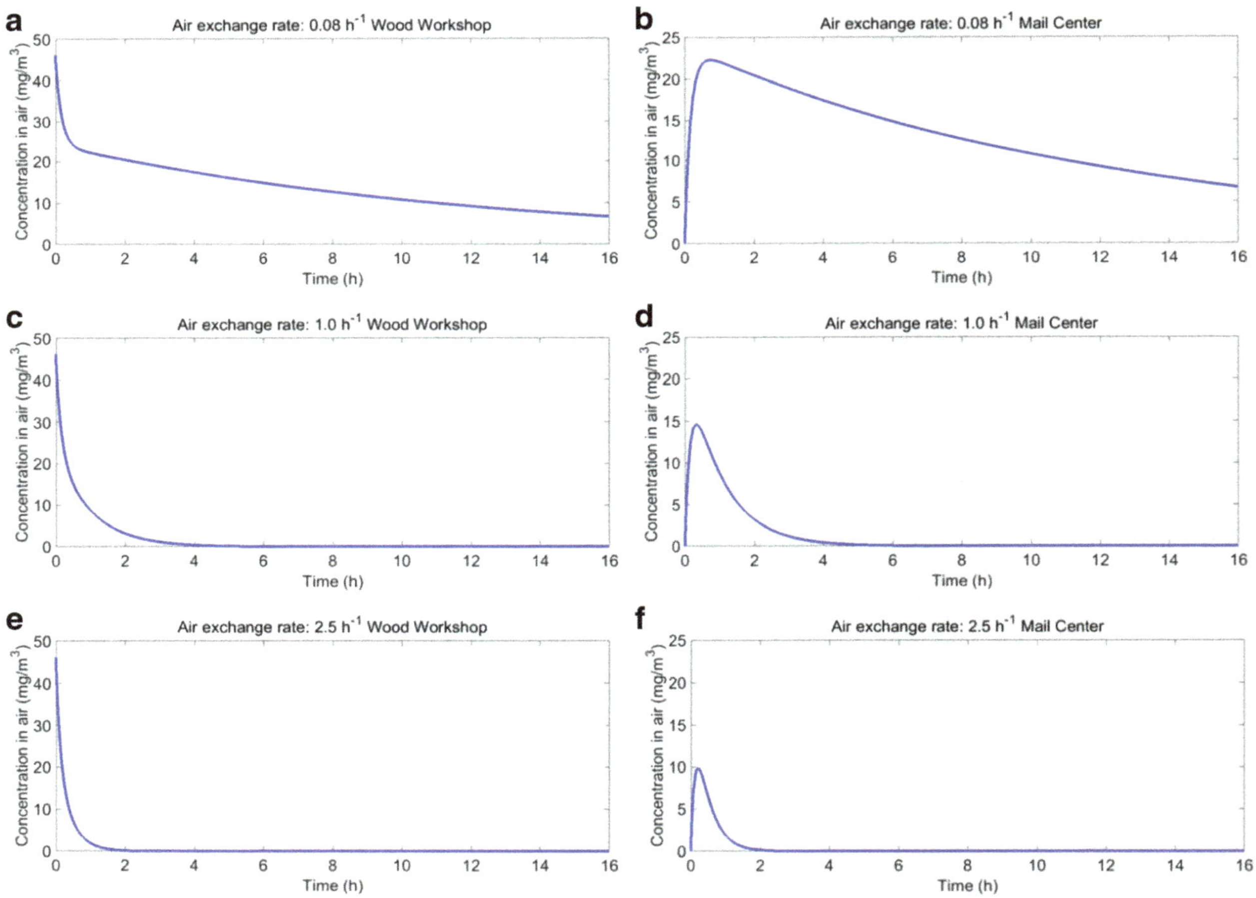

Fig. 7 Concentration time pattern for the most abundant VOC (glycol ether) for three scenarios with different air exchange rate for both the wood workshop (**a**, **c** and **e**) and the post sorting room (**b**, **d**, **f**). The assumed air exchange rates were 0.08 h^{-1} (**a**, **b**), 1.0 h^{-1} (**c**, **d**) and 2.5 h^{-1} (**e**, **f**)

(ARDS). One worker died of pneumonia and four surviving workers showed bilateral ground-glass opacities on their initial CT scans and displayed interstitial pneumonia, which gradually improved, similar to our case. No information on exposures to airborne particulate matter was reported. In addition to the direct exposure to polymer fumes, the smoking history and its effects on bronchial or alveolar inflammation or surfactant composition, may also interact with the exposure to the waterproofing product. In similar cases it was seen that exposure to a water repellent product, interacted with underlying idiopathic pulmonary fibrosis, resulting in a fatality [40]. To our knowledge there were no pre-existing health issues that may have contributed to condition of our patient. As he was 40 years old at the time of the event, pre-existing idiopathic pulmonary fibrosis is very unlikely. Furthermore, during his last outpatient visit the chest X-ray demonstrated no remaining abnormalities (a HR-CT scan however was not repeated).

In our case, respiratory symptoms were also reported by the group of postal workers, who were exposed 15 h after application of the product. It is suggested that the draft caused by an outdoor wind speed of 3-4 m/s from the South to South East (see Additional file 1: Table S2 for a full account of the weather report) pushed the overspray cloud of particles from the wood workshop to the mail sorting centre through the 2.0 m^2 open air connection in the wall separating the two adjacent rooms. Such behavior of waterproofing product aerosols was observed in other studies [23]. Based on our observations in Experiment 2 these particles must have deposited within the hour on tables and floors in the mail sorting centre. On the treated table top the aerosols would merge and polymerize and form a hard top coating. However, in this case the aerosols were dispersed over a wide surface, lost water and remained droplets with polymer and residual fluoro-compounds potentially absorbed on other deposited dust particles. When the workers entered in this work area on the next morning it is likely that when they started working, these deposited particles became airborne through resuspension and were subsequently inhaled. Exposure to coarse dust from hard floors is known to cause particles exposure peaks when they are resuspended from the floor by persons entering an indoor environment [41, 42]. It is suggested that these particles (that were initially derived from the aqueous product) had completely dried out and became water insoluble solid fluoropolymer cores that may have been causative of the effects in the airways as described (see Additional file 1: Figure S7). If the dust particles penetrated deeply into the lungs, they may have inhibited lung surfactant function, causing the workers symptoms. In their case Tan et al. [28] indicated that the pyrolysis products that had been released in open air 'entered the workshop through ventilation holes on the top of the building's wall'; thus the workers had been exposed during the night and were then admitted to hospital after their shift (an exact time was not reported) [17]. It was indicated that (similar to our case) the workers were not warned by odor or visual smoke, and they had been exposed for several hours during their shift before symptoms occurred. The first symptoms of dry cough and increasing dyspnea symptoms indicated hospital admittance. There are some similarities with our case, e.g. the setting (smoker entering a work space, no alert, latency in onset of symptoms, type of symptoms); however, an important difference is that Tan et al. reported emissions from pyrolysis products, including hydrogen fluoride and much smaller fluorocarbon monomers as much smaller gas phase components [29], than we identified in our reconstruction [17]. Moreover, both the exposure type and level and the spectrum of health effects, including a fatal outcome, indicate a much more severe incident.

In a recently reported incident a group of 43 persons were exposed to a tile coating product that was applied using a high pressure airless spray gun in a supermarket in Greenland [23]. Of this group 39 were admitted to the hospital in Nuuk for evaluation. The product contained C_9-C_{13} alkanes and alkylsiloxanes but no fluorinated compounds. Similar to our case most of the victims were exposed in the same building for less than 2.5 h and some far from the primary source of application (on another floor). Some of them entered the building after cessation of the spray event. They were not warned by odor or by irritating properties of the product. In contrast to our case on the day after the use of the product, surfaces in most of the building were visibly contaminated. In this incident half of the victims were workers and most of them smoked. The spray gun operator and two other workers with high exposure had more severe respiratory symptoms with a decreased oxygen saturation and in two bilateral perihilar infiltrates on CXR were observed. The most common health effects were an onset of dry cough (39/39) and shortness of breath (29/39) within 1-12 h after the incident but with normal oxygen saturation.

An interesting observation in our case is the complete lack of health effects in the applicant. The over spray did not cause any complaints. It must be assumed that the freshly sprayed product consisted primarily of coarse aqueous aerosols with 5% of organic substances (consistent with the product formulation, see Additional file 1: Table S1), and, thus, was not causing an airway response.. We suggest that this situation differed from the situation in the mail sorting centre in the sense that in this case the workers inhaled the (presumably much smaller) dried solid water-insoluble fluoro copolymer particles (see Additional file 1: Figure S7).

In conclusion, we have investigated reported health effects occurring ca. 3 and 15 h after use of a wood impregnation product, respectively. We believe that the lung trauma in the by-stander can be explained by inhalation of pyrolysis products from smoking contaminated cigarettes. The secondary exposure was most likely caused by inhalation of fluoropolymers adsorbed on paper dust particles that became airborne after deposition. This product was marketed as a consumer product not intended for spraying. The product label did not contain any safety sentences and did not refer to possible health or environmental risks. Afterwards, the manufacturer changed the label to include a warning not to spray the product. Also the producer informed the authors that the product in its current composition was withdrawn from the market by the end of 2012.

Abbreviations

CID: Collision induced dissociation; CRP: C-reactive protein; CT: Computer tomography; CXR: Chest X-ray; FEV1: Forced expiratory volume in one second; FVC: Forced vital capacity; HRCT: High resolution computed tomography; IOM: Institute of Occupational Medicine; NIST: National Institute of Standardization and Testing; SIM: Selected ion monitoring; SOA: Secondary organic aerosol; SVOC: Semivolatile organic compounds; TD-GC-MS: Thermal desorption gas chromatography mass spectrometry; TLCO: Carbon monoxide transfer factor of the lung; VC: Vital capacity; VOC: Volatile organic compounds

Acknowledgements

The authors would like to acknowledge the workers who helped to understand what happened. We are indebted to the fire brigade officer, labor inspector and occupational physician who shared their views with the authors. We would like to thank Thom Oostendorp who assisted with the modelling work.

Funding

This was a shared cost project of the Radboud Institute for Health Sciences, Nijmegen, The Netherlands and the National Research Centre for the Working Environment, Copenhagen, Denmark.

Authors' contributions

PS investigated the occupational incident and wrote the case report. LMP and BB described the medical history and treatment of the patient. EvD performed a literature study of previous reported cases. HL supported the physicochemical characterization of the product. RC performed sample collection and data analysis for Experiment 1. AN, IK, IP, STL and PW performed Experiment 2 with related sample collection and chemical and data analysis. AO and PS performed the modelling. PW, JBS and FvR participated in discussions during the preparation of the manuscript. All authors read and approved the final manuscript.

Competing interests

The authors declare that they have no competing interests.

Author details

[1]Research Lab Molecular Epidemiology, Radboud Institute for Health Sciences, Radboudumc, PO Box 9101, 6500 HB Nijmegen, The Netherlands. [2]Department of Lung Diseases, Jeroen Bosch Hospital, 's-Hertogenbosch, The Netherlands. [3]Arbo Unie Expert Centre for Chemical Risk Management, Utrecht, The Netherlands. [4]Oxility BV, Best, The Netherlands. [5]The National Research Centre for the Working Environment, Copenhagen, Denmark. [6]Present address: Ministry of Social Affairs and Employment, The Hague, The Netherlands. [7]Present address: Witteveen+Bos Consulting, The Hague, The Netherlands.

References

1. Woo OF, Healey KM, Sheppard D, Tong TG. Chest pain and hypoxemia from inhalation of a trichloroethane aerosol product. J Toxicol Clin Toxicol. 1983; 20:333–41.
2. Testud F, Gabrielle L, Paquin ML, Descotes J. Acute alveolitis after using a waterproofing aerosol: apropos of 2 cases. Rev Med Interne. 1998;19:262–4.
3. Burkhart KK, Britt A, Petrini G, O'Donnell S, Donovan JW. Pulmonary toxicity following exposure to an aerosolized leather protector. J Toxicol Clin Toxicol. 1996;34:21–4.
4. Heinzer R, Ribordy V, Kuzoe B, Lazor R, Fitting JW. Recurrence of acute respiratory failure following use of waterproofing sprays. Thorax. 2004;59:541–2.
5. Vernez D, Bruzzi R, Kupferschmidt H, De-Batz A, Droz P, Lazor R. Acute respiratory syndrome after inhalation of waterproofing sprays: a posteriori exposure-response assessment in 102 cases. J Occup Environ Hyg. 2006;3:250–61.
6. Laliberté M, Sanfaçon G, Blais R. Acute pulmonary toxicity linked to use of a leather protector. Ann Emerg Med. 1995;25:841–4.
7. Daubert GP, Spiller H, Crouch BI, Seifert S, Simone K, Smolinske S. Pulmonary toxicity following exposure to waterproofing grout sealer. J Med Toxicol. 2009;5:125–9.
8. Tanino M, Kamishima K, Miyamoto H, Miyamoto K, Kawakami Y. Acute respiratory failure caused by inhalation of waterproofing spray fumes. Nihon Kokyuki Gakkai Zasshi. 1999;37:983–6.
9. Tagawa A, Ikehara K, Tsuburai T, Nishiyama H, Miyazawa N, Hashiba T, Suzuki M, Suzuki S, Ishigatsubo Y. Acute lung injury caused by inhalation of waterproofing spray. Nihon Kokyuki Gakkai Zasshi. 2003;41:123–6.
10. Bonte F, Rudolphus A, Tan KY, Aerts JG. Severe respiratory symptoms following the use of waterproofing sprays. Ned Tijdschr Geneeskd. 2003; 147:1185–8.
11. Kobayashi K, Tachikawa S, Horiguchi T, Kondo R, Shiga M, Hirose M, Sasaki Y, Torigoe H. A couple suffering acute respiratory illness due to waterproofing spray exposure. Nihon Kokyuki Gakkai Zasshi. 2006;44:647–52.
12. Hashimoto K, Arita K, Kajihara T, Nitta T, Mito A, Awaya H, Yamasaki M, Ohashi N. Two cases of lung injury due to inhalation of waterproofing spray with special reference to pulmonary function disorder. Nihon Kokyuki Gakkai Zasshi. 2009;47:367–71.
13. Wallace GMF, Brown PH. Horse rug lung: toxic pneumonitis due to fluorocarbon inhalation. Occup Environ Med. 2005;62:414–6.
14. Lazor-Blanchet C, Rusca S, Vernez D, Berry R, Albrecht E, Droz PO, Boillat MA. Acute pulmonary toxicity following occupational exposure to a floor stain protector in the building industry in Switzerland. Int Arch Occup Environ Health. 2004;77:244–8.
15. Yamashita M, Tanaka J. Pulmonary collapse and pneumonia due to inhalation of a waterproofing aerosol in female CD-1 mice. J Toxicol Clin Toxicol. 1995;33:631–7.
16. Hubbs AF, Castranova V, Ma JY, Frazer DG, Siegel PD, Ducatman BS, Grote A, Schwegler-Berry D, Robinson VA, Van Dyke C, Barger M, Xiang J, Parker J. Acute lung injury induced by a commercial leather conditioner. Toxicol Appl Pharmacol. 1997;143:37–46.
17. Sørli JB, Hansen JS, Nørgaard AW, Levin M, Larsen ST. An in vitro method for predicting inhalation toxicity of impregnation spray products. ALTEX. 2015;32(2):101–11.
18. Nørgaard AW, Larsen ST, Hammer M, Poulsen SS, Jensen KA, Nielsen GD, Wolkoff P. Lung damage in mice after inhalation of nanofilm spray products: the role of perfluorination and free hydroxyl groups. Toxicol Sci. 2010;116:216–24.
19. Nørgaard AW, Hansen JS, Sørli JB, Levin M, Wolkoff P, Nielsen GD, Larsen ST. Pulmonary toxicity of perfluorinated silane-based nanofilm spray products: solvent dependency. Toxicol Sci. 2014;137:179–88.
20. Yamashita M, Tanaka J, Yamashita M, Hirai H, Suzuki M, Kajigaya H. Mist particle

diameters are related to the toxicity of waterproofing sprays: comparison between toxic and non-toxic products. Vet Hum Toxicol. 1997;39:71–4.

21. Yamashita M, Yamashita M, Tanaka J, Hirai H, Suzuki M, Kajigaya H. Toxicity of waterproofing spray is influenced by the mist particle size. Vet Hum Toxicol. 1997;39:332–4.
22. Larsen ST, Dallot C, Larsen SW, Rose F, Poulsen SS, Nørgaard AW, Hansen JS, Sørli JB, Nielsen GD, Foged C. Mechanism of action of lung damage caused by a Nanofilm spray product. Toxicol Sci. 2014;40(2):436–44.
23. Duch P, Nørgaard AW, Hansen JS, Sørli JB, Jacobsen P, Lynggard F, Levin M, Nielsen GD, Wolkoff P, Ebbehøj NE, Larsen ST. Pulmonary toxicity following exposure to a tile coating product containing alkylsiloxanes. A clinical and toxicological evaluation. Clin Toxicol (Phila). 2014;52(5):498–505.
24. Fischer M, Koch W, Windt H, Dasenbrock C. 2012. A pilot study on the refinement of acute inhalation toxicity studies: the isolated perfused rat lung as a screening tool for surface-active substances. Altern Lab Anim. 2012;40(4):199–209.
25. Tashiro K, Matsumoto Y, Nishizuka K, Shibata K, Yamamoto K, Yamashita M, Kobayashi T. Mechanism of acute lung injury caused by inhalation of fabric protector and the effect of surfactant replacement. Intensive Care Med. 1998;24:55–60.
26. Pauluhn J, Hahn A, Spielmann H. Assessment of early acute lung injury in rats exposed to aerosols of consumer products: attempt to disentangle the "magic Nano" conundrum. Inhal Toxicol. 2008;20(14):1245–62.
27. Fagan DG, Forrest JB, Enhorning G, Lamprey M, Guy J. Acute pulmonary toxicity of a commercial fluorocarbon–lipid aerosol. Histopathology. 1997;1:209–23.
28. Tan D, Wang C, Ling J, Xia Z, Xu J. Acute respiratory distress syndrome after accidental inhalation of fluorocarbon monomers and pyrolysis products. Occup Environ Med. 2016;3:287–8.
29. NIST Standard Reference Database 1A. NIST/EPA/NIH Mass Spectral Database (NIST 11) and NIST Mass Spectral Search Program (Version 2.0g) National Institute for Standards and Technology, Gaithersburg MD, 2011. https://www.nist.gov/sites/default/files/documents/srd/NIST1a11Ver2-0Man.pdf Accessed 25 Jul 2017.
30. Vernez DS, Droz PO, Lazor-Blanchet C, Jaques S. Characterizing emission and breathing-zone concentrations following exposure cases to fluororesin-based waterproofing spray mists. J Occup Environ Hyg. 2004;1:582–92.
31. Hays HL, Spiller H. Fluoropolymer-associated illness. Clin Toxicol (Phila). 2014;52:848–55.
32. Schmid O, Möller W, Semmler-Behnke M, Ferron GA, Karg E, Lipka J, Schulz H, Kreyling WG, Stoeger T. Dosimetry and toxicology of inhaled ultrafine particles. Biomarkers. 2009;14:67–73.
33. Donaldson K, Stone V. Current hypotheses on the mechanisms of toxicity of ultrafine particles. Ann Ist Super Sanita. 2003;39:405–10.
34. Zuo YY, Veldhuizen RA, Neumann AW, Petersen NO, Possmayer F. Current perspectives in pulmonary surfactant–inhibition, enhancement and evaluation. Biochim Biophys Acta. 2008;1778:1947–77.
35. Warheit DB, Seidel WC, Carakostas MC, Hartsky MA. Attenuation of perfluoropolymer fume pulmonary toxicity: effect of filters, combustion method, and aerosol age. Exp Mol Pathol. 1990;52:309–29.
36. Wegman DH, Peters JM. Polymer fume fever and cigarette smoking. Ann Intern Med. 1974;81:55–7.
37. Albrecht WN, Bryant CJ. Polymer-fume fever associated with smoking and use of a mold-release spray containing polytetrafluoroethylene. J Occup Med. 1987;29:817–9.
38. Silver MJ, Young DK. Acute noncardiogenic pulmonary edema due to polymer fume fever. Cleve Clin J Med. 1993;60:479–82.
39. Clayton JW. Fluorocarbon toxicity and biological action. In: Tarant P, editor. Fluorine chemistry reviews. New York: Dekker; 1967. p. 197–252.
40. Bennett D, Bargagli E, Refini RM, Pieroni MG, Fossi A, Romeo R, Volterrani L, Mazzei MA, Rottoli P. Acute exacerbation of idiopathic pulmonary fibrosis after inhalation of a water repellent. Int J Occup Med Environ Health. 2015;28:775–9.
41. Scheepers PTJ, Cremers R, van Hout SPR, Anzion RBM. Influence of a portable air treatment unit on health-related quality indicators of indoor air in a classroom. J Environ Monit. 2011;14:429–39.
42. Scheepers PT, de Hartog JJ, Reijnaerts J, Beckmann G, Anzion R, Poels K, Godderis L. Influence of combined dust reducing carpet and compact air filtration unit on the indoor air quality of a classroom. Environ Sci Processes Impacts. 2015;17:316–25.

2

Prevalence of latent tuberculosis infection among foreign students in Lübeck, Germany tested with QuantiFERON-TB Gold In-Tube and QuantiFERON-TB Gold Plus

Elia Noemi Gallegos Morales[1*], Johannes Knierer[1], Anja Schablon[1], Albert Nienhaus[1,2] and Jan Felix Kersten[1]

Abstract

Background: The tuberculosis (TB) incidence rate in foreign-born individuals has been increasing in Germany in recent years. Foreign students may be an important source of latent tuberculosis infection (LTBI) in low-incidence countries. In Germany, there are no guidelines for LTBI screening of foreign students. The aim of the study was to estimate LTBI prevalence and evaluate associated risk factors among foreign students in Germany. The second purpose of our study was to compare the results of the new generation of QuantiFERON-TB Gold Plus (QFT-Plus) to those of its predecessor QuantiFERON-TB Gold In-Tube (QFT-GIT).

Methods: This cross-sectional study was conducted between February 2016 and March 2016. Foreign students and young professionals attending the university and higher education institutes in Lübeck, Germany were tested with QFT-Plus and QFT-GIT. Participants filled out a questionnaire for the purpose of LTBI risk assessment and analysis. Variables associated with a positive test result were analyzed using logistic regression.

Results: One hundred thirty four students participated in the study. The overall prevalence as regards positive results from both tests, QFT-Plus and QFT-GIT, was 9.7%, and the prevalence of positive QFT-Plus results was 8.2%. The main independent variables associated with a positive QFT-Plus result were a) being born in a high-incidence country (OR = 6.7, 95% CI: 1.3–34.3) and b) previous contact with a person with active TB (OR = 4.5, 95% CI: 1.1–18.3). Higher age (OR = 2.8, 95% CI: 0.7–11.3) and male gender (OR = 1.6, 95% CI: 0.4–6.7) showed a tendency toward positive QFT-Plus results but this was not statistically significant. Agreement between QFT-Plus and QFT-GIT results was $\kappa = 0.85$, $p < 0.001$.

Conclusions: The LTBI prevalence among foreign students was about 10%. We recommend implementing a policy whereby all foreign students are screened by means of a questionnaire about LTBI risk factors, so that only students with present risk factors are tested for LTBI. The agreement between the new QFT-Plus and the QFT-GIT ($\kappa = 0.85$) was good. QFT-Plus might be used in the same format as its predecessor.

Keywords: Foreign students, Latent tuberculosis infection, Risk factors, QuantiFERON-TB Gold Plus

* Correspondence: e.gallegos-morales@uke.de
[1]Center of Excellence for Health Services Research in Nursing (CVcare), University Medical Center Hamburg-Eppendorf (UKE), Hamburg, Germany
Full list of author information is available at the end of the article

Background

The downward trend of tuberculosis (TB) incidence in Germany has come to an end. TB incidence in Germany had decreased over the last decades, reaching its lowest level in 2012, with 4217 reported TB cases (TB incidence of 5.2 new TB cases a year per 100,000 inhabitants (hereinafter 5.2:100,000 for short)). Since then, TB incidence has been increasing and reached 5865 reported cases of active TB in 2015, 1648 more TB cases than in 2012. Nevertheless, Germany is still a low TB incidence country with a TB incidence of 7.3:100,000 in 2015 [1].

The overall TB incidence in Germany increased in recent years, mainly due to the increased number of TB cases in foreign-born people residing in Germany. All TB cases considered, the proportion of foreign-born people increased from 43.1% in 2007 to 72.1% in 2015. TB incidence in foreign-born subjects (50.3:100,000) was 20 times higher than the incidence in the native population (2.5:100,000) in 2015. (TB incidence rate 2007 in foreign-born residents: 22.8:100,000 and in native population: 4.3:100,000). Among foreign-born subjects with active TB, the peak age for TB was between 15 and 19 years [1].

Diel et al. [2] explained the considerable increase of TB incidence in Germany during recent years by the higher numbers of asylum seekers entering the country since 2014. However, not only has the number of asylum seekers increased in recent years, but also the number of foreign students attending universities and higher education institutions in Germany. The German Federal Statistical Office revealed in a press release that in the 2014/2015 winter term 236,000 foreign students were registered at German higher education institutions and universities. The number of foreign students has been increasing for the past ten years (2004/2005 winter term: 187,000 foreign students) [3].

The main goal of the World Health Organization (WHO) End TB Strategy is to end the global TB epidemic by 2035. One of the three pillars of this strategy is TB prevention. An important component in TB prevention is the management of latent tuberculosis infection (LTBI) in countries with a lower TB incidence (<100:100,000) by preventive treatment of persons at risk. A large proportion of TB cases in these countries are due to LTBI reactivation. Preventive therapy could reduce the risk of developing active TB by 60–90% [4, 5].

In the United States, the American College Health Association (ACHA) has developed guidelines for incoming students that recommend screening and targeted testing of college and university students to control and prevent infection by *Mycobacterium tuberculosis* [6]. Collins et al. found that in the U.S., students accounted for 30% of the TB cases among temporary visa holders [7]. This suggests that students might make up a significant proportion of residents with TB in the U.S. Ogiwara et al. proposed that early LTBI screening among foreign students could reduce the spread of TB [8]. Ricks et al. implied that four out of five active TB cases among foreign-born persons in the U.S. are attributed to the reactivation of LTBI. Preventing LTBI reactivation represents a big challenge to TB elimination [9].

Currently, no policy exists that recommends systematic testing for LTBI among foreign students prior to or during the process of entering Germany. To our knowledge, the prevalence and risk factors for LTBI among students and young professionals recently migrated to Germany has not yet been studied.

The WHO recommends using either tuberculin skin test (TST) or interferon-gamma release assay (IGRA) to test for LTBI in high-income and upper middle-income countries with an estimated TB incidence of ≤100:100,000 [10]. Until recently two IGRAs were commercially available, T-SPOT.TB (Oxford Immunotec, Abingdon, UK) and QuantiFERON-TB Gold In-Tube (QFT-GIT) (Qiagen, Hilden, Germany). In 2015 Qiagen released the QuantiFERON-TB Gold Plus (QFT-Plus), which according to the manufacturer offers a higher sensitivity and specificity [11].

The aim of this cross-sectional study is to estimate the prevalence and the associated risk factors of a positive IGRA as a marker for LTBI among students and young professionals with a migration background in Lübeck, Germany. The second purpose of our study is to compare the results of the new generation IGRA, QFT-Plus, to those of its predecessor, QFT-GIT.

Methods

Study design, setting and subjects

This cross-sectional study was conducted between February 2016 and March 2016. The target population for this cross-sectional study was foreign students and young professionals attending courses offered by the university and two higher education institutions in Lübeck, Germany. Students were recruited by word-of-mouth advertising, flyers on notice boards and e-mails sent from the international office of each institution. Students attending universities other than those in Lübeck were not directly recruited, but their participation in this study was allowed.

Students participated in this study on a voluntary basis and their contribution was remunerated. The inclusion criteria were: age ≥ 18 years, being a student or a young professional attending a German university/higher education institution, having signed the consent form and being born in or being a national of a country with a TB incidence ≥10:100,000 according to the WHO [12]. Participants without a migration background fulfilling the nationality criteria only because of their parents' nationality were excluded. Students fulfilling the inclusion criteria attended an appointment at the University of Lübeck where data was collected and blood was drawn. A Palestinian participant was included in the study, although there is no TB incidence data for that country according to the WHO.

We declared as a high-incidence country all those countries with a TB incidence of ≥125:100,000. The participants' nationality was classified by WHO regions.

Data collection

After signing the consent form, participants filled out a standard questionnaire asking about risk factors. The questionnaire included questions about socio-demographic aspects (gender, age, country of birth, nationality, time living in Germany), subject studied, previous contact with TB, TB in the participants' own history, previous TB test results (IGRA and TST), BCG (*Bacille Calmette-Guérin*) vaccination, previous chest X-rays and other diseases or medications that compromise the immune system.

Test method: IGRA

The participants' blood samples were tested by two IGRA methods: QFT-GIT and QFT-Plus (both: Qiagen, Hilden, Germany).

Students were tested at the University of Lübeck, where rooms were booked for study purposes only. Blood sampling was performed by two study physicians using lithium heparin tubes. The blood samples were stored in a room temperature box and transported to the laboratory within max. 8 h. In the laboratory, medical lab technicians decanted an exact amount of blood from the heparin tubes into the QFT-GIT and the QFT-Plus tubes. The samples were incubated for at least 16 h and Interferon-gamma (IFN-γ) ELISA (Enzyme-linked Immunosorbent Assay) was performed directly afterwards.

Results were considered positive if the IFN-γ value was ≥0.35 IU/ml after correction for negative control in any of the two tests. A result was considered negative if the IFN-γ value was <0.35 IU/ml and if the mitogen (positive response control) was ≥0.5 IU/ml. Since the QFT-Plus has two tubes, TB-antigen 1 and TB-antigen 2, the maximum of the two was taken as the result, as per the manufacturer's suggestion [13].

Management of IGRA-positive participants

All participants were informed about their results. Participants with a positive test result in at least one of the two IGRAs were advised by the study physicians to repeat the tests in order to verify the test result (costs for follow-up tests were covered by the study). If the test kept being positive, participants were advised to take a chest X-ray in order to rule out active TB. Repetition of the IGRA was performed one week after the first positive test was performed in the scope of a four week variability study. Results of this study are reported else were [14]. Participants who had had prior contact with a person with active TB during the last 2 years were offered specialist advice. Participants with a positive test result were informed about the symptoms of active TB and about risk factors leading to LTBI reactivation.

Data analysis

Categorical variables were expressed as counts and corresponding rates and continuous variables were expressed as means with standard deviation (SD) or with a 95% confidence interval (95%-CI). Associations between the IGRA result and categorical variables were investigated using chi-squared tests. The variables (gender, age, country of birth and previous TB contact) that were associated univariate with the QFT-Plus result in the chi-squared test were included in a logistic regression model with stepwise backward selection. Agreement between the QFT-GIT and QFT-Plus was assessed using the Cohen's kappa coefficient. All data was analyzed with SPSS Version 22 (IBM Corp., Armonk, NY). Two-tailed P-value of <0.05 was considered statistically significant.

Results

The study involved 134 foreign students and young professionals. Four out of 134 participants were enrolled in other universities than those in Lübeck. Questionnaires were filled in completely, there was no missing data. The study population is described in Table 1. In our sample the mean age was 25.1 years (SD 3.8) with an age range from 19 to 39 years. Gender was almost equally distributed, with a slightly higher proportion of female participants (53.7%). Participants migrated to Germany at ages ranging from 17 months (1.4 years) to 36 years. The mean age in which students migrated was 20.9 years.

A total of 11 positive QFT-Plus results (8.2%) were observed. When both tests (QFT-GIT and QFT-Plus) are taken into account the number of participants with a positive test result in either QFT increases to a total of 13 (9.7%).

As the agreement between QFT-Plus and QFT-GIT was high, presentation of IGRA results by putative risk factors was limited to the QFT-Plus (Table 1). The prevalence of positive QFT-Plus results was higher among male participants (11.3% versus 5.6%, p = 0.34) and among participants born in a TB high-incidence country (18.8% versus 2.3%). The participants with a positive QFT-Plus were nationals of three WHO regions, Africa, South-East Asia and the Western Pacific, each region accounting for about one-third of positive results. None of the participants from Europe was QFT-Plus positive. Subjects reporting a previous contact with a person with active TB were more often QFT-Plus

Table 1 Description of the study population and QFT-Plus results by putative risk factors

Variable	N (Col-%)	QFT-Plus positive N (Row-%)	QFT-Plus negative N (Row-%)	*P*-Value
Gender				0.345
Female	72 (53.7)	4 (5.6)	68 (94.4)	
Male	62 (46.3)	7 (11.3)	55 (88.7)	
Age				0.050
19–25 years	87 (64.9)	4 (4.6)	83 (95.4)	
26–39 years	47 (35.1)	7 (14.9)	40 (85.1)	
Country of birth classified by TB-Incidence				0.002
< 125:100,000	86 (64.2)	2 (2.3)	84 (97.7)	
≥ 125:100,000	48 (35.8)	9 (18.8)	39 (81.3)	
Nationality classified by WHO regions				<0.001
Africa	15 (11.2)	4 (26.7)	11 (73.3)	
The Americas	16 (11.9)	0 (0)	16 (100)	
South-East Asia	20 (14.9)	3 (15.0)	17 (85.0)	
Europe	49 (36.6)	0 (0)	49 (100)	
Eastern Mediterranean	20 (14.9)	0 (0)	20 (100)	
Western Pacific	14 (10.4)	4 (28.6)	10 (71.4)	
Time living in Germany				0.808
< 2 years	53 (39.6)	4 (7.5)	49 (92.5)	
2–10 years	71 (53.0)	7 (9.9)	64 (90.1)	
> 10 years	10 (7.5)	0 (0)	10 (100)	
Previous TB contact				0.007
Yes	35 (26.1)	7 (20.0)	28 (80.0)	
No	99 (73.9)	4 (4.0)	95 (96.0)	
Type of TB contact				0.009
Relatives	9 (25.7)	5 (55.6)	4 (44.4)	
Friends/acquaintances	7 (20.0)	1 (14.3)	6 (85.7)	
Professional	14 (40.0)	0 (0)	14 (100)	
Other type	5 (14.3)	1 (20.0)	4 (80.0)	
TB in own history				0.082
Yes	1 (0.7)	1 (100)	0 (0)	
No	133 (99.3)	10 (7.5)	123 (92.5)	
BCG vaccination				0.064*
Yes	66 (49.3)	2 (3.0)	64 (97.0)	
No	18 (13.4)	3 (16.7)	15 (83.3)	
Unknown	50 (37.3)	6 (12.0)	44 (88.0)	
Previous TST				0.306
Positive	11 (8.2)	2 (18.2)	9 (81.8)	
Negative	18 (13.4)	0 (0)	18 (100)	
Unknown	6 (4.5)	0 (0)	6 (100)	
No TST	99 (73.9)	9 (9.1)	90 (90.9)	
Study subject				0.350
Medicine	47 (35.1)	5 (10.6)	42 (89.4)	
Engineering	49 (36.6)	3 (6.1)	46 (93.9)	
Natural sciences	21 (15.7)	3 (14.3)	18 (85.7)	
Other subject	17 (12.7)	0 (0)	17 (100)	

*For BCG vaccination variable, *P*-Value was calculated between participants whose BCG status was known

positive than those with no known contact (20% versus 4%). In most cases (5 of 7; 71%) the contact person was a relative. One participant had suffered from active TB two years before participating in the study.

Out of the 13 participants with positive IGRA results in at least one of the two IGRA test methods, 11 participants consented to retesting. Upon second testing, positivity was confirmed in at least one of the two IGRA test methods in all cases. None of the chest X-rays of participants with a positive IGRA showed signs of ongoing active TB. Despite the study physicians' advice, four of the participants refused to take a chest X-ray. As none of the participants showed clinical signs of ongoing active TB, we assumed that no participant was suffering from active TB.

As shown in Fig. 1, we found that statistically significant risk factors for having a positive QFT-Plus as an LTBI marker were: being born in a high-incidence country (OR = 6.7, 95% CI: 1.3–34.3) and having had previous contact with a person with active TB (OR = 4.5, 95% CI: 1.1–18.3). A higher age (OR = 2.8, 95% CI: 0.7–11.3) and male gender (OR = 1.6, 95% CI: 0.4–6.7) showed a tendency to have a higher risk of acquiring LTBI, however these factors showed no statistical significance.

The participants were tested simultaneously with QFT-Plus and QFT-GIT. Fig. 2 shows the concordance of these two test methods. Nine participants showed positive results in both tests. Two participants were only positive in the QFT-Plus test while another two participants, who were also born in a TB high-incidence country, had a positive QFT-GIT result (Fig. 2). The concordance between QFT-Plus and QFT-GIT was estimated as $\kappa = 0.85$ ($p < 0.001$).

Discussion

This cross-sectional study is to our knowledge the first to determine the prevalence of LTBI among foreign students and young professionals in Germany. We found an overall prevalence of positive QFT-Plus of 8.2%, which is considerably higher than with students in low-incidence countries. In Italy, Durando et al. conducted two studies in which LTBI prevalence among medical students was 0.1% (test method IGRA) in 2015 [15] and among healthcare students 0.5% (test method IGRA) in 2013 [16]. Schablon et al. found an LTBI prevalence of 2.1% (test method IGRA) among nursing students working in Germany [17]. In South Korea LTBI prevalence according to Jung et al. was 5.2% (test method IGRA) among medical students [18]. Ogiwara et al. showed that in different years the LTBI prevalence (test method IGRA) among Japanese healthcare students ranged from 0.7 to 1.0% while among foreign students the LTBI prevalence was 4.3 to 8.6% [8].

Four studies among high TB burden countries were conducted. In students from Rio de Janeiro, Brazil, the LTBI prevalence was 6.9% (test method TST) according to Teixeira et al. [19]. Du et al. showed that LTBI prevalence among Chinese students was 40.7% (test method IGRA) [20]. LTBI prevalence among Ugandan medical students was 44.8% and 35.2% among veterinary students according to Mugerwa et al. [21] and 45.1% according to Lou et al. [22], which is considerably higher than our numbers. Nevertheless, in the Ugandan studies TST was used as a test method for investigating LTBI prevalence. This might have led to an overestimation of LTBI prevalence due to cross reactivity of TST with the BCG vaccination [20, 23]. The latter three studies conducted in Uganda and in China imply that the LTBI prevalence in students from high TB burden countries is much higher than in other countries (e.g. Italy, Germany, etc.).

As there is no data available on LTBI prevalence among students from Lübeck no comparison is possible. However the TB incidence of the district Lübeck was 4.7:100,000 in 2015 and therefore lower than the TB incidence in Germany (7.3:100,000). We assume that LTBI prevalence is lower in students from Lübeck than in foreign students [1].

Our risk assessment analysis demonstrated that being born in a country with a high TB incidence (TB incidence ≥125:100,000) is a major risk factor for IGRA positivity and therefore for an LTBI among foreign students. This association has also been demonstrated in Italy [16] and in Japan [8], though the definition of a

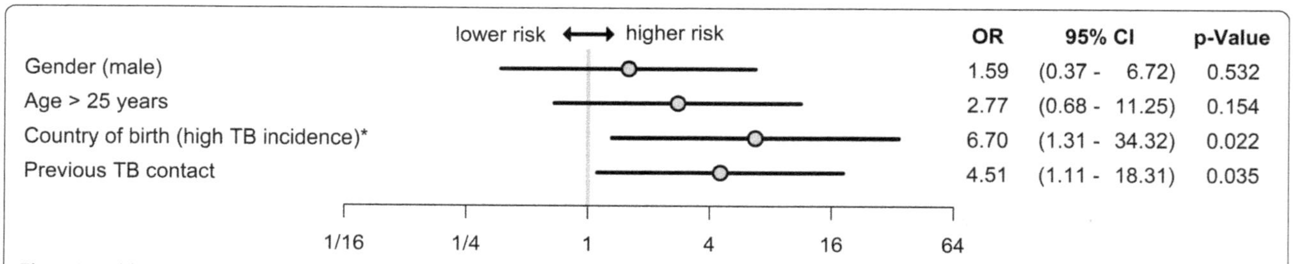

Fig. 1 Variables associated with positive QFT-Plus. The variables were analyzed using logistic regression models to identify independent variables associated with a positive QFT-Plus result. * Countries with an annual TB incidence of ≥125:100,000

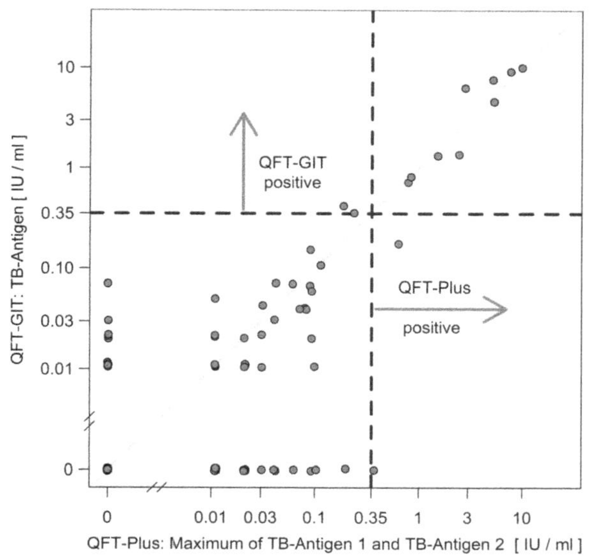

Fig. 2 Concordance between QFT-Plus and QFT-GIT. For QFT-Plus the highest IFN-γ value of antigen tubes TB-1 and TB-2 was taken as the result

high-incidence country in these two studies was a TB incidence of ≥20:100,000. As a second risk factor for IGRA positivity we identified previous contact with a person infected with active TB. This was also demonstrated in students from Uganda and Italy [15, 21, 22].

Fournier et al. described in their study that family TB contact leads to a higher LTBI rate than professional contact in low-incidence and in high-incidence countries [24]. This corresponds to our results, since in our population the majority of participants with a positive QFT-Plus test that reported previous contact with TB had had contact with an infected family member.

In other studies male gender [19, 21, 22] and a higher age [22] were a significant predictor for an LTBI. Our data shows the same tendency for a higher risk for these two variables. However, due to the small number of participants and therefore limited power it was not statistically significant.

Our secondary assessment showed that the agreement between the new QFT-Plus and the QFT-GIT ($\kappa = 0.85$) was far greater than that between TST and QFT-GIT found by Jung et al. ($\kappa = 0.34$), which is poor [18]. This agreement is expected because QFT-GIT and QFT-Plus are based on the same testing methods and principles.

Studies have demonstrated that active TB might be attributed to reactivation of LTBI [9, 25]. This reactivation was shown to be higher among foreign-born than among natives in the U.S. [26]. Ricks et al. showed that the odds of TB reactivation were higher among foreign-born people from countries with a TB incidence of ≥150:100,000 [9]. Diel et al. showed that in Germany the majority (58.1%) of all immigrants developed the disease within the first 5 years [25]. Since students stay in Germany for several years, LTBI reactivation might occur during their residence in Germany. In a review, Ai et al. stated that the LTBI reactivation rate is especially high for persons who had been recently infected (15 times greater within the first 2 years after infection) [27].

As LTBI is an important source of active TB infection in low-incidence countries, the WHO has released guidelines specifically for the management of LTBI. The WHO found evidence for increased prevalence of LTBI, higher risk of progression (LTBI reactivation) and higher incidence of active TB among immigrants from high TB burden countries. Therefore they recommend countries with a TB incidence of <100:100,000 to consider systematic testing and treatment of LTBI for immigrants from high TB burden countries [10] (currently: Afghanistan, Bangladesh, Brazil, Cambodia, China, DR Congo, Ethiopia, India, Indonesia, Kenya, Mozambique, Myanmar, Nigeria, Pakistan, Philippines, the Russian Federation, South Africa, Thailand, Uganda, UR Tanzania, Vietnam and Zimbabwe [5]).

Although some countries such as the UK and Canada have already implemented LTBI screening policies for incoming immigrants [28–30], there are no similar regulations in Germany. Diel et al. suggested that public health policies should focus on TB prevention with LTBI testing of all immigrants applying for a resident visa in Germany [25]. In the U.S., the ACHA guidelines recommend screening all incoming students for TB by using a questionnaire inquiring about six different risk factors for TB infection. Students showing at least one risk factor (e.g. students who were born in or had visited a country with a TB incidence of ≥20:100,000, exposure to TB, including professional contact) should be tested with TST or IGRA [6]. We suggest creating a similar policy to the ACHA Guidelines with targeted testing. Since everyone has a different risk profile for LTBI, untargeted systematic testing would include testing of low-risk persons which may lead to a reduction in the positive predictive value of IGRAs [31]. In order to preserve the positive predictive value of IGRAs, only risk groups should be undergoing LTBI testing with IGRAs.

According to our findings we recommend that foreign students should be screened with a questionnaire inquiring about risk factors before the decision to test is taken. Those who are screened as having had prior contact with a person with active TB or who come from a high-incidence country (≥125:100,000 inhabitants) or a high TB burden country should be tested for LTBI. We agree with the WHO recommendation to ask students about active TB symptoms before LTBI testing. If someone suffers from these symptoms, active TB should be investigated [10].

Countries with a TB incidence of <100:100,000 should test with either TST or IGRA [10]. It is known that the

TST shows cross reactivity with the BCG vaccination [20, 23] and the majority of TB high incidence countries carry out BCG vaccination [32]. Therefore IGRAs are more useful for LTBI evaluation in BCG vaccinated individuals [33] and should be preferred when testing migrants in Germany with positive risk factors.

Pareek et al. showed in a review that successful LTBI screening involves key steps e.g. accurate identification of migrants, appropriate screening and initiation as well as completion of chemotherapy [28]. LTBI reactivation and thus the spread of the disease can be averted by means of preventive chemotherapy [10]. Nevertheless, Diel et al. in 2004 note that preventive therapy might not be useful in some immigrant groups in Germany, such as those originating from Eastern Europe, since people from those countries are more likely to be infected with resistant *Mycobacterium tuberculosis* [25].

Strengths and limitations

Participants in this study with a positive QFT-Plus result came from three WHO regions: Africa, South-East Asia and Western Pacific. The WHO global report 2015 showed that over 80% of new TB cases came from these three regions [5]. We found those regions well represented in our study.

This study recruited a fairly small number of participants (n = 134), who may not be representative of other bodies of foreign students in Germany. Caution must be exercised in drawing general conclusions from the results of these studies.

Nevertheless this was the first study describing LTBI prevalence in foreign students in Germany. More studies should be conducted to better determine if and how policies should be developed to screen and test for LTBI in order to achieve better control of the disease.

Conclusions

In Germany, no specific policies exist for systematic LTBI screening among foreign students in universities and higher education institutions. Considering the steady increase in the proportion of foreigners with active TB compared to the native population and the increasing TB incidence in Germany for the last three years, a policy for LTBI screening and targeted testing among foreign students should be considered to prevent a further increase in TB incidence caused by LTBI reactivation. Our data implies that systematic LTBI testing should be preceded by a questionnaire with a view to testing only those students with risk factors (e.g. previous contact with TB or being born in a high-incidence country).

Our secondary assessment showed that the agreement between the new QFT-Plus and the QFT-GIT was good, which suggests that QFT-Plus might be used in the same format as its predecessor.

Abbreviations

95% CI: 95% Confidence interval; ACHA: American College Health Association; BCG: Bacille Calmette-Guérin; BGW: Institute for Statutory Accident Insurance and Prevention in the Health and Welfare Services; CVcare: Center of Excellence for Health Services Research in Nursing, Hamburg, Germany; ELISA: Enzyme-linked Immunosorbent Assay; IFN- γ: Interferon-gamma; IGRA: Interferon-gamma release assay; LIST: Lübecker International Student Tutorium; LTBI: Latent tuberculosis infection; OR: Odds ratio; QFT- Plus : QuantiFERON-TB Gold Plus; QFT-GIT: QuantiFERON-TB Gold In-Tube; SD: Standard deviation; TB: Tuberculosis; TST: Tuberculin skin test; U.S.: United States of America; UKE: University Medical Center Hamburg-Eppendorf; WHO: World Health Organization

Acknowledgements

We thank the University of Lübeck for allowing us to test participants on its premises. We thank the Lübecker International Student Tutorium (LIST) for helping with recruitment of participants and the students for taking part in this study. We also thank all CVcare workers, especially Peter Koch for helping with the data mask, Elisabeth Muth for helping with the literature and Olaf Kleinmüller for helping with the ethics application. We thank the Fenner Laboratory for its prompt processing of samples.

Funding

No special funds were received for this study. However, the Institute for Health Services Research in Dermatology and Nursing of the University Medical Centre Hamburg-Eppendorf (UKE) receives an unrestricted fund from the Institution for Statutory Accident Insurance and Prevention in the Health and Welfare services (BGW) on an annual basis to maintain the working group at the UKE. The funds are provided by a non-profit organization that is part of the social security system in Germany. The funder had no role in study design, data collection and analysis, decision to publish, or preparation of the manuscript.

Authors' contributions

Conceived and designed the experiments: ENGM, JK, AS, JFK, AN. Performed the experiments: ENGM, JK. Analyzed the data: ENGM, JFK, JK, AS, AN. Created figures and tables: JFK, ENGM, JK. Wrote the paper: ENGM, JK, JFK, AS, AN. All authors read and approved the final manuscript.

Competing interests

The authors have declared that no competing interests exist.

Author details

[1]Center of Excellence for Health Services Research in Nursing (CVcare), University Medical Center Hamburg-Eppendorf (UKE), Hamburg, Germany. [2]Institute for Statutory Accident Insurance and Prevention in the Health and Welfare Services (BGW), Hamburg, Germany.

References

1. Brodhun B, Altmann D, Hauer B, Fiebig L, Haas W. Bericht zur Epidemiologie der Tuberkulose in Deutschland für 2015. Berlin: Robert Koch-Institut; 2016.
2. Diel R, Loddenkemper R, Nienhaus A. Consequences of tuberculosis among asylum seekers for health care workers in Germany. J Occup Med Toxicol. 2016;11:4.
3. Statistisches Bundesamt: 134 500 Deutsche studierten 2013 im Ausland, press release Wiesbaden 16 Dec 2015, 469/15 [cited 16 June 2016]. Available: https://www.destatis.de/DE/PresseService/Presse/Pressemitteilungen/2015/12/PD15_469_217.html.

4. WHO. Implementing the end TB strategy: the essentials. Geneva, World Health Organization WHO; 2015.
5. WHO. Global Tuberculosis Report 2015. Geneva: World Health Organization; 2015.
6. ACHA. Tuberculosis Screening and Targeted Testing of College and University Students. In: ACHA guidelines. Hanover: ACHA; 2016. p. 1–9.
7. Collins JM, Reves RR, Belknap RW. High Rates of Tuberculosis and Opportunities for Prevention among International Students in the U.S. Annals of the American Thoracic Society. 2016;13(4):522–8.
8. Ogiwara T, Kimura T, Tokue Y, Watanabe R, Nara M, Obuchi T, et al. Tuberculosis screening using a T-cell interferon-gamma release assay in Japanese medical students and non-Japanese international students. Tohoku J Exp Med. 2013;230(2):87–91.
9. Ricks PM, Cain KP, Oeltmann JE, Kammerer JS, Moonan PK. Estimating the burden of tuberculosis among foreign-born persons acquired prior to entering the U.S., 2005-2009. PLoS One. 2011;6(11):e27405.
10. WHO. Guidelines on the management of latent tuberculosis infection. Geneva: World Health Organization WHO; 2015.
11. Qiagen: QIAGEN launches QuantiFERON®-TB Gold Plus – a new generation of the most accurate test for detecting tuberculosis infections 2015, press release 7 Jan 2015 [cited 16 June 2016]. Available: https://www.qiagen.com/de/about-us/press-releases/pressreleaseview?ID={C861949E-DF50-475B-8148-B4C70034C49E}&lang=en
12. Incidence Data by country (2007 - present) [cited 30 May 2016]. In: WHO. Global Health Observatory data repository. Geneva. 2015. Available: http://apps.who.int/gho/data/node.main.1320?lang=en.
13. QuantiFERON®-TB Gold Plus (QFT®-Plus) ELISA Package Insert [cited 16 June 2016]. Available: http://www.quantiferon.com/irm/content/PI/QFT/PLUS/2PK-Elisa/UK.pdf .
14. Knierer J, Gallegos Morales EN, Schablon A, Nienhaus A, Kersten JF. QFT-Plus: a plus in variability? - Evaluation of new generation IGRA in serial testing of students with a migration background in Germany. J Occup Med Toxicol. 2017;12:1.
15. Durando P, Alicino C, Orsi A, Barberis I, Paganino C, Dini G, et al. Latent tuberculosis infection among a large cohort of medical students at a teaching hospital in Italy. Biomed Res Int. 2015;2015:746895.
16. Durando P, Sotgiu G, Spigno F, Piccinini M, Mazzarello G, Viscoli C, et al. Latent tuberculosis infection and associated risk factors among undergraduate healthcare students in Italy: a cross-sectional study. BMC Infect Dis. 2013;13:443.
17. Schablon A, Diel R, Diner G, Anske U, Pankow W, Ringshausen FC, et al. Specificity of a whole blood IGRA in German nursing students. BMC Infect Dis. 2011;11:245.
18. Jung da H, Jo KW, Shim TS. Prevalence of Latent Tuberculosis Infection among Medical Students in South Korea. Tuberc Respir Dis (Seoul). 2012; 73(4):219–23.
19. Teixeira EG, Menzies D, Comstock GW, Cunha AJ, Kritski AL, Soares LC, et al. Latent tuberculosis infection among undergraduate medical students in Rio de Janeiro State, Brazil. Int J Tuberc Lung Dis. 2005;9(8):841–7.
20. Du F, Zhang Z, Gao T, Liu Z, Jia H, Xing A, et al. Diagnosis of latent tuberculosis by ELISPOT assay and tuberculin skin test. Med Mal Infect. 2016;46(3):150–3.
21. Mugerwa H, Byarugaba DK, Mpooya S, Miremba P, Kalyango JN, Karamagi C, et al. High Prevalence of tuberculosis infection among medical students in Makerere University, Kampala: results of a cross sectional study. Arch Public Health. 2013;71(1):7.
22. Lou JK, Okot-Nwang M, Katamba A. Prevalence of positive tuberculin skin test and associated factors among Makerere medical students, Kampala, Uganda. Afr Health Sci. 2015;15(4):1247–55.
23. Diel R, Goletti D, Ferrara G, Bothamley G, Cirillo D, Kampmann B, et al. Interferon-gamma release assays for the diagnosis of latent Mycobacterium tuberculosis infection: a systematic review and meta-analysis. Eur Respir J. 2011;37(1):88–99.
24. Fournier A, Antoun F, Larnaudie S. Recent latent tuberculous infection (LTBI) in different sub-groups of contacts. Rev Mal Respir. 2012;29(9): 1079–87.
25. Diel R, Rüsch-Gerdes S, Niemann S. Molecular epidemiology of tuberculosis among immigrants in Hamburg, Germany. J Clin Microbiol. 2004;42(7):2952–60.
26. Shea KM, Kammerer JS, Winston CA, Navin TR, Horsburgh CR Jr. Estimated rate of reactivation of latent tuberculosis infection in the United States, overall and by population subgroup. Am J Epidemiol. 2014;179(2):216–25.
27. Ai JW, Ruan QL, Liu QH, Zhang WH. Updates on the risk factors for latent tuberculosis reactivation and their managements. Emerg Microbes Infect. 2016;5:e10.
28. Pareek M, Greenaway C, Noori T, Munoz J, Zenner D. The impact of migration on tuberculosis epidemiology and control in high-income countries: a review. BMC Med. 2016;14:48.
29. Greenaway C, Kamran K, Schwartzman K. Canadian Tuberculosis Standards. In: Chapter 13: Tuberculosis surveillance and screening in selected high-risk populations. 7th ed. Ottawa: Centre for Communicable Diseases and Infection Control,Public Health Agency of Canada; 2014.
30. Public Health England. Latent TB Testing and Treatment for Migrants. A practical guide for commissioners and practitioners. London: Public Health England, NHS England; 2015.
31. Nienhaus A, Ringshausen FC, Costa JT, Schablon A, Tripodi D. IFN-gamma release assay versus tuberculin skin test for monitoring TB infection in healthcare workers. Expert Rev Anti-Infect Ther. 2013;11(1):37–48.
32. Zwerling A, Behr MA, Verma A, Brewer TF, Menzies D, Pai M. The BCG World Atlas: a database of global BCG vaccination policies and practices. PLoS Med. 2011;8(3):e1001012.
33. Diel R, Nienhaus A, Lange C, Meywald-Walter K, Forssbohm M, Schaberg T. Tuberculosis contact investigation with a new, specific blood test in a low-incidence population containing a high proportion of BCG-vaccinated persons. Respir Res. 2006;7:77.

3

Contamination of health care workers' coats at the University Teaching Hospital in Lusaka, Zambia: the nosocomial risk

Susan Mwamungule[1], Henry Mwelwa Chimana[1], Sydney Malama[2*], Geoffrey Mainda[3], Geoffrey Kwenda[1] and John Bwalya Muma[3]

Abstract

Background: Health care Associated Infections (HAIs) are a major public health problem in both developed and developing countries. They pose a severe impact in resource-poor settings, where the rate of infection is estimated to be relatively high. Therefore, this study was conducted to establish empirical evidence related to HAIs in Zambia.

Method: This was a prospective cross-sectional study conducted from October, 2013 to May 2014 at the University Teaching Hospital (UTH) in Lusaka. A total of 107 white coats worn by health care-workers at UTH were sampled for possible bacteriological contamination.

Results: Of the 107 white coats screened, 94 (72.8 %) were contaminated with bacteria. There was no difference in the contamination levels between white coats worn for more than 60 min (47.8 %) compared to those worn for 30–60 min (46.7 %) ($p = 0.612$). Further, the antibiotic sensitivity tests indicated that the bacterial isolates were resistant to some of the antibiotics assessed. Isolates of *Staphylococcus aureus* and *Klebsiella pnumoniae* exhibited the highest resistance to most of the antibiotics assessed.

Conclusion: This study has shown that white coats worn by health care-workers at the University Teaching Hospital generally have high microbial contaminations and hence pose a nosocomial risk. It is therefore, recommended that white coats be regularly sanitized, and health care workers also be sensitized on public health risk of HAIs associated with contaminated coats.

Keywords: Health-worker, Nosocomial, Bacteria, Antibiotic- resistance, Zambia

Introduction

Health-care Associated Infections (HAIs) are a major public health problem in both developed and developing countries [1, 2]. They pose a severe impact in resource-poor settings, where the rate of infection is estimated to range from 25 to 40 % (WHO 2005, 2008). Studies have shown that HAIs exert a tremendous toll on patients, families and systems of care, resulting in increased morbidity and mortality, and eventually increasing healthcare costs [2]. An estimated 1.4 million people worldwide suffer from infections acquired in hospitals [3]. Prevention of health care associated infections has increasingly received attention in recent years due to the ever–increasing health care costs, as well as the escalating problem of antibiotic resistance [4]. Previous studies have shown that up to 37 % of nosocomial infections in intensive care units (ICUs) are directly attributable to transmission of resistant organisms across patients [5]. Standard infection control practices have focused on universal hand hygiene and barrier precautions for patients infected or colonized with resistant organisms.

The role of bacterial contamination of uniforms of health care workers (HCWs) in the horizontal transmission of bacteria remains poorly understood. Despite their efforts, healthcare workers may serve as potential vectors of disease, disseminating virulent microorganisms among their patients [6]. Health care workers are at risk of contracting infectious microorganisms by

* Correspondence: sydneymalama1971@gmail.com
[2]Health Promotions Unit, Institute of Economic and Social Research, University of Zambia, Lusaka, Zambia
Full list of author information is available at the end of the article

virtue of being in constant contact with patients. Therefore, both patients and health care workers can transmit infection through direct contact, as well as through indirect contact with inanimate objects.

In 2005, WHO Patient Safety Initiative launched the First Global Patient Safety Challenge to galvanize international focus and action on the critical issue of HAIs. Since then, there has been a growing body of data implicating HCWs' uniforms as a potential reservoir of pathogenic organisms [7].

A recent study in Israel isolated pathogenic bacteria on uniforms of 85 of 135 (63 %) physicians and nurses [8]. These contaminated uniforms might have acted as vectors for the continued dissemination of bacteria from patients to HCWs and vice versa. Healthcare-associated infections represent a heavy social and financial burden. Another study on white coats reported 95 % contamination, while others found presence of *Staphylococcus aureus* in 23 % of the white coats [8, 9]. These bacteria appear to be found more specifically around sleeves and pockets [10]. In the USA, it was estimated that 1.7 million cases of HAIs occurred every year, with almost 99,000 deaths related to these cases [10].

The WHO Patient-Safety Initiative indicated that any potential source of HAIs that could threaten the well-being of individuals within healthcare facilities should be investigated and mitigated (WHO, 2005). There is however, no documented evidence indicating that similar studies have been done in Zambia. Therefore, this study was conducted to establish empirical evidence related to HAIs in Zambia.

Materials and methods

Study site and design

This was a prospective cross-sectional study conducted at the University Teaching Hospital (UTH) in Lusaka from October, 2013 to May 2014. The hospital is the largest hospital in Zambia and often serves as a national referral center for people needing specialized medical treatment.

Study population

The study population included health care workers at UTH from the following departments based on their unique mode and levels of contamination: Obstetrics and Gynaecology, the Outpatient (OPD), Pathology & Microbiology, Intensive Care Unit, Medical, Paediatrics and Surgical wards.

Inclusion and exclusion criteria

The study included health workers coming in direct contact with patients who wore white coats from the laboratory, intensive care unit, and paediatrics, surgical, obstetrics and gynecology and OPD departments. Health workers who wore white coats but did not deal directly with patients were excluded from the study. It was estimated there were approximately 133 persons in the selected units who wore white coats and came in direct contact with patients which thus form our study population.

Sample size

There was no data on the prevalence of microbiological contamination of health workers coats in Zambia. Therefore, in order to estimate the prevalence within 5 % allowable error and considering a 95 % confidence level, the calculation was based on the assumption that 50 % of health workers' coats in Zambia had microbiological contamination. Based on these assumptions, the number of persons to be sampled were estimated using the simple random formula as indicated by Dohoo et al. [11]. Therefore, the number of persons to be included in the study was calculated to be 384 health workers, given that sampling would be done from an infinite population. This sample size was adjusted taking into account there was a finite population of 133 HCWs who wore white coats in the target operative units distributed as follows: obstetrics and gynecology (24), the out-patient department (14), laboratory department (16), intensive care unit (12), medical (22), pediatrics (25) and surgery (20). Therefore, the adjusted sample size, estimated according to the formula provided by Dohoo et al. [11], was 99 HCWs. We therefore targeted to 99 HWCs from distributed in the various eligible department.

Sampling of coats

Each white coat was sampled using two sterile saline-moistened swabs with Peptone water (Oxoid). The first swab was taken from the cuff and second from the side pocket mouth. These sites were chosen because they are known to harbour microorganisms in highest concentration [12, 13]. Sampling was qualitatively done were the wet swab was rubbed against the coats and the swab was placed back into a sterile contained. Sampling was done after a written consent from the participants. The samples were labeled and transferred to the medical microbiology laboratory located with the UTH in cool boxes (+4 °C). All laboratory analyses were carried out within 1 h of sample collection.

Culture and drug susceptibility testing

The swabs collected were directly inoculated in duplicate on blood agar, (Oxoid) Mac Conkey agar and Muller Hinton agar (Oxoid). The pairs of inoculated media were incubated aerobically at 37 °C for 24 h and then examined for bacteria growth according to standard protocol [14]. The positive culture growths were examined for colony characteristics, Gram-reaction and biochemical characteristics as described by Cheesbrough (2000) [14]. The biochemical characteristics tested were: (i) catalase, (ii) coagulase, (iii) oxidase, (iv) hemolysis, (v) sugar fermentation, (vi) indole production, (vii) citrate utilization, (viii) urease activity, (ix) triple sugar iron and (x) hydrogen sulphide production.

Purified bacterial isolates were subjected to drug susceptibility tests using the Kirby Bauer disc diffusion method [14]. Commercially available antibiotic discs that were used include: ciprofloxacin, norfloxacin, gentamycin, erythromycin, clindamycin, cephalexin, co-trimoxazole, tetracycline, cefoxitin, ampicillin, vancomycin and chloramphenicol (Hi Media Laboratories Pvt. Ltd, India). These antibiotics were chosen based on the type of microorganisms frequently isolated and their availability at University Teaching Hospital.

Collection of epidemiological data

A pretested structured questionnaire was used to collect data needed for evaluation of the relationship between white-coat contamination and usage/handling practices by health workers. Participants interviewed were drawn from different medical specialties and units listed above and only those persons who volunteered to participate were enrolled into the study. The data collected included information on demographics, history, and duration of usage and personal hygiene practices. Each participant completed an anonymous study questionnaire soliciting information regarding his or her specialty/unit, and white-coat usage practices (e.g., length of usage, frequency of washing, number of white coats possessed, type of cleaning agents used and frequency of usage in the hospital). For the purpose of this study, the usage of a white coat was defined as the approximate length of time the health workers wore the coat while on duty.

Data analysis

After collection, the data was coded and was checked for completeness, and the Statistical Package for Social Sciences (SPSS®) version 16.0 was used to process and analyze the data. A coat was considered contaminated if any bacterial was isolated on culture regardless of quantity. Frequency tables and other statistical presentations were done using Microsoft Excel® 2007. The Chi-square's exact test was used to test for associated between categorical variables and the outcome of interest (coat contamination); and also between two predictor variables. The p-value of less than 0.05 was considered as statistically significant.

Ethics approval

Ethical approval was sought from the University of Zambia, School of Medicine Research Ethics Committee and written consents were obtained from all the study participants.

Results

A total of 107 health care workers participated in this study and had their coats sampled. The distribution of workers whose coats were sampled, according to work department is as follows: obstetrics and gynecology (18), the out-patient department (10), laboratory department (15), intensive care unit (9), medical (20), pediatrics (20) and surgery (15).

Of the 107 white coats screened, 94 (72.8 %) were contaminated with bacteria. There was no difference in the contamination levels between white coats worn for more than 60 min (47.8 %) compared to those worn for 30–60 min (46.7 %) ($p = 0.612$). Further, there was no statistical difference in contamination levels by number of coats owned. Similarly, there was no statistical difference in contaminations between coats washed once a week compared to those washed more than once ($p = 0.7$). Contamination of coats among those who used disinfectants was slightly lower (33.3 %) compared to those never did (58.1 %), although this was not statistically significant ($p = 0.1$). Coats stored at home were more likely to be contaminated (62.9 %) compared to those stored within the hospital premises (26.7 %) ($p = 0.03$). On the other hand, white coats worn just within departments were more likely to be contaminated (52.7 %) compared to those worn both inside and outside the respective department (36.4 %). Coat contamination rate by type of usage was higher for those used in clinical duties only than for those used in both clinical and non-clinical duties (Table 1).

As measured by profession, coats worn by labaratory officers were observed to have slightly higher contamination rates (50 %) than medical officers (47 %). Contamination rates of coats worn by male health workers was observed to be higher (49.4 %) as compared to those worn by female health workers (40.9 %).

The results further showed that *Staphylococcus aureus* contamination had the highest isolation frequency (17.8 %) followed by *Pseudomonas spp.* (3.7 %) whereas *E. coli* and *Enterobacter spp.* had the least isolation frequencies of 0.9 % each. Gram negative bacterial (GNB) were isolated from 5.6 % of the coats.

Drug susceptibility testing

The antibiotic sensitivity tests indicated that the bacterial isolates were resistant to some of the antibiotics assessed. Isolates of *Staphylococcus aureus* and *Klebsiella pnumoniae* exhibited the highest resistance to most of the antibiotics assessed. The most effective antibiotics were ciprofloxacin, chloramphenicol and gentamycin. Clindamycin, cotrimozaxole, ampicilin and cefoxitin exhibited some measures of resistant against GNB, *Pseudomonas spp*, *Escherichia coli*, *Klebsiella pnumoniae* and *Staphylococcus aureus*, respectively (Table 2).

Table 1 Relationship between white-coat usage/handling practices and bacterial contamination of white coats among health workers ($n = 107$) at UTH (2014)

Parameter assessed	No. of white coats examined	No. of white coats contaminated	Contamination rate (%)
Length of time of white coat is in use			
30–60 mins	15	7	46.7
>60 mins	92	44	47.8
Total	107	51	47.7
Number of white coats possessed			
1	18	8	44.4
2	49	23	46.9
>2	40	20	50.0
Total	107	51	47.7
Frequency of laundering of white coat per week			
Once	29	12	41.4
>Twice	78	39	50.0
Total	107	51	47.7
Places worn			
Within department	74	39	52.7
Outside department	33	12	36.4
Total	107	51	47.7
Professional			
Medical officer	83	39	47.0
Lab personnel	24	12	50.0
Total	107	51	47.7
Gender			
Male	85	42	49.4
Female	22	9	40.9
Total	107	51	47.7
Storage			
Within hospital	45	12	26.7
Home	62	39	62.9
Total	107	51	47.7
Disinfectant used			
Yes	45	15	33.3
No	62	36	58.1
Total	107	51	47.7

Pseudomonas spp. and *E. coli* were both highly resistant against cephalexin (100 %). *Enterobacter spp.* and most GNB were also highly resistant against cephalexin (75 and 83.3 %), respectively. Similarly, *S. aureus* was highly resistant against ampicillin (75 %), then co-trimoxazole and cefoxitin at 68.4 % each. The least resistance was observed against chloramphenicol (15.8 %). *Klebsiella Pneumoniae* was highly resistant to co-trimoxazole (100 %), with 50 % resistance observed against cephalexin, tetracycline and chloramphenicol, respectively (Table 2).

Discussion

The aim of this study was to establish empirical evidence related to HAIs in Zambia. This study has shown that white coats used by health care workers at the University Teaching Hospital generally harbor substantive loads of bacterial agents and could play an important role in the transmission of nosocomial infections in health-care settings.

This study has also demonstrated that up to 72.8 % of the white coats screened were contaminated with bacteria. This result was similar to what was observed elsewhere, where white-coats contamination ranged from 23 to 95 % [15, 16]. The rate of bacterial contamination of health care workers' white coats may be associated with patients' continuously shedding off infectious microorganisms in the hospital environment. Other studies have suggested that a patient's skin can be a source of contamination for the health care workers' white coat [17, 18]. As the health care worker attends to patients, there is great possibility of cross-contamination. It has been demonstrated that microorganisms can survive between 10 and 98 days on most fabrics found in hospitals, such as those used for white coats, as well as cotton and polyester, or polyester materials [19]. In line with above research reports, this study has shown that health care workers' white coats could contribute to the transmission of pathogenic microorganisms in a hospital environment.

The white coats of health care workers from the Paediatrics and Medical units were more contaminated than those of health care workers from the surgical wards. This study has also shown that *staphylococcus aureus*, contamination of white coats in medical, paediatrics and surgical ward was 3 % in all these units. However, Wong et al. [13] and Srinivasan et al. [20], reported that *Staphylococcus aureus* was less likely to be isolated from the white coats of health workers in a medical unit than those from a health worker in surgical or other units which was attributed to lower patient contact in the medical wards as compared to other units. However, based on the findings in this study, the low level of contamination in surgical wards could be attributed to the presence of infection prevention and control strategies at the time the study was undertaken. The medical officers' white coats were the least contaminated compared to that of laboratory officers. Although the difference in the levels of contamination was not statistically significant, the fact that laboratory officers deal with patients' specimens directly could explain this apparent difference. Furthermore, the laboratory is likely to harbor a high concentration of organisms within the environment

Table 2 Antimicrobial susceptibility test of bacterial isolates from white coats

Antibiotics	*S. aureus*			*K. pneumoniae*			*Pseudomonas spp.*			*E. coli*			*Enterobacter* spp.			GNB			Total		
	N	*R*	%R	N	R	%R	N	R	%R	N	R	%R	N	R	%R	N	R	%R	N	R	%R
Ciprofloxacin (5 mcg)	3	1	33				4	1	25	2	0	0	4	2	50	6	1	16.7	19	5	26.3
Norfloxacin (10 mcg)	13	6	46.2																13	6	46.2
Gentamycin (10 mcg)	4	2	50	2	0	0	4	1	25	2	0	0	4	2	50	6	1	16.7	22	6	27.3
Erythromycin (15 mcg)	19	10	52.6																19	10	52.6
Clindamycin (10 mcg)	19	8	42.1																19	8	42.1
Cefalexin (30 mcg)	4	2	50	2	1	50	4	4	100	2	2	100	4	3	75	6	5	83.3	22	17	77.3
Co-trimoxazole (25 mcg)	19	13	68.4	2	2	100													21	15	71.4
Tetracyclin (30 mcg)	4	2	50	2	1	50	4	1	25	2	0	0	4	3	25	6	4	66.7	22	11	50
Chloramphenicol (30 mcg)	19	3	15.8	2	1	50	4	1	25	2	0	0	4	2	50	6	2	33.3	37	9	51.5
Cefoxitin (30 mcg)	19	13	68.4																19	13	68.4
Vancomycin (30 mcg)	19	11	57.9	2	0	0													21	11	57.9
Ampicillin (10 mcg)	4	3	75				4	3	75	2	1	50	4	1	25	6	4	66.7	20	12	60.0

since it is the place where specimen containers are opened and processing of cultures is done.

Lower rates of white-coat contaminations were observed among health workers who laundered their coats daily with disinfectants, while higher rates were observed in those who used coats for more than 60 min compared to those used between 30 and 60 min. These results were similar to what other studies had observed in the similar arrangement [15, 20]. In this study, higher contamination rates were observed in white coats used only during clinical duties when compared to those used both during clinical and non-clinical duties, suggesting a strong relationship between coat usage and patient care management. There has been controversy over whether white coats should be worn in nonclinical areas such as the canteen and libraries. This is beyond the scope of this study since transmission of infection from contaminated coats to other people was not investigated. However, it is suffice to say wearing contaminated coats could pose a risk of nosocomial infections to susceptible individuals.

Staphylococcus aureus and some Gram-negative bacilli were the most frequently isolated microorganisms from the white coats of health workers' in this study. This was similar to the spectrum of bacterial agents isolated in similar investigations [16, 20]. These microorganisms are frequently found in the hospital environment and are mainly skin commensals, but they have also been implicated as causative agents of nosocomial infection [21]. In one study, it was reported that up to 65 % of nurses had methicillin-resistant *Staphylococcus aureus* (MRSA) contaminated uniforms after being in contact with patient's wound during care activities [17]. Generally, health care workers' hands are the other principal source of white-coat contamination with pathogens frequently found in the hospital environment. A study has shown that compliance with hand-hygiene protocols among health workers was poor in some health facilities [22].

In this study, *Staphylococcus aureus* and *Klebsiella pnumoniae* exhibited the highest rates of resistance against ampicillin and co-trimoxazole, respectively. *Escherichia coli, Pseudomonas spp., Enterobacter spp.* and some GNB exhibited resistance against cephalexin. The high levels of antibiotic resistance exhibited by bacterial isolates from the coats in this study are of concern to public health [23]. These antibiotic-resistant microorganisms are particularly important because they are capable of initiating severe nosocomiasis in a hospital environment which often require contact isolation and aggressive treatment to prevent their spread [21, 24].

Conclusion

This study has shown that white coats worn by health workers at the University Teaching Hospital generally have high microbial contaminations, especially those worn by laboratory personnel and those worn for a longer time. This study has further established that there is a relationship between white-coat usage/handling practices and bacterial contamination, suggesting that the manner in which the white coat is used or handled by a health worker can largely determine the likelihood of its harboring and potentially transmitting pathogens. It is therefore, recommended that white coats be regularly sanitized, and health care workers also be sensitized on public health risk of HAIs associated with contaminated coats.

Competing interests

The authors declare that they have no competing interests.

Authors' contributions

Contribution SM designed the study, conducted laboratory analysis and also drafted the manuscript; HMC interpreted the results, edited and corrected the manuscript and assisted with supervision; SM analysed the data and revised the manuscript. GM analysed the data and revised the manuscript. GK organized the laboratory specimen and also revised the manuscript and helped with supervision. JBM interpreted the results, edited and corrected the manuscript and supervised the research. All authors read and approved the final manuscript.

Acknowledgement

The authors wish to thank the participants and the management at the University Teaching Hospital for their cooperation. The authors' further wish to thank the technical personnel in the Microbiology laboratory for the assistance rendered during the study period. This research received no specific grant from any funding agency, commercial or not-for-profit.

Author details

[1]Department of Biomedical Sciences, School of Medicine, University of Zambia, Lusaka, Zambia. [2]Health Promotions Unit, Institute of Economic and Social Research, University of Zambia, Lusaka, Zambia. [3]Department of Disease Control, School of Veterinary Medicine, University of Zambia, Lusaka, Zambia.

References

1. Priya H, Acharya S, Bhat M, Ballal M. Microbial contamination of the white coats of dental staff in the clinical setting. J Dent Res Dent Clin Dent Prospects. 2009;3:136.
2. Pittet D, Donaldson L. Clean care is safer care: A worldwide priority. Lancet. 2005;366:1246–7.
3. Levy MM, Fink MP, Marshall JC, Abraham E, Angus D, Cook D, et al. 2001 sccm/esicm/accp/ats/sis international sepsis definitions conference. Intensive Care Med. 2003;29:530–8.
4. Boucher HW, Talbot GH, Bradley JS, Edwards JE, Gilbert D, Rice LB, et al. Bad bugs, no drugs: no ESKAPE! an update from the infectious diseases society of America. Clin Infect Dis. 2009;48:1–12.
5. Weist K, Pollege K, Schulz I, Rüden H, Gastmeier P. How many nosocomial infections are associated with cross-transmission? A prospective cohort study in a surgical intensive care unit. Infect Control Hosp Epidemiol. 2002;23:127–32.
6. Saloojee H, Steenhoff A. The health professional's role in preventing nosocomial infections. Postgrad Med J. 2001;77:16–9.
7. Pittet D, Allegranzi B, Boyce J, World Health Organization World Alliance for Patient Safety First Global Patient Safety Challenge Core Group of Experts. The World Health Organization guidelines on hand hygiene in health care and their consensus recommendations. World Health. 2009;30:611–22.
8. Wiener-Well Y, Galuty M, Rudensky B, Schlesinger Y, Attias D, Yinnon AM. Nursing and physician attire as possible source of nosocomial infections. Am J Infect Control. 2011;39:555–9.
9. National Nosocomial Infections Surveillance System. National Nosocomial Infections Surveillance (NNIS) System Report, data summary from January 1992 through June 2004, issued October 2004. Am J Infect Control. 2004;32:470.
10. Pinon A, Gachet J, Alexandre V, Decherf S, Vialette MI. Microbiological Contamination of Bed Linen and Staff Uniforms in a Hospital. *Advances in Microbiology*. 2013: 2013.
11. Dohoo IR, Martin W, Stryhn HE. Veterinary epidemiologic research. 2003.
12. Loh W, Ng W, Holton J. Bacterial flora on the white coats of medical students. J Hosp Infect. 2000;45:65–8.
13. Fang G, Keys TF, Gentry LO, Harris AA, Rivera N, Getz K, et al. Prosthetic valve endocarditis resulting from nosocomial bacteremia: a prospective, multicenter study. Ann Intern Med. 1993;119:560–7.
14. Cheesbrough M. *District laboratory practice in tropical countries*. Cambridge university press. 2006.
15. Treakle AM, Thom KA, Furuno JP, Strauss SM, Harris AD, Perencevich EN. Bacterial contamination of health care workers' white coats. Am J Infect Control. 2009;37:101–5.
16. Pilonetto M, Rosa EAR, Brofman PRS, Baggio D, Calvário F, Schelp C, et al. Hospital gowns as a vehicle for bacterial dissemination in an intensive care unit. Braz J Infect Dis. 2004;8:206–10.
17. Boyce JM, White RL, Spruill EY. Impact of methicillin-resistant Staphylococcus aureus on the incidence of nosocomial staphylococcal infections. J Infect Dis. 1983;148:763.
18. Muto CA, Jernigan JA, Ostrowsky BE, Richet HM, Jarvis WR, Boyce JM, et al. SHEA guideline for preventing nosocomial transmission of multidrug-resistant strains of Staphylococcus aureus and enterococcus. Infect Control Hosp Epidemiol. 2003;24:362–86.
19. Chacko L, Jose S, Isac A, Bhat KG. Survival of nosocomial bacteria on hospital fabrics. Indian J Med Microbio. 2003;21:291.
20. Srinivasan A, Wolfenden LL, Song X, Mackie K, Hartsell TL, Jones HD, et al. An outbreak of Pseudomonas aeruginosa infections associated with flexible bronchoscopes. N Engl J Med. 2003;348:221–7.
21. An Expert A, Healthcare P, Lewis S. The potential for nosocomial infection transmission by white coats used by physicians in Nigeria: implications for improved patient-safety initiatives. World Health Popul. 2010;11:44–54.
22. Harris AD, Samore MH, Nafziger R, DiRosario K, Roghmann MC, Carmeli Y. A survey on handwashing practices and opinions of healthcare workers. J Hosp Infect. 2000;45:318–21.
23. Jones RN. Global epidemiology of antimicrobial resistance among community-acquired and nosocomial pathogens: a five-year summary from the SENTRY Antimicrobial Surveillance Program (1997–2001). Semin Respir Crit Care Med. 2003;24(1):121–34.
24. Lee N, Lee H, Ko N, Chang C, HsinΓÇÉI Shih MD, Wu C, et al. Clinical and economic impact of multidrug resistance in nosocomial Acinetobacter baumannii bacteremia. Infect Control Hosp Epidemiol. 2007;28:713–9.

4

Lung function and fractional exhaled nitric oxide among petroleum refinery workers

Sultan Ayoub Meo[1,2*], Abdulrahman Hamad Alrashed[1], Abdulrahman Abdulaziz Almana[1], Yazeed Ibrahim Altheiban[1], Mohammed Saud Aldosari[1], Nawaf Faleh Almudarra[1] and Sulaiman Ali Alwabel[1]

Abstract

Background: Occupational and environmental exposure to petroleum refinery products poses a great threat to human health. This study aimed to assess the lung function and Fractional Exhaled Nitric Oxide (FeNO) among petroleum refinery workers.

Methods: In this cross-sectional study, 112 participants (56 petroleum refinery workers with mean age 35.20 ± 1.62 years, and 56 age, weight, height, ethnicity and socioeconomically matched control subjects with mean age 30.02 ± 1.76 years) were recruited. A comprehensive clinical history and examination was conducted to decide whether to include in the study or not. Ventilatory lung function test parameters were recorded by using a Spirometer and Fractional Exhaled Nitric Oxide (FeNO) was measured by Niox Mino.

Results: A significant decline in lung function parameters FEV1 ($p = 0.0001$), FEV1/FVC Ratio ($p = 0.01$), PEF ($p = 0.0001$), FEF 25 % ($p = 0.0001$), FEF-50 % ($p = 0.012$) was observed among oil refinery workers compared to their matched controls. However, there was no difference in the mean values of FeNO between the groups.

Conclusion: Subjects working in the petroleum refinery have significantly impaired lung functions. However, there was no change in the values of FENO between the groups. The lung function impairment pattern provide evidence in the favor of an obstructive lung disease.

Keywords: Crude oil, Lung functions, Fractional exhaled nitric oxide (FeNO)

Introduction

In Middle East, large number of petrochemical refineries are located mainly in the Gulf Cooperation Council (GCC) countries including Saudi Arabia, UAE, Qatar, Kuwait and Bahrain. These countries have added the most incremental petrochemical refinery capacity. People working in oil refineries are exposed to crude oil and wide variety of other petrochemical compounds. Crude oil is a complex combination of many chemical compounds; composed mainly of para-phenol, aromatic hydrocarbons [1], benzene, chromium, mercury, nickel, nitrogen, oxygen, iron, sulfur, toluene and xylene [2]. The fragrant hydrocarbons of toxicological attention are benzene, poly nuclear aromatic hydrocarbons [3] and traces of metals. Crude oil also contains large quantity of sulfur, light naphtha, heavy naphtha, and gasoline. The aromatic hydrocarbons are the main airborne exposure [1]. The petrochemical hydrocarbons compounds possess toxico-kinetc properties which become a cause of health risk [4, 5]. A large number of professionals work in the petrochemical industries. Oil refinery workers are prone to various pulmonary diseases secondary to inhalation of petrochemical compounds and lead to an immunological response mechanism causing hypersensitivity [4, 5]. Occupational and environmental exposure to petrochemical products pose threat to human health and have caused world-wide concerns.

Spirometry and Fractional Exhaled Nitric Oxide (FeNO) are mainly important in the workplace where occupational and environmental inhalation exposures can affect and cause respiratory diseases such as bronchial asthma and chronic obstructive pulmonary disease (COPD). Lung functions along with FENO are essential in the diagnosis

* Correspondence: sultanmeo@hotmail.com
[1]Department of Physiology, College of Medicine, King Saud University, Riyadh, Kingdom of Saudi Arabia
[2]Clinical Physiology, Department of Physiology (29), College of Medicine, King Khalid University Hospital, King Saud University, P.O. Box 2925, Riyadh 11461, Saudi Arabia

of respiratory problems. Lung function and FENO measurements could be used for clinical settings especially for the early diagnosis of COPD development [6, 7]. Respiratory functions in addition to Fractional Exhaled Nitric Oxide (FeNO) in subjects working in petrochemical refineries have not been collectively and extensively studied. Therefore, this study aimed to determine the lung functions and Fractional Exhaled Nitric Oxide (FeNO) among petrochemical refinery workers.

Subjects and methods

The present study was conducted in the Department of Physiology, College of Medicine, King Saud University, Riyadh, Saudi Arabia during the period Oct 2014 to April 2015. Ethical approval was obtained from the Department of Community Medicine, College of Medicine, KSU and informed consent was obtained from all the participants.

In this study, 112 participants (56 petroleum refinery workers and 56 control subjects) were selected. The refinery workers worked 8 h a day, five days in a week. The mean duration of exposure in the petrochemical refinery was 12.44 ± 1.49 years. All the subjects were adjusted for age, weight, height, ethnicity and socioeconomic and demographic status without history of any other occupational or industrial exposure known to cause respiratory illness. A comprehensive clinical history and examination of each of the subjects was conducted to decide whether to include in the research study or not. The control group was also selected in a similar way. The control group consisted of technicians working at the university, receptionists, secretaries and porters.

Exclusion criteria

Subjects with identified cases of anemia, blood diseases, diabetes mellitus, chronic obstructive pulmonary diseases, bronchial asthma, malignancy and drug addicts were excluded from the study. Subjects who smoke cigarette or shisha were also excluded from the study [8, 9].

Spirometry

The ventilatory lung function parameters were measured by using an electronic spirometer SPIROVIT SP-1 (Schiller, Switzerland). Lung function test parameters were recorded including Forced Vital Capacity (FVC), Forced Expiratory Volume in first second (FEV1), Forced Expiratory Ratio (FEV1/FVC %), Peak Expiratory Flow (PEF), Forced Expiratory Flow (FEF-25 %), Forced Expiratory Flow (FEF-50 %) and Forced Expiratory Flow (FEF-75 %). The established techniques in performing the various lung function tests for this study were based on the American Thoracic Society of Standardization 2005 [10]. After taking a comprehensive clinical history and anthropometric data, subjects were informed about the entire process. The subjects were encouraged to practice the procedure at their best possible efforts before doing the actual pulmonary function test. The participants performed the test in standing position without a nose clip and best values were recorded.

Fractional exhaled Nitric Oxide [FeNO]

The Fractional Exhaled Nitric Oxide [FeNO] was determined by using a Niox Mino, Aerocrine, Solna, Sweden. The FeNO device was pre-calibrated for a programmed tests for 300 measurements. Tests were recorded at a fixed time of the day to minimize the diurnal variation [11]. The established procedures in performing FeNO test was based on the American Thoracic Society/ERS Standardization procedure for FENO [11]. Tests for the oil refinery worker were performed in the adjacent room in the oil industry and for control group all measurements were conducted in Physiology Department.

Statistical analysis

The data were computed into the computer, analyzed by using the Statistical Package for Social Sciences [SPSS for Windows, version 21.0]. Unpaired student's t-test (parametric test) was applied to test the difference in the means between the variables. The level of significance was considered at $p < 0.05$.

Results

Table 1 presents the comparison of anthropometric and ventilatory lung function parameters between petroleum refinery workers compared to their matched control. Mean age of control subjects was 30.02 ± 1.76 (mean ± SEM) years, height 174 ± 0.93 cm (mean ± SEM) cm and weight 80.25 ± 2.68 (mean ± SEM) kg. On the other hand, for oil refinery workers, mean age was 35.20 ± 1.62 (mean ± SEM) years, height 170.75 ± 0.83 (mean ± SEM) cm and weight 78.36 ± 1.55 (mean ± SEM) kg. There was no difference in anthropometric parameters age, height and weight among the groups (Table 1). There was a significant decrease in lung function parameters among oil refinery workers including FEV1 ($p = 0.0001$), FEV1/FVC Ratio ($p = 0.013$), PEF ($p = 0.0001$), FEF 25 % ($p = 0.0001$), FEF-50 % ($p = 0.012$) compared to their age, height, weight, ethnicity and socioeconomic status matched control subjects (Table 1). No change in the mean value of FENO was found between the groups (Table 2).

Discussion

Oil refineries produce a wide range of volatile agents and particulate matter into the environment. Subjects exposed to oil refinery substances have been associated with adverse outcomes and respiratory illnesses [12, 13]. In the current study, we found a significant decrease in lung function parameters including FEV1, PEF, FEV1/FVC %,

Table 1 Comparison of anthropometric and lung function parameters between the oil refinery workers and control group

Parameter	Control (n=56)	Oil refinery workers (n=56)	p-value
Age (years)	30.02±1.76	35.20±1.62	0.320
Height (cm)	174±0.93	170.75±0.83	0.100
Weight (kg)	80.25±2.68	78.36±1.55	0.543
FVC (lit)	5.21±0.15	4.76±0.20	0.083
FEV1 (lit/sec)	3.99±0.14	3.08±0.16	0.0001
FEV1/FVC (%)	76.66±2.01	67.19±3.15	0.013
PEF (lit/ sec)	6.89±0.34	4.80±0.37	0.0001
FEF 25% (lit/sec)	6.39±0.33	4.45±0.36	0.0001
FEF 50% (lit/sec)	4.62±0.25	3.65±0.28	0.012
FEF 75% (lit/sec)	2.24±0.16	1.92±0.15	0.151

Note: Values are presented in Mean ± SEM

FEF-25 % and FEF-50 % in petroleum refinery workers relative to their matched control group. Although, there was no change in the mean value of FENO between the groups.

In 2007, a Greek oil-tanker ran aground, resulting in a huge oil spill along the coastal areas of Karachi, and large number of people were involved in oil cleanup operation. Meo et al., [14] conducted a study on the subjects who were involved in the cleaning of oil at the costal belt side. Subjects involved in oil cleanup operation had significant decline in Forced Vital Capacity (FVC), Forced Expiratory Volume in first second (FEV1), Forced Expiratory Flow (FEF (25–75%)) and Maximum Voluntary Ventilation (MVV) compared to their matched controls. This impairment was reversible and lung functions parameters were improved when the subjects were withdrawn from the oil cleanup sites.

In another study, Meo et al., [15] reported a duration-response effect and shows that long term exposure to crude oil distinctly decreased the pulmonary function and subjects who were exposed to crude oil spill for more than 15 days showed a significant reduction in FVC, FEV1, F7EF25–75 % and MVV relative to their matched controls. In the present study, we found that subjects exposed to oil refinery had a significant decrease in lung function parameters including FEV1, PEF, FEV1/FVC %, FEF-25 % and FEF-50 % relative to their control group. Similarly, Jung et al., [16] reported that, adolescents who lived close to the oil spill area showed a decrease in FEV1. Our findings are in agreement to the previous studies conducted by Meo et al., [14], Meo et al., [15], and Jung et al., [16].

Kesavachandran et al. [17] reported that the pulmonary function parameters (FVC and FEV1) were decreased among petrol pump (or also named as gas stations) workers compared to predicted value. Similarly, Singhal et al., [18] assessed the respiratory ventilatory functions in petrol pump workers who were exposed to petrol vapors during the duty hours. The ventilatory functions including FVC and FEV1 were found to be decreased in the study group. Sandip et al., [19] found a significant reduction in FEV1, FVC, FEF 25–75 %, PEFR and PIFR in petrol pump workers. Furthermore, Madhuri et al., [20] measured the pulmonary function test in petrol pump workers (filling attendants) who were exposed to petrol vapors during duty hours. FVC, FEV1, FEV1/FVC %, FEF25, FEF75 % and PEFR were significantly decreased in petrol pump workers. Similarly, Sushil et al., [21] showed that the lung functions FVC, FEV1, MVV and PEFR were decreased in petrol pump workers as compared to controls. The studies conducted by Kesavachandran et al. [17], Singhal et al., [18], Sandip et al., [19], Madhuri et al., [20] and Sushil et al., [21] supported our point of view that subjects exposed to petroleum substances have impaired lung function parameters.

Minov et al., [22] conducted a cross sectional study in subjects employed in the coking unit of a petroleum refinery compared to an equal number of age, gender, and smoking habits matched office workers. The lung

Table 2 Comparison of anthropometric and FeNO between the oil refinery workers and control group

Parameter	Control (n=56)	Oil refinery workers (n=56)	p-value
Age (years)	30.02±1.76	35.20±1.62	0.320
Height (cm)	174±0.93	170.75±0.83	0.100
Weight (kg)	80.25±2.68	78.36±1.55	0.543
FeNO (ppb)	28.14±2.53	22.98±1.74	0.096

Note: Values are presented in Mean ± SEM

function tests results showed significantly lower MEF-50 and MEF-75 among petroleum refinery workers. Moitra et al., [23] reported that, subjects involved in manual cigarette lighter refilling with liquefied petroleum gas (LPG) have decrement in FEV1, FEV1/FVC Ratio. The adverse effect may be relevant to occupational group exposed to volatile hydrocarbons especially in employment sectors. Rusconi et al., [24] conducted a study on the effects of exposure to petroleum refinery emissions on lung function in children and adolescents living in a petrochemical polluted area. Children living in the reference zone showed an impaired lung function parameters FEV1 and FEF (25–75%). Petro-chemical substances are a complex mixture of aromatic hydrocarbons with high volatility. These substances reach the deeper parts of the lungs. Workers exposed to petro- chemical substances are at risk of petro-chemical vapour inhalation and they have more chances of chronic involvement of lungs as indicated by the results in the present study. The petro-chemical pollutants may alter the properties and concentration of surfactant and may thus contribute to the closure of small airways [25].

In the present study, we found a significant decrease in lung function parameters including FEV1, PEF, FEV1/FVC %, FEF-25 % and FEF-50 % in petroleum oil refinery workers compared to their matched control group. However, we did not find any difference in the mean value of FENO between the petroleum refinery workers and control group. While the reason for non significant FeNo is not known, it might be due to the difference in the subject selection. In the present study, we selected the petroleum refinery workers who were involved in the lab inside the refinery plant. These workers were exposed for a short time to crude oil as they were, most of the time, work inside the lab and were exposed to crude oil only while taking the samples or during their visit to the site. We believe that the level of exposure to petroleum compounds for the outdoor workers particularly who were involved in digging, cleaning and shifting the oil, would be much higher than that for indoor workers such as inside the lab. Hence we did not find any significant difference in FeNo values between the groups.

Study limitations

The present study has few limitations that must be mentioned. One of the limitations of the present study is its cross-sectional nature that hampers to find any cause-and-effect relationships. We considered the subjects who were involved in the lab of the oil refinery, these subjects were not very appropriate subjects as most of the time they were inside the lab in the industry which reduces their actual exposure time in oil refinery. We calculate the power of the study, our study sample size is slightly low. Therefore we suggest that, in future large sample sized lung function along with FeNO measurement studies on the subjects with appropriate exposure to the petrochemical substances should be conducted to get the better inference.

Conclusion

It is concluded that, subjects exposed to petrochemical refinery have significantly decreased in lung function parameters. However, our study could not detect any change in the mean value of FENO between the groups. The lung function pattern observed in this study provide an evidence in the favor of an obstructive lung disease. We believe, that, workplace exposure among petroleum refinery workers lead to lung function impairment. Kingdom of Saudi Arabia is one of the world largest oil producing countries, large numbers of people are involved in oil refinery. This study gives great insight into the health problems faced by oil refinery workers and there is a need to take more preventive measures to minimize the health hazards to the workers who are involved in the petroleum industries.

Competing interests

The authors declare that they have no competing interests.

Authors' contribution

SAM, conceived and designed the study, analyzed the data, supervised the overall research project and wrote the manuscript. AHA, AAA, YIA, involved in getting IRB approval, literature review, data collection and data analysis: MSA, NFA, SAA were involved in developing the research proforma, literature review, data collection and helped to draft the manuscript. All authors read and approved the final manuscript.

Acknowledgement

The authors are thankful to the Deanship of Scientific Research, King Saud University, Riyadh, Saudi Arabia for supporting the work through research group project (RGP-VPP 181). The authors are also thankful to Dr. Shafi and Dr Armen for their guidance and the management of the oil industry and the workers for their cooperation.

References

1. Smith HM. Qualitative and quantitative aspects of crude oil compositions. Bulletin Bureau Mines. 1968;445–54.
2. King RW. Petroleum: its composition, analysis and processing. In: Weaver NK, editor. Occupational Medicine state of art reviews. Philadelphia: Henley and Belfus; 1988. p. 409–30.
3. Mac Farland HN. Toxicology of petroleum hydrocarbons. In: Weaver NK, editor. Occupational Medicine state of art reviews. Henley and Belfus: Philadephia; 1988. p. 445–54.
4. Carrasco JM, Lope V, Perez-Gomez B, Aragones N, Suarez B, Lopez-Abente G, et al. Association between health information, use of protective devices and occurrence of acute health problems in the Prestige oil spill clean-up in Asturias and Cantabria (Spain): A cross-sectional study. BMC Public Health. 2006;36(1):1.
5. Best O, Seiyefa B. The human health implications of crude oil spills in the Niger delta, Nigeria: An interpretation of published studies. Niger Med J. 2013;54(1):10–6.
6. Olivieri M, Talamini G, Corradi M, Perbellin L, Mutti A, Tantucci C, et al. Reference values for exhaled nitric oxide (reveno) study. Respir Res. 2006;30(7):94.1–6.
7. Malerba M, Radaeli A, Olivini A, Damiani G, Ragnoli B, Montuschi P, et al. Exhaled nitric oxide as a biomarker in COPD and related comorbidities. Biomed Res Int. 2014;2014:271918.

8. Meo SA, Al-Drees AM, Al Masri AA, Al Rouq F, Azeem MA. Effect of duration of exposure to cement dust on respiratory function of non-smoking cement mill workers. Int J Environ Res Public Health. 2013;10(1):390–8.
9. Meo SA, AlShehri KA, AlHarbi BB, Barayyan OR, Bawazir AS, Alanazi OA, et al. Effect of shisha (Waterpipe) smoking on lung functions and Fractional Exhaled Nitric Oxide (FeNO) among Saudi Young Adult Shisha Smokers. Int J Environ Res Public Health. 2014;11(9):9638–48.
10. Miller MR, Hankinson J, Brusasco V, Burgos F, Casaburi R, Coates A, et al. Standardisation of spirometry. Eur Respir J. 2005;26(2):319–38.
11. Dweik RA, Boggs PB, Erzurum SC, Irvin CG, Leigh MW, Lundberg JO, et al. An official ATS clinical practice guideline: interpretation of exhaled nitric oxide levels (FENO) for clinical applications. Am J Respir Crit Care Med. 2011;184(5):602–15.
12. Yang CY, Chang CC, Chuang HY, Ho CK, Wu TN, Chang PY. Increased risk of preterm delivery among people living near the three oil refineries in Taiwan. Environ Int. 2004;30:337–42.
13. Brender JD, Maantay JA, Chakraborty J. Residential proximity to environ- mental hazards and adverse health outcomes. Am J Public Health. 2011;101 Suppl 1:S37–52.
14. Meo SA, Al-Drees AM, Meo IM, Al-Saadi MM, Azeem MA. Lung function in subjects exposed to crude oil spill into sea water. Mar Pollut Bull. 2008;56(1):88–94.
15. Meo SA, Al-Drees AM, Rasheed S, Meo IM, Khan MM, Al-Saadi MM, et al. Effect of duration of exposure to polluted air environment on lung function in subjects exposed to crude oil spill into sea water. Int J Occup Med Environ Health. 2009;22(1):35–41.
16. Jung SC, Kim KM, Lee KS, Roh S, Jeong WC, Kwak SJ, et al. Respiratory effects of the hebei spirit oil spill on children in taean Korea. Allergy Asthma Immunol Res. 2013;5(6):365–70.
17. Kesavachandran C, Rrastogi SK, Anand M, Mathur N, Dhawan A. Lung function abnormalities among petrol-pump workers of Lucknow North India. Curr Sci. 2006;90(9):1177–8.
18. Singhal M, Khaliq F, Singhal S, Tandon OP. Pulmonary functions in petrol pump workers: a preliminary study. Indian J Physiol Pharmacol. 2007;51(3):244–8.
19. Sandip Meghnad H, Patil PM, Thakare AE, Yuganti Prabhakar V. Lung function test in petrol pump workers. Natl J Physiol Pharm Pharmacol. 2012;2(1):71–5.
20. Madhuri BA, Chandrashekar M, Ambareesha K. A study on pulmonary function test in petrol pump workers in kanchepuram population. Int J Biol Med Res. 2012;3(2):1712–4.
21. Dube S, Mungal SU, Kulkarni M. Evaluation of Respiratory Functions in Petrol Pump Workers at Nanded. Int J Recent Trends Sci Technol. 2013;8(2):149–52.
22. Minov J, Karadzinska-Bislimovska J, Vasilevska K, Trajceva L, Risteska-Kuc S, Stoleski S, et al. Respiratory and nasal symptoms, immunological changes and lung function among petroleum refinery workers. Med Lav. 2010;101(5):364–74.
23. Moitra S, Blanc PD, Brashier BB. Airflow obstruction among street vendors who refill cigarette lighters with liquefied petroleum gas. Int J Tuberc Lung Dis. 2014;18(9):1126–31.
24. Rusconi F, Catelan D, Accetta G, Peluso M, Pistelli R, Barbone F, et al. Asthma symptoms, lung function, and markers of oxidative stress and inflammation in children exposed to oil refinery pollution. J Asthma. 2011;48(1):84–90.
25. Cotes JE. Lung function assessment and application in medicine. 5th ed. Boston: Oxford Blackwell Scientific Publications. 1993. P-122.

5

Multiple subcutaneous granulomas and severe rhinitis after intradermal deposition of epoxy

Steffen Roth[1,2] and Anne Kristin Møller Fell[1*]

Abstract

Background: We present an unusual case of subcutaneous granulomas that also highlights the importance of assessing possible associations between exposure and symptoms early in the diagnostic approach to prevent further adverse health effects. Granulomas of the skin are seen in association with several diseases and after foreign body penetration of soft tissue, but have not been described after contact with epoxy. Epoxy resins are commonly used in paints and other protective coatings, including flooring materials.

Case presentation: We report a case of granulomatous inflammation in a 58-year-old man after accidental intradermal deposition of unhardened epoxy. Multiple subcutaneous nodules were present on his right forearm, from hand to elbow, for a period of 6 months after the incident. Biopsies and histological analysis showed a granulomatous inflammation without necrosis. Microscopic analysis of the biopsies did not show mycobacterium tuberculosis, other bacteria, or fungal elements. Standard patch testing was negative. The nodules disappeared gradually, but intense pruritus remained. The patient returned to exposure and developed severe work related rhinitis.

Conclusions: This case report describes an unusual case of multiple subcutaneous granulomas after a small injury with an epoxy-contaminated tool. Initially no association between the granulomas and exposure was established and the patient returned to work and epoxy exposure. He subsequently developed severe work related rhinitis. The case highlights the challenges of establishing an association between exposure and dermal reactions and that exposure should be reduced or avoided when sensitisation to allergens may have occurred

Keywords: Granuloma, Skin, Rhinitis, Work-related, Occupation, Epoxy

Background

Granulomas of the skin are seen in association with several diseases and after foreign body penetration of soft tissue, but have not been described following contact with epoxy. The granulomatous response is chronic inflammation characterized by focal collections of macrophages, epithelioid cells, and multinucleated giant cells, and may be accompanied by necrosis and fibrosis [1]. Granuloma formation is usually regarded as a means of defending the host from persistent exogenous or endogenous irritants that cannot be eliminated. Several diseases are characterized by the formation of granulomas, including rheumatoid arthritis, sarcoidosis, and leprosy [2]. Infections can result in the formation of granulomas, as in tuberculosis, schistosomiasis, histoplasmosis, and cryptococcosis. Granulomas are also associated with vasculitis [3] and can be found when a foreign body (such as glass, wood, or metal) penetrates the soft tissues of the body [4]. In 2012, a subset of severe asthma with granulomatous pathology was described for the first time [5].

Epoxy has a wide range of industrial applications, including metal coatings, use in electronic and electrical components, high-tension electrical insulators, fiber-reinforcing materials, and structural adhesives. Epoxy resins, also known as polyepoxides, are reactive prepolymers and polymers containing epoxide groups. Epoxy resins may self-react through catalytic homopolymerization, or combine

* Correspondence: annfel@sthf.no
[1]Department of Occupational and Environmental Medicine, Telemark Hospital, Ulefossveien 55, Skien 3710, Norway
Full list of author information is available at the end of the article

with a wide range of coreactants including polyfunctional amines, acids, phenols, alcohols, and thiols. These coreactants are often referred to as hardeners or curatives. Reactions of polyepoxides with themselves or with polyfunctional hardeners form polymers that may have strong mechanical properties as well as high temperature and chemical resistance, and are thus widely used. The epoxy resin itself may be formed by a reaction between the substances bisphenol A diglycidyl and epichlorohydrin; these account for about 75 % of the epoxy resins used worldwide. Depending on the producer, the coreactants vary. Polyepoxides as highly reactive substances are known to be associated with work-related allergic contact dermatitis and occupational asthma [6]. A possible association between rhinitis and exposure to epoxy has been reported but is not well described in the literature [7]. We present an unusual case of subcutaneous granulomas that also highlights the importance of assessing possible associations between exposure and symptoms early in the diagnostic approach to prevent the development of further adverse health effects.

Case presentation

A 58-year-old man presented with multiple lesions of the skin on his right forearm from the hand to the elbow. His medical history did not include any diseases associated with granulomatous inflammation or immunosuppression, and there was no family history of granulomatous disease. Prior to the patient's current work, he had worked with epoxy resins for 4 years, repairing concrete constructions, in the period from 1988 to 1992. He had no exposure to epoxy in the period from 1992 to 1998 and had since then worked for 15 years as an industrial flooring specialist constructing epoxy floors. He had daily contact with polyepoxides, which he first would use as a coating on concrete floors. After hardening, he would use a primer over the first layer and add a final layer of epoxy compound. The patient blended the compounds together directly before he applied the mixture to the floor with a mason's trowel. He reported sporadic use of gloves and a filter mask while working with epoxy compounds.

In August 2013, he accidentally cut himself on the second digit of the right hand with the mason's trowel contaminated with unhardened epoxy. During the following 10 days, he developed swelling with redness and pain of the digit, which spread to his palm. Because of the increasing symptoms, the patient contacted his general practitioner, 20 days after the accident. The level of C-reactive protein (CRP) was then < 5 mg/L. The wound was cleaned but the patient reported that some of the hardened compound remained in the depth of the wound. The patient was given dicloxacillin (500 mg × 4). The wound swabs did not show any growth of aerobic or anaerobic pathogens. In the following days, after another visit to the emergency ward because of an increase of the swelling, he was given erythromycin (250 mg × 2). At this point, the level of CRP was still < 5 mg/L. Thereafter, during the next weeks, the swelling and pain of his finger and palm disappeared. At the same time, multiple nodules (Fig. 1) appeared on the dorsal side of his right forearm. The nodules were surrounded by swelling and redness and the patient reported pruritus. He was referred to the internal medicine ward. CRP, erythrocyte sedimentation rate, leukocytes, and angiotensin-converting enzyme were within normal limits. Two biopsies were taken from the nodules, and the patient was given cetirizine hydrochloride (10 mg × 2) and prednisolon (20 mg × 1, two weeks treatment) with minor effect. The first biopsy showed granulomatous inflammation without necrosis/necrobiosis and no signs of vasculitis, while the second biopsy showed lymphohistocytic inflammation with mild eosinophilic involvement. Microscopic analysis of the biopsies did not show mycobacterium tuberculosis, other bacteria, or fungal elements (Periodic acid-Schiff and Ziehl-Neelsen stains) and the patient was released. The nodules increased in size during the subsequent weeks and varied between 1 and 3 cm in diameter. The patient was referred to a dermatologist for standard patch testing including epoxy, which was negative. The patient had no variation in his general well-being, but several more nodules appeared proximal of the first ones.

During the period of medical investigation, the patient did not work and had no further exposure. He reported that he manipulated the granulomas by squeezing, whereby they would disappear some days later. The granulomas did not spread proximal of his right elbow. All granulomas had disappeared six months after the day of intradermal deposition of epoxy resins (Fig. 2).

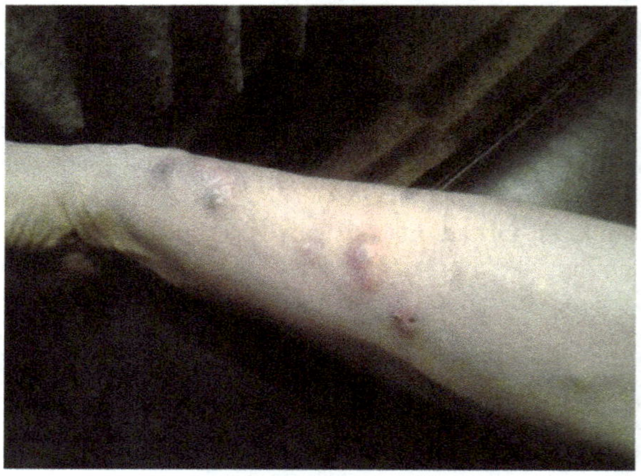

Fig. 1 The patients right arm two weeks after the intradermal deposition of unhardend epoxy

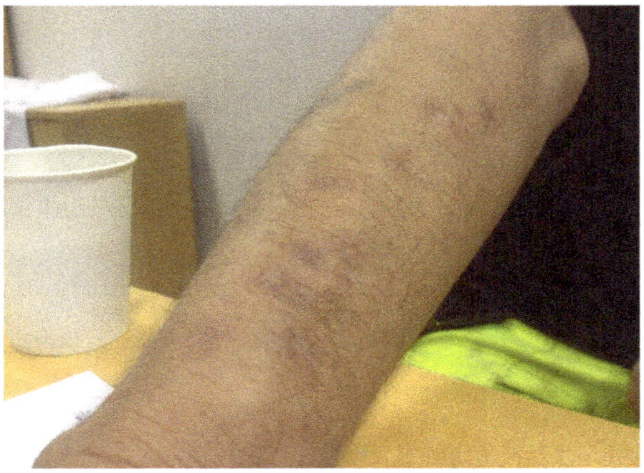

Fig. 2 The patients arm six months after the intradermal deposition of epoxy

However, pruritus in the previously affected area remained. The patient then returned to his work and epoxy exposure continued. Shortly thereafter, he developed rhinitis with symptoms limited to exposure at work and was referred to the department of occupational and environmental medicine. The patient reported that the rhinitis symptoms had increased during the past weeks and that frequent sneezing and a constantly runny nose affected his ability to work. The symptoms improved when he was absent from work, indicating that the patient had developed occupational rhinitis. The patients' medical history did not include any information on former allergic reactions. Standard allergy testing (inhalation panel IP-6 and IP-7) did not reveal any allergies, but the patients total serum immunoglobulin-E (IgE) level increased (from 325 to 435 units) between two visits in our department. We wanted to send the patient to a centre specialized in specific inhalation challenge tests (SiC). However, because such testing requires several hours of traveling and the patient feared worsening of his rhinitis, he refused further testing.

Discussion

Epoxy resins can cause both immediate and delayed allergic reactions, but immediate reactions are rare [8–10]. It is known also that components associated with epoxy resins such as acid anhydrides have potent direct irritant effects on the skin [7] and thus may induce irritant dermatitis. Our patient developed granulomas in a large area around the wound, thus embolization of material from the contaminated tool may be considered as a possible mechanism of the granulomas. Displacement of bisphenol A polycarbonate, a polymer commonly used in biomedical devices such as indwelling catheters and granulomas of the lung [11], has been described in one case report. It is also known that indwelling biomedical devices can disintegrate and embolize into lymphatic vessels. As an example, foreign body granulomas may occur locally after injection of silicone in cosmetic procedures [12].

In the present case, allergy to epoxy was suspected and standard patch testing performed. However, no allergy against epoxy was revealed and the patient returned to his workplace. His IgE level increased between two visits in our department. This may indicate an allergic response, but could not be directly attributed to the epoxy exposure because we had no evidence of a specific allergic reaction. Most commonly, epoxy exposures will result in irritant or allergic contact dermatitis that will not result in elevations of total IgE. Exposure to low molecule weight chemicals such as epoxy can, however, result in mixed immunological responses which may be IgE-mediated [8].

It is known that testing for epoxy allergy can be challenging and that epicutan tests may give false-negative results, thus testing with workplace substances is recommended [7, 13]. Unfortunately, our patient was not referred to the department of occupational and environmental medicine before he returned to work and continued his epoxy exposure. When further approaches were made to establish an association between exposure and his dermal reactions, he had already developed severe rhinitis. The patient then did not want to perform specific challenge testing because he feared worsening of symptoms. In Norway, patch tests with workplace substances can be performed in hospitals with a department of dermatology, nonetheless SiC-testing is limited to one specialist center only. Because attention has been drawn to possible adverse effects from the lower respiratory tract induced by SiC-testing [14], this limits the use of such testing further. In our case, the assessment of work relation thus had to rely on specialist assessment alone. Although questions that identify rhinitis symptoms at work, which improve on days away from work, may have a high sensitivity for detecting occupational disease, the specificity may be relatively low as shown for work-related asthma [15]. Thus, it is important to stress that exposure is reduced or avoided until assessment of possible work relation has been made.

Since specific IgE was not examined, and taking the limitations of the skin prick test into consideration, it is possible also that that the patient's rhinitis was caused by another work related exposure. His work as an industrial flooring specialist may have involved mixed and multiple chemical exposures. For our patient, early recognition of an association between the dermal reactions and exposure probably could have secured the use of personal protective equipment or other means to stop or reduce exposure. Instead, the worker returned to exposure and developed severe work related upper airway symptoms. It is difficult to know if avoidance of exposure at an earlier stage could have prevented the development of respiratory symptoms for this worker. However, after the establishment of the diagnosis, the patient avoided further exposure to epoxy products and reported improvement of symptoms from the nose.

Conclusions

We report an unusual case of multiple subcutaneous granulomas and severe work related rhinitis after a small injury with an epoxy-contaminated tool. It remains unclear whether the development of rhinitis in our patient may be a result of sensitization after intradermal deposition of epoxy or other irritants, or represents a delayed response to long-term airborne occupational exposure. However, the case highlights the challenges of establishing the association between exposure and dermal reactions. It may also be a reminder of the potential major role for the skin in respiratory allergy and that efforts should be made to prevent sensitization through skin exposure.

Abbreviations

CRP, C-reactive protein; IgE, immunoglobulin-E; SiC, specific inhalation challenge test

Funding

Financial support for writing the manuscript was provided by Telemark Hospital, Skien, Norway.

Authors' contributions

SR examined the patient in the outpatient clinic at the Department of Environmental and Occupational Medicine, Telemark Hospital and was the first author of the manuscript. AKMF supervised the patient care and revised the manuscript. Both authors have approved the final version of the manuscript.

Authors' information

SR: MD and specialist in occupational and environmental medicine. AKMF: MD, PhD, specialist in occupational and environmental medicine.

Competing interests

The authors declare that they have no competing interests.

Author details

[1]Department of Occupational and Environmental Medicine, Telemark Hospital, Ulefossveien 55, Skien 3710, Norway. [2]Department of Occupational and Environmental Medicine, University Hospital of North Norway, Tromsø, Norway.

References

1. Williams GT, Williams WJ. Granulomatous inflammation-a review. J Clin Pathol. 1983;36:723–33.
2. Iannuzzi M, Rybicki BA, Teirstein AS. Sarcoidosis. N Engl J Med. 2007;357: 2153–65.
3. Falk RJ, Gross WL, Guillevin L, Hoffman GS, Jayne DR, Jenette JC, et al. Granulomatosis with polyangiitis (Wegener's): an alternative name for Wegener's granulomatosis. Arthritis Rheum. 2011;63:863–4.
4. Joyce S, Rao Sripathi BH, Mampilly MO, Firdoose Nyer CS. Foreign body granuloma. J Maxillofac Oral Surg. 2014;3:351–4.
5. Wenzel SE, Vitari CA, Shende M, Strollo DC, Larkin A, Yousem SA. Asthmatic granulomatosis: a novel disease with asthmatic and granulomatous features. Am J Respir Crit Care Med. 2012;186:501–7.
6. Bray PG. Epoxy resins. Occup Med. 1999;14:743–58.
7. Hox V, Steelant B, Fokkens W, Nemery B, Hellings PW. Occupational upper airway disease: how work affects the nose. Allergy. 2014;69:282–91.
8. Hannu T, Frilander H, Kauppi P, Kuuliala O, Alanko K. IgE-mediated occupational asthma from epoxy resin. Int Arch Allergy Immunol. 2009;148:41–4.
9. Scherer-Hofmeier K, Bircher A, Tamm M, Miedinger D. Occupational rhinitis and asthma. Ther Umsch. 2012;69:261–7.
10. Crépy MN, Bensefa-Colas L. News on occupational contact dermatitis. Rev Prat. 2014;64:342–9.
11. Baydur A, Koss MN, Sharma OP, Dalgleish GE, Nguyen DV, Mullick FG, et al. Microscopic pulmonary embolisation of an indwelling central venous catheter with granulomatous inflammatory response. Eur Respir J. 2005;26: 351–3.
12. Schwartzfarb EM, Hametti JM, Romanelli P, Ricotti C. Foreign body granuloma formation secondary to silicone injection. Dermatol Online J. 2008;14:20.
13. Aalto-Korte K, Pesonen M, Suuronen K. Occupational allergic contact dermatitis caused by epoxy chemicals: occupations, sensitizing products, and diagnosis. Contact Dermatitis 2015; doi:10.1111/cod.12445.
14. Vandenplas O, D'Alpaos V, Evrard G, Jamart J. Incidence of severe asthmatic reactions after challenge exposure to occupational agents. Chest. 2013;143: 1261–8.
15. Baur X, Sigsgaard T, Aasen TB, Burge PS, Heederik D, Henneberger P, et al. Guidelines for the management of work-related asthma. Eur Respir J. 2012; 39:529–45.

6

What do healthcare workers in elderly care know about occupational health and safety? An explorative survey

Stefanie Schönrock[1], Anja Schablon[1], Albert Nienhaus[1,2*] and Claudia Peters[1]

Abstract

Background: Demographic changes will lead to a growing demand for healthy, motivated healthcare workers (HCW) in the years ahead. Along with well-targeted prevention, knowledge of occupational health and safety and infection precaution is essential for a healthy working life. In this context back-friendly working methods and protection from infectious diseases are necessary in elderly care.

Methods: In 2012, a survey was conducted in nine residential and two semi-residential nursing homes, as well as in one home care service in the Schwerin area of northeast Germany. Four hundred and seventy three HCWs were asked to fill in a questionnaire on what they knew about aspects of occupational health and safety such as vaccinations and preventative measures administered by occupational physicians, hygiene, back-friendly working methods and infection prevention. The statistical evaluation was descriptive, with a comparison between job title. Differences were examined with chi square or Fisher's exact test.

Results: The response rate was 28 % ($n = 132$). The largest group of respondents (36 %) were qualified geriatric HCWs. More than 74 % of employees felt well informed about opportunities for precautionary checks and vaccination by occupational physician, and 93 % utilized these opportunities. When it came to assigning modes of transmission to specific infectious diseases, only 23 % of participants were well informed, and one in three (31 %) care assistants was inadequately informed. Fewer than half of participants could correctly name the indications for hand disinfection. Only 66 % of the HCWs said they were aware of training offers for the management of multidrug-resistant organisms in their institution. They did know about possible aids to back-friendly working, although gaps in knowledge were apparent. Only 59 % of respondents knew that care utensils should preferably be stored at working height so as to reduce awkward body postures.

Conclusions: Employees in elderly care are well informed about the range of precautionary occupational medical examinations and take advantage of this offering. Questions in the survey regarding hygiene management were answered in a competent manner. On the other hand some gaps in the knowledge about infection prevention and occupational safety became apparent. Differences between qualified and unqualified participating professionals occurred only in the knowledge of infectious diseases and pathogens and the associated path of infection. The extent to which training can help to improve infection prevention and occupational health and safety should be investigated.

Keywords: Healthcare workers, Infection prevention, Elderly care, Occupational health

* Correspondence: a.nienhaus@uke.de
[1]University Medical Center Hamburg-Eppendorf (UKE), Institute for Health Services Research in Dermatology and Nursing (CVcare), Martinistrasse 52, 20246 Hamburg, Germany
[2]Department of Occupational Health Research, Institute for Statutory Accident Insurance and Prevention in the Health and Welfare Services (BGW), Hamburg, Germany

Background

Healthy employees are the most important resource for a healthy business. The implementation of measures to ensure occupational safety and the improvement of safety and health protection for employees is covered by the German Occupational Health and Safety [1].

The purpose of the Occupational Health and Safety Act [1] and its regulations (i.e., Ordinance on Biological Substances [2] is the health improvement of all employees in Germany. Especially in professional sectors like care work, a preservation of the employee's health in the long run becomes increasingly important. As a result of demographic changes in Germany, the number of people in need of care will increase significantly in the years ahead. According to Hackmann [3] there will be approximately 4.4 million nursing cases by 2050. In other words, the proportion of individuals needing professional nursing care will increase by 270 %. In future, care will be provided less frequently by families and increasingly by professional institutions such as nursing homes and home care services. This means that an additional five hundred thousand healthcare workers (HCW) will be needed in the care sector [4].

Moreover, extending the length of time that is spent in a profession in a working life could help to meet the additional need alongside recruiting and training new healthcare staff. The average period worked by HCWs in elderly care is only 8.4 years to date, which is less than in medical healthcare and nursing [5]. The risk of HCWs in elderly care quitting their jobs prematurely is higher than in other fields [6]. People often leave the profession for "family" and "health" reasons. The health aspects could be countered by training and education in health protection and prevention. Moreover, general working conditions must be improved in order to prevent people from leaving the profession because of low income, physical workload, lack of flexible working hours, stress at work, retirement expectations and lack of recognition of the work accomplished by the profession [7]. Musculoskeletal disorders are the most common reasons for incapacity to work. The prevalence of back complaints in the population of HCWs for the elderly is almost 50 % [8]. The proportion of HCWs with an increased risk of long-term work incapacity due to musculoskeletal disorders has been estimated at 30 % [7]. Improved occupational safety and health protection for elderly-care workers could therefore make an important contribution toward prolonging the time people spend in the profession.

In 2012, HCWs in elderly care reported 899 spinal disc–related disorders of the lumbar spine to the Institution for Statutory Accident Insurance and Prevention in Healthcare and Welfare Services (BGW) [9]. High pressure loads on spinal discs when moving patients are often the probable cause of these disorders [10]. However, the pressure load on spinal discs when moving patients can be reduced considerably by using various working techniques and aids [11]. In addition to pressure loads, awkward body postures are common in elderly care [12]. These can be reduced considerably by adopting ergonomic measures such as raising bed heights [13].

Even more frequent than spinal disc–related disorders were reports of skin diseases (1,738 reports) and infections (1,250 reports) by geriatric HCWs [9]. The number of blood-borne virus infections has declined in recent years [14]. However, the number of tuberculosis infections reported has increased, as has the number of reported cases of methicillin-resistant *Staphylococcus aureus* (MRSA) colonization or infection [15]. In Germany, the risk of tuberculosis increases with age, so geriatric HCWs run a higher risk of infection [16]. The same applies to the risk of MRSA colonization, which is twice as high for nursing staff as for other healthcare staff [17].

The number of skin disease cases reported in elderly care is still high. The proportion of employees who have to quit the profession on account of a skin disease has fallen considerably thanks to the success of secondary individual prevention [18]. Nevertheless, skin diseases can result in long periods of absence. A controlled study showed that workplace seminars could lead to prevention of or improvement in skin-disorders [19].

Therefore, along with preventing skin diseases, occupational health and safety for HCWs in elderly care should concentrate on infection precautions and musculoskeletal disorders, an important task that can be covered, for instance, by occupational physicians. However, apart from medical attention, the employees' ability to maintain their own health and avoid work-related health risks is a major prerequisite for successful occupational health and safety.

The aim of our study was to examine the employees' knowledge of occupational health and safety issues and to determine differences between the participating professional groups.

Methods

Study population

In September and October 2012 we selected a convenience sample of the geriatric residential homes and their employees in the Schwerin area of Mecklenburg-Western Pomerania, Germany. All employees work for one employer in nine residential and two semi-residential nursing homes and for one homecare service. These institutions have a total of 820 residential places. We surveyed all employees in the institutions with direct contact with residents at work. A total of 473 employees received a questionnaire about infection prevention and occupational safety in elderly care. In order to preserve anonymity, no information on the study participants' own residential areas was collected.

The institutions were recruited by presenting the project in person to the company's board of directors. Participation in the study was voluntary. The questionnaire was accompanied by a letter explaining data privacy.

The survey instrument

Based on the Occupational Health and Safety Act [1] the Ordinance on Biological Substances [2] regulations for precautionary medical examinations [20] and recommendations of Germanys central federal institution for disease control and prevention [21], we developed the questionnaire that was to be filled in by the employees themselves. Along with questions on socio-demographic data, it contains questions on the place of work, multidrug resistant organisms (MDRO) and infectious diseases. The closed questions have two (yes, no) or three (yes, no, not known) answer categories, or permitted multiple responses. Part A of the questionnaire, "Personal information about you", solicits socio-demographic data such as gender, age, professional status and experience in (elderly) care work. Part B "General information on your workplace in respect of occupational health and safety" asks about the availability of an occupational physician at the workplace, implementation of a risk assessment and about preventive occupational healthcare and facilities that support back-friendly working. Part C "Infection control at your place of work" contains questions on hygiene training, a hygiene plan and on indications for and approaches to hand disinfection. The fourth set of questions, Part D "Multidrug resistant organisms in elderly care", deals with training sessions on MDROs, the preventative measures required and with personnel screening. Part E "Infectious diseases: modes of transmission and protective measures" required multiple answers in its two sections. In the first table the participants are asked to identify the transmission modes of seven different infectious diseases or pathogens (Table 4). In the second table, respondents are asked to mark appropriate infection prophylaxis measures for three paths of infection (Table 5).

Table 4 suggests 28 possible answers, of which 12 are correct. Table 5 has 27 possible answers, of which 18 are correct and 9 either wrong or correct only in special situations. The number of correct answers is presented in Table 6.

A respondent with at least 10 out of 12 correct answers in Table 4 was assessed as having good knowledge, while a score of 8 to 9 was deemed satisfactory, 6 to 7 adequate, and fewer than 6 correct answers inadequate. Knowledge was also rated as inadequate if there were more wrong answers than correct ones.

Respondents with a score of at least 15 out of 18 possible correct answers in Table 5 were rated as having a good knowledge, while the knowledge of those with 13 to 14 was assessed as satisfactory, 11 to 12 as adequate and of those with fewer than 11 correct answers as inadequate.

The WHO lists five typical indicators for hand disinfection [22]. We added a sixth (wrong) indication to this list and asked participants to state which situation typically requires hand disinfection. The questionnaire also contains six images of hand disinfection procedures. Four images show a correct procedure (images 2, 3, 4 and 6) and two an incorrect procedure (images 1 and 5, Fig. 2).

Nine measures have been specified for dealing with MDROs, of which the German Recommendations suggest six as obligatory [21]. Three measures are not wrong, but not obligatory and usually unnecessary. The following measures should always be adopted when dealing with MDROs: strict adherence to hygiene regulations, hand disinfection, use of protective clothing (disposable gloves and nose and mouth protection where contact with infectious material is possible, protective gowns in the event of close contact with MRSA-positive residents) [21]. The following are useful in certain situations, but not always necessary: displaying warning notices on residents' rooms, strict isolation of infected persons, wearing of protective goggles.

The questionnaire was tested by some nurses in elderly care. To increase the response rate we reminded all participants after four weeks to complete and return the questionnaires.

The questionnaires were analysed descriptively using the SPSS statistics program (Version 21). For the comparison of occupational groups the classification in qualified geriatric and medical HCWs and care assistants was used. Differences between professional groups were ascertained by means of the Chi-square test or Fisher's exact test. The level of significance was specified as $p < 0.05$.

Ethical consideration

All data in this trial was collected, analyzed and disclosed anonymously, following the terms of the Hamburg Medical Association and the Data Protection Act of the City of Hamburg (HmbDSG).

Results

Of the 473 questionnaires sent out, 132 were completed and returned, equivalent to a response rate of 28 %. The study population is described in Table 1. Eighty-four per cent of the participants were women. The largest age group was those under 30 years (29 %), followed by the 40- to 49-year-olds (28 %). Thirty-six per cent of respondents were qualified geriatric HCWs, 16 % medical HCWs, and 27 % were care assistants. The majority of

Table 1 Description of study population

	N	%
Total	132	100
Gender		
Female	111	84.1
Male	21	15.9
Age		
Under 30 years	38	28.8
30–39 years	26	19.7
40–49 years	37	28.0
50–59 years	28	21.2
Over 59 years	3	2.3
Professional status		
Geriatric HCWs (qualified)	48	36.4
Medical HCWs (qualified)	21	15.9
Care assistants	35	26.5
Others	28	21.2
Years in elderly care		
0–5 years	48	36.4
6 –10 years	25	18.9
11–15 years	18	13.6
16–20 years	18	13.6
>20 years	23	17.4

respondents had up to 5 years' experience of elderly-care work (36 %), and 17 % more than 20 years' experience.

Workplace and occupational health and safety in the institution

Eighty-three per cent of respondents said that regular precautionary checks and vaccinations against infectious diseases were offered (Table 2). Of those, 93 % took advantage of such offers. Three quarters (74 %) of respondents felt well informed about precautionary checks and vaccinations against infectious diseases. Eighty per cent of respondents knew the on-site occupational physician. Just over half of employees (51 %) did not know whether a risk assessment had been carried out at their workplace. Asked whether a needle-stick injury was followed up with a check by the occupational physician, 66 % chose "Yes". Asked the main things to which attention should be paid to assist back-friendly moving and handling of residents, 99 % ticked "Use of aids" and "Adjusting bed to working height", while 84 % saw "Working in pairs" and 59 % "Keeping care utensils at working height" as important.

Infection control

Asked whether there were regular infection control training offers, 92 % of respondents chose "Yes" (Fig. 1).

Table 2 Knowledge of healthcare staff about occupational safety in their institution

	Yes	No	Not known	Total
	N (%)	N (%)	N (%)	N (%)
Occupational physician on site	106 (80.3)	25 (18.9)	1 (0.8)	132 (100.0)
Risk assessment conducted	48 (36.4)	16 (12.1)	68 (51.1)	132 (100.0)
Regular precautionary checks and vaccinations on offer	110 (83.3)	11 (8.3)	11 (8.3)	132 (100.0)
Precautionary check accepted	102 (92.7)	8 (7.3)	-	110 (83.3)
Informed about precautionary check	98 (74.2)	34 (25.8)	-	132 (100.0)
Occupational physician consulted after needle-stick injury	87 (65.9)	45 (34.1)	-	132 (100.0)

All respondents (100 %) agreed that the hygiene plan was available to all employees at any time. Asked when hands should be disinfected, 98 % opted for "After contact with residents", 96 % for "After contact with potentially infectious material", 94 % for "Before contact with residents", 74 % for "Before an aseptic activity" and 46 % "After contact with patients' immediate surroundings". Eighty-one per cent ticked "Before septic activities", the only answer that does not appear in the WHO list of five indications for hand disinfection [22] (Fig. 1). All five correct indications were selected by 42 % of respondents, while 21 % selected three indications, and 7 % only two (no table).

Regarding the images of correct procedures of hand disinfection, 97 % chose Image 2 and/or Image 3, 86 % Image 4 and 82 % Image 6, while approximately 2 % of respondents classed Image 1 and around 8 % Image 5 as correct procedures (Fig. 2).

Multidrug resistance organisms in elderly care

Sixty-six per cent of respondents said that MDROs training took place; 92 % agreed that employees were informed if a resident had an MDRO infection, and 91 % stated that their institution had a standard procedure for dealing with MDRO infections. (Table 3).

Regarding protective measures to be taken in such cases, all respondents chose "Hand disinfection", 99 % selected "Disposable gloves", and 97 % "Mouth protection" and/or "Disposable gowns" (Fig. 3). Fourteen per cent opted for "Protective goggles". The six options that are always advisable were chosen by 76 % of participants. A further 11 % placed a cross by five of the six measures (no Table).

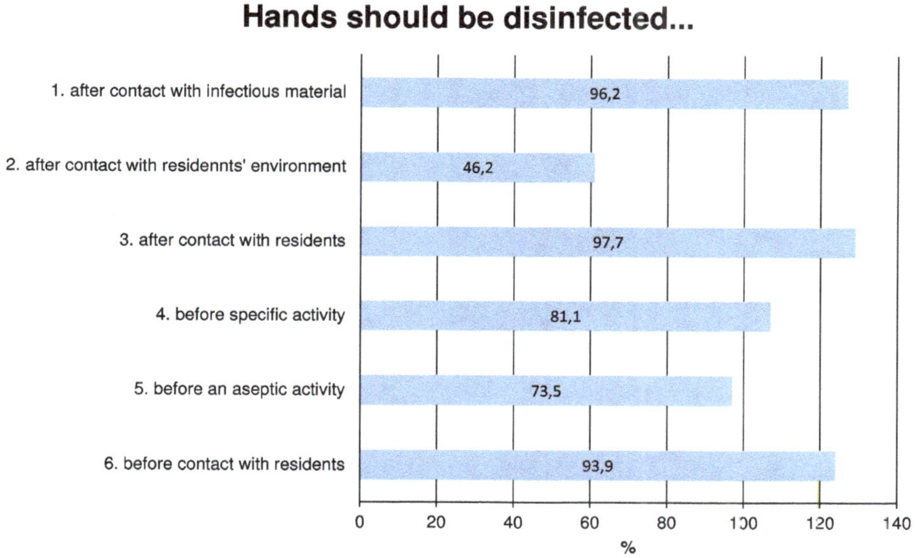

Fig. 1 When should hands be disinfected: 5 Indications for hand disinfection [17]. Numbers 1–3 and 5–6 are correct

Infectious diseases: transmission modes and protective measures

With these questions, employees were asked to match seven different infectious diseases or pathogens with their mode(s) of transmission. The study participants' responses are shown in Table 4. The proportion of correct answers ranges from 94 % for droplet infection in the case of influenza to 29 % for droplet infection with adenoviral conjunctivitis. More than 80 % of respondents marked a cross by seven of the 12 correct answers. In terms of school-type grades for the quality of knowledge, 23 % of participants had good knowledge and 33 % had satisfactory knowledge (Table 6).

Table 5 shows the responses on protective measures by mode of transmission. The proportion of correct answers ranges from 100 % for hand disinfection to prevent contact and smear infection to 34 % for protective vaccination against contact and smear infection. More than 80 % of participants who answered chose eleven of the 18 correct answers, while 32 % had a good knowledge and 33 % had a satisfactory knowledge of protective measures (Table 6).

Here, no significant difference occurred between the professional groups. However, the only statistically significant difference between qualified and assistant staff showed in the knowledge of infection paths. Almost one third (31 %) of care assistants had inadequate knowledge about protective measures (Table 6).

Discussion

No previous questionnaire-based survey of geriatric HCWs' knowledge of infection prevention and occupational health and safety had been undertaken, making this the first study to explore the subject. The available literature tends to refer to existing knowledge about how to improve the care of patients [21]. Consequently, despite the small sample size and the moderate response rate of 28 %, our study represents the first indication of geriatric HCWs' degree of knowledge. The participating HCWs answered questions regarding infection control in a competent manner. On the other hand our survey showed some gaps in the knowledge about infection prevention and occupational health. Differences between qualified and unqualified participating professionals occurred only in the knowledge of infectious diseases.

Occupational-medical coverage, including preventive and precautionary measures are one of the major elements of the German Occupational Health and Safety Act [1]. While most employees were acquainted with the occupational physician on site, around half did not know whether a risk assessment had been conducted at their workplace. The frequency of risk assessments in nursing homes for the elderly and whether employees are adequately informed about them should be investigated. On a positive note, 90 % of those who were aware of the precautionary offers available also utilised them. According to Kromark et al. [23] there is no difference between older and younger employees as regards their participation in preventive measures. Sixteen per cent of respondents did not know that regular precautionary checks and vaccinations were on offer.

Back-friendly working is another important aspect of occupational health. Looking after elderly, immobile residents places great physical strain on healthcare staff, who often work in awkward body postures [24]. Older

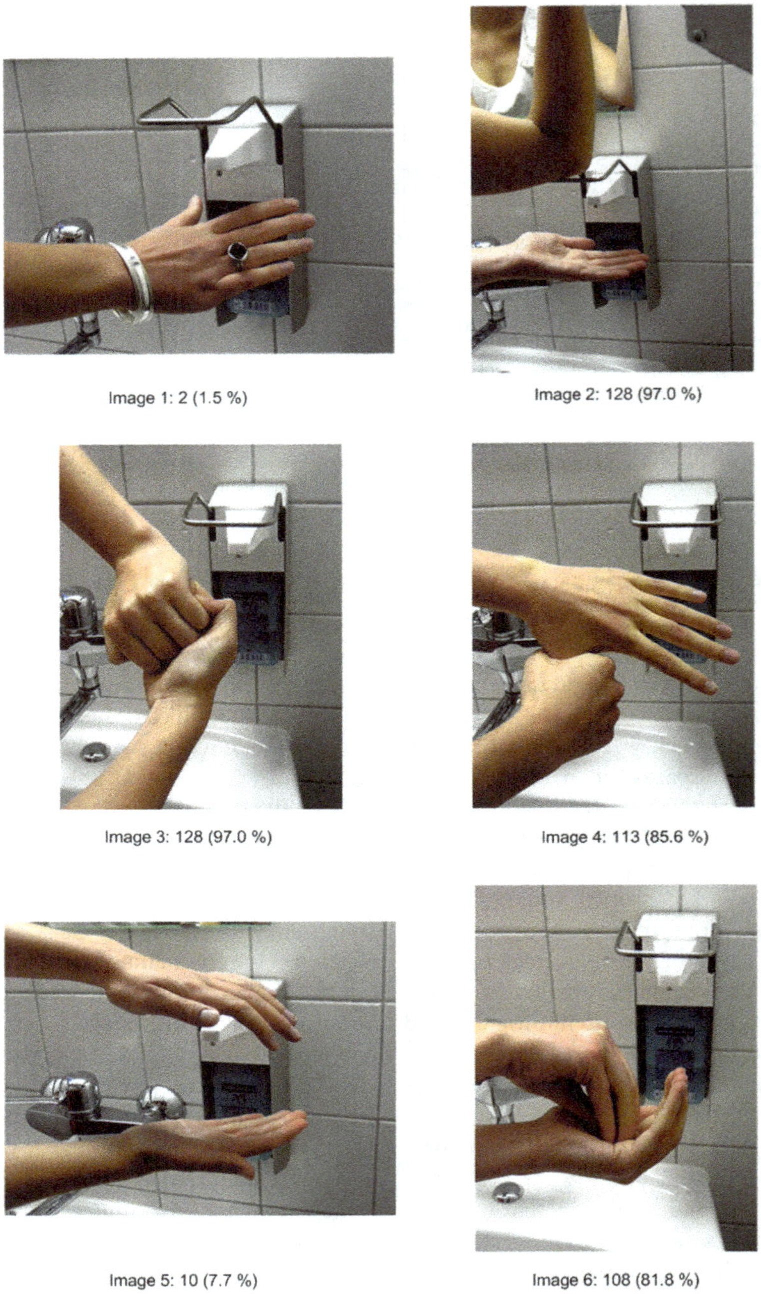

Fig. 2 Which steps form part of correct hand disinfection? Multiple answers possible. Images 2, 3, 4, 6 are correct.

Table 3 Dealing with multidrug resistant organisms (MDRO) in nursing homes for the elderly

	Yes	No	Not known	Total
	N (%)	N (%)	N (%)	N
MDRO training	86 (65.6)	14 (10.7)	31 (23.7)	131
Informed about MDRO cases	120 (91.6)	11 (8.4)		131
Personnel screened for MDROs	13 (9.9)	58 (44.3)	60 (45.8)	131
MDRO standard exists	118 (90.8)	12 (9.2)		130

geriatric HCWs are more likely to suffer from complaints of the cervical spine and lumbar spine than their younger colleagues [23]. Dulon et al. [25] determined a prevalence of 48 % for lumbar-spine complaints and of around 17 % for complaints concerning the neck and shoulder area [25]. They concluded that increasing age and career length in the nursing profession–along with earlier back problems and psychological stress at work–were significant risk factors. Nearly all respondents

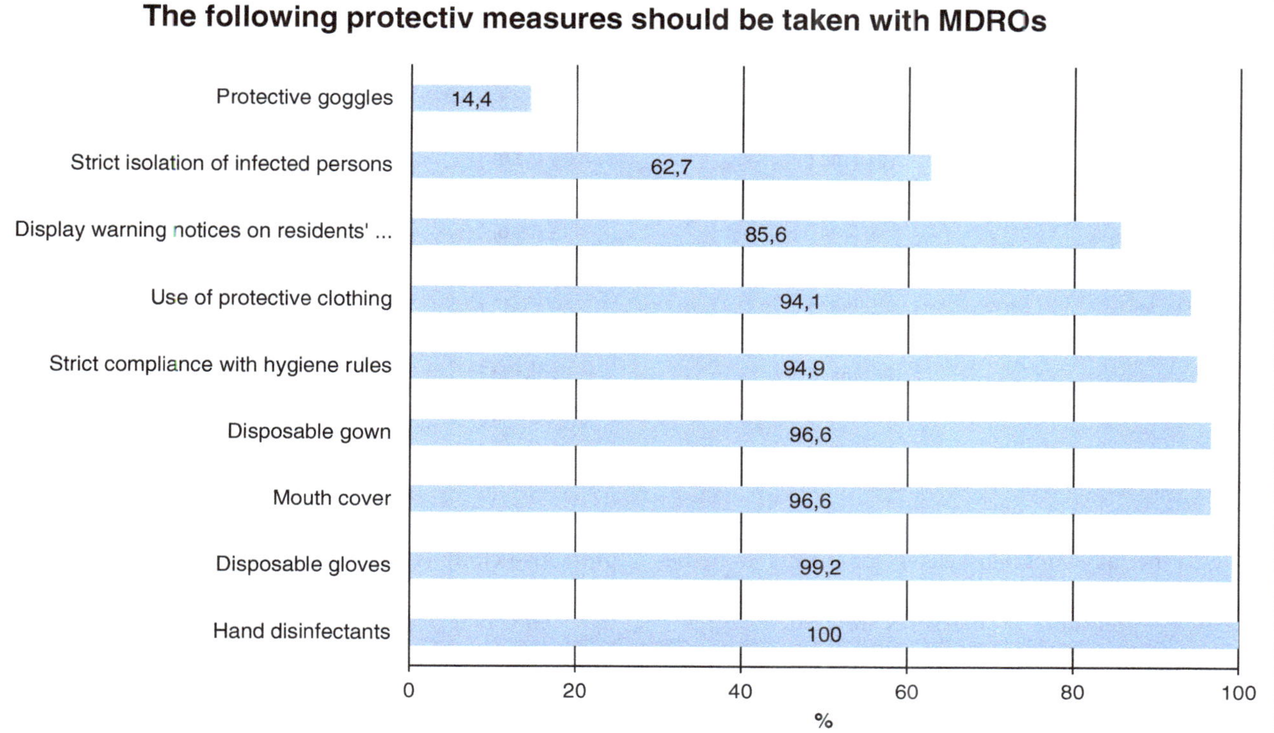

Fig. 3 What protective measures are required for dealing with residents with an MDRO infection?

chose "Adjusting beds to working height" and "Use of aids" as important for practising back-friendly working. Next came "Working in pairs", though this can hardly be guaranteed because of the staffing situation. Only 60 % regarded "Keeping care utensils at working height" as important. This highlights a gap in knowledge that should be dealt with in training courses. Employees in nursing homes for the elderly have a significant advantage over outpatient HCWs in terms of the availability of aids and help from colleagues. However, orthopaedic complaints were more frequently found among employees in residential institutions [8]. With any measures, however, it is important to ask how theoretical knowledge is put into practice. Too few staff, too much work, too little time, an absence of aids, aids that are difficult to use, or possibly even staff complacency can be reasons these important measures for back-friendly working are not or only partly adopted. In order to prevent

Table 4 Employees' knowledge of infectious diseases and/or pathogens and their paths of infections

Infections[a]	Paths of infection				
	Contact/smear infection (faecal/oral)	Droplet infection (aerogenous)	Food and water (alimentary)	Blood (haemato-genous)	Total
	N (%)	N (%)	N (%)	N (%)	N
Conjunctivitis (Adenoviral)	**100 (88.5)**	**33 (29.2)**	2 (1.8)	2 (1.8)	113
Flu (Influenza)	**39 (32.8)**	**112 (94.1)**	5 (4.2)	1 (0.8)	119
Hepatitis (B and C)	29 (24.4)	16 (13.4)	17 (14.3)	**107 (89.9)**	119
MRSA	**102 (84.3)**	**83 (68.6)**	6 (5.0)	35 (28.9)	121
Norovirus infection	**96 (81.4)**	**53 (44.9)**	39 (33.1)	5 (4.2)	118
Salmonella infection	**61 (49.6)**	13 (10.6)	**107 (87.0)**	3 (2.4)	123
Lung tuberculosis	23 (19.7)	**96 (82.1)**	9 (7.7)	32 (27.4)	117

[a]Multiple answers possible, correct answers are bold

Table 5 Employees' knowledge of protective measures by modes of transmission

	Mode of transmission[a]			
	Contact/smear infection (faecal/oral)	Droplet infection (aerogenous)	Blood (haemato-genous)	Total
	N (%)	N (%)	N (%)	N
Hand disinfection	**121 (100.0)**	**75 (62.0)**	**69 (57.0)**	121
Protective vaccination	**39 (34.2)**	**89 (78.1)**	**81 (71.1)**	114
Mouth and nose cover	58 (47.9)	**115 (95.0)**	17 (14.0)	122
Single room	**92 (83.6)**	**86 (78.2)**	27 (24.5)	110
Disposable glove	**119 (96.7)**	94 (76.4)	**113 (91.9)**	123
Protective goggles	37 (39.4)	**84 (89.4)**	26 (27.7)	94
Disposable materials	**113 (93.4)**	**97 (81.8)**	**99 (80.2)**	121
Protective gown	**110 (94.0)**	**88 (75.2)**	71 (60.7)	117
Surface disinfection	**119 (97.5)**	105 (86.1)	101 (82.8)	122

[a]Multiple answers possible, correct answers are bold

existing especially musculoskeletal complaints from becoming chronic – thereby leading employees to quit the profession – precautionary measures are needed [26].

An increase of multiresistant pathogens in hospitals and care facilities for the elderly requires the awareness of and the adherence to infection control guidelines. Appropriate knowledge is therefore of central significance for the prevention of infection. All respondents agreed that the hygiene plan was accessible to all, reflecting results from a study by Peters et al. [27]. They performed a cross sectional study on infection control in residential geriatric nursing facilities in Germany 2012. The questionnaire recorded important parameters of hygiene, resident and staff protection and actions in case of existing MDROs. Most of the residential geriatric nursing homes had standards for MDROs and regular hygiene training for staff. The facilities provided adequate protective clothing, affected residents are usually isolated and hygienic laundry processing conducted [27]. A further important aspect is the knowledge about correct hand disinfection. It appears that most employees disinfect their hands "After contact with residents", "After contact with potentially infectious material" and "Before contact with residents". They tend to see the risk of infections in activities involving direct contact with residents or patients rather than from the environment. Respectively, further training in this area seems advisable. However, one must also question the extent to which these indications are acknowledged in practice. Aiello et al. [28] showed that employees' knowledge of hygiene measures and infection sources led them to carry out preventive measures, but that they did not always know the correct way of doing so. According to a study by Ashraf et al. [29], reasons employees do not

Table 6 Employees' knowledge of infectious diseases and/or pathogens and their paths of infection, and employees' knowledge of protective measures by mode of transmission, classified and analysed

Knowledge of pathogens**	Geriatric HCWs (qualified)	Medical HCWs (qualified)	Care assistants	Social service, supervisors, trainees, community service	Total
	N (%)	N (%)	N (%)	N (%)	N (%)
Good	12 (25.0)	9 (42.9)	6 (17.1)	3 (10.7)	30 (22.7)
Satisfactory	17 (35.4)	7 (33.3)	11 (31.4)	9 (32.1)	44 (33.3)
Adequate	14 (29.2)	5 (23.8)	7 (20.0)	12 (42.9)	38 (28.8)
Inadequate	5 (10.4)	0 (––)	11 (31.4)	4 (14.3)	20 (15.2)
Protective measures					
Good	16 (33.3)	10 (47.6)	9 (25.7)	7 (25.0)	42 (31.8)
Satisfactory	15 (31.3)	6 (28.6)	14 (40.0)	8 (28.6)	43 (32.6)
Adequate	8 (16.7)	2 (9.5)	2 (5.7)	6 (21.4)	18 (13.6)
Inadequate	9 (18.8)	3 (14.3)	10 (28.6)	7 (25.0)	29 (22.0)
Total	48 (100.0)	21 (100.0)	35 (100.0)	28 (100.0)	132 (100.0)

**$P = 0.023$

follow guidelines when carrying out hygiene measures include a lack of equipment such as alcohol-based disinfectants in the vicinity of employees in long-term care facilities. The same study also found that although the majority of employees were familiar with the existing hygiene guidelines and considered them important, only one third answered the relevant questions correctly. The authors came to the conclusion that training courses should be used to help employees understand existing hygiene guidelines so as to eliminate obstacles to applying them. Sound knowledge contributes toward better compliance and thus more effective protection. However, 31 % of respondents said that despite having guidelines they would not change their hand hygiene practices [29].

Larson et al. [30] found that various methods of influencing employees' hand hygiene, such as feedback, training courses or provision of better technical equipment, had only a minimal long-term effect on the frequency of hand washing. Yet 40 % of healthcare staff took the view that "six to ten hand-cleaning units per hour" were necessary to avoid nosocomial infections. In fact, those carers often washed their hands less than five times per hour [31]. The study by Alvaran et al. [32] showed that although HCWs in elderly care had more theoretical knowledge, care assistants had better subjective knowledge of hygiene techniques. However, it was unable to show an association between the mention of more frequent hand hygiene and the current degree of knowledge or a positive attitude to hand hygiene [32]. Our study did not examine whether knowledge is relevant to daily behaviour. Parmeggiani et al. [33] found in a questionnaire-based survey of emergency departments in Italian hospitals that, despite good knowledge and a positive attitude toward the usual ways of protecting against nosocomial infections, the level of compliance with those measures was rather low.

In Germany the recommendations [21] for "Infection Prevention in Long-term Care Facilities" are regarded as an important model for dealing with and preventing infections. The recommendations also include measures relating to residents, personnel, visitors and the surroundings in the event that residents are infected with MDROs, especially with MRSA. As regards MDROs in elderly care in our study, approximately two thirds of respondents were aware of training offers, while most said that they were informed if a resident had an MDRO infection. This information should always be provided so that healthcare staff can adapt to the new, potentially infectious situation. Residential nursing homes for the elderly should also inform the hospital if one of their residents with a (known) MDRO infection has to be transferred to hospital. However, only 10 % of employees said that nursing homes screened their personnel if there were frequent cases of MDRO infection. Employees can be MDRO infection carriers, and this would be a way of identifying possible carriers and of preventing further infections both among residents and staff.

Sowirka et al. [34] revealed that twenty-nine per cent of healthcare staff in a nursing home were tested positive for *Staphylococcus aureus* in a non-epidemic situation, and 14 % of these were MRSA carriers. No significant association was found between MRSA carriage and age, length of service or professional position. However, another study found that women were more frequently affected than men [35]. One study showed that bags and work clothing were especially heavily contaminated with MRSA; almost all of respondents marked "Use of protective clothing" as a possible protection against this [36]. The German recommendations [21] advise that disposable gloves and a mask for the mouth and nose be worn in the event of possible contact with infectious materials, and gowns in the event of close contact with MRSA-positive residents. It also recommends disinfecting the hands after direct contact with residents, after removing protective clothing and on leaving the patient's room. Our results show that nearly all of the HCWs agreed with the use of disposable gloves and with wearing a mouth cover and/or disposable gown. The employees regarded the use of hand disinfectants as an important measure for protection from MDRO infections and as an important way of avoiding transmission. Two thirds opted for strict isolation of infected persons. Since this requires appropriate rooms, it is hard to implement in some nursing institutions for the elderly, especially when they are fully occupied and have multi-bed rooms. According to the recommendations, isolation of MRSA-positive residents in nursing homes is not obligatory. Cohort isolation of a group of MRSA-positive residents may be considered. It must also be ensured that there is no risk of transmission to or infection of MRSA-negative fellow residents, for example, through open wounds or devices [21]. In the event of isolation, it would be desirable to have additional personnel to cope with the more demanding requirements. According to Furuno et al. [37] the majority of HCWs see isolation as the greatest aid to reducing the transmission of resistant pathogens. Yet one must consider the negative consequences of isolation, including adverse psychological effects such as depression and anxiety [38]. Whether these protective measures should be adopted in the event of MDRO incidences requires investigation.

In assessing the study findings it should be borne in mind that the method used was subjective (employee survey in writing). Thus the answers to questions depend both on the respondents' state of mind at the time and on their individual perception and way of thinking. Self-reported information may entail distortions in response behaviour, e.g., along the lines of what is socially desirable. The employees who completed the questionnaire may be those who were already intensely preoccupied with the topics of hygiene and occupational health and safety or who had experienced problems in this connection at the workplace. Moreover, the questionnaire is a measuring instrument developed specially for this survey and used for the first time. Since the response rate was only 28 %, the results should be interpreted with caution. The survey was not directed to scrutinize why existing knowledge is not being applied and it can only be assumed that the discrepancy between knowledge and application of hygiene standards is often influenced by lack of time and staff at the workplace.

In addition, the employees surveyed all worked for the same employer, so the findings may not be transferable to other institutions. In this respect, this study should be seen as an explorative study that attempts for the first time to record what HCWs in elderly care know about infection prevention and occupational health and safety.

Conclusion

Our study concludes that geriatric HCWs in our sample are well informed about the range of preventive occupational medical examinations and answered questions regarding infection control in a competent manner. No significant differences between qualified and unqualified participating professionals occurred. On the other hand there are some gaps in geriatric HCWs' knowledge of occupational health and safety and infection control. Further efforts to improve employees' knowledge are required. Systematic investigation of the knowledge, attitude and associated behaviour of HCWs in care of the elderly is needed, so as to improve understanding of how to positively influence employees' behaviour.

Abbreviations

BGW: Statutory Accident Insurance and Prevention in Healthcare and Welfare Services; HCW: Healthcare workers; MRSA: Methicillin-resistant staphylococcus aureus; MDRO: Multidrug resistant organism.

Competing interests

The authors declare that they have no competing interests.

Authors' contributions

SS was involved in designing the study, performed data collection, made the statistical analysis and interpretation of the data and drafted the manuscript. AS participated in the design of the study and has been involved drafting the manuscript. AN participated in the design of the study and helped to draft the manuscript. CP participated in the design of the study and has been involved drafting the manuscript. All authors read and approved the final version of the manuscript.

Acknowledgements

We thank the HCWs for their participation in the study.

References

1. Gesetz über die Durchführung von Maßnahmen des Arbeitsschutzes zur Verbesserung der Sicherheit und des Gesundheitsschutzes der Beschäftigten bei der Arbeit (Arbeitsschutzgesetz - ArbSchG). Bundesgesetzblatt. 2013;2013.
2. Verordnung zur Neufassung der Verordnung über Sicherheit und Gesundheitsschutz bei Tätigkeiten mit Biologischen Arbeitsstoffen und zur Änderung der Gefahrstoffverordnung. Bundesgesetzblatt. 2013;2013:2514–2534.
3. Hackmann T. Entwicklung der professionellen Pflege vor dem Hintergrund des demografischen Wandels. In: Nienhaus A, editor. Gefährdungsprofile-Unfälle und arbeitsbedinte Erkrankungen ind Gesundheitsdienst und Wohlfahrtspfleg. 2010.
4. Harling M, Schablon A, Nienhaus A. Validierung der Nurse-Work-Instability-Scale-Ergebnisse der Baseline-Befragung einer prospektiven Studie an einer Kohorte von Altenpflegekräften. In: Nienhaus A, editor. RiRe - Risiken und Ressourcen in Gesundheitsdienst und Wohlfahrtspflege. Heidelberg: Ecomed; 2014. p. 115–35.
5. Hackmann T. Arbeitsmarkt Pflege: Bestimmung der künftigen Altenpflegekräfte unter Berücksichtigung der Berufsverweildauer. Sozialer Fortschritt. 2010;59:235–44.
6. Harling M, Schablon A, Nienhaus A. Abgeschlossene medizinische Rehabilitationen und Erwerbsminderungsrenten bei Pflegepersonal im Vergleich zu anderen Berufsgruppen. In: Gesundheit, Migration und Einkommensgleichheit. Bericht vom siebten Workshop des Forschungsdatenzentrums der Rentenversicherung (FDZ-RV) im Wissenschaftszentrum Berlin für Sozialforschung (WZB) - Band 55/2010. Berlin: Deutsche Rentenversicherung Bund; 2010. p. 72–85.
7. Harling M, Schablon A, Peters C, Nienhaus A. Predictive values and other quality criteria of the German version of the Nurse-Work Instability Scale (Nurse-WIS) - follow-up survey findings of a prospective study of a cohort of geriatric care workers. J Occup Med Toxicol. 2014;9:30.
8. Kromark K, Dulon M, Beck BB, Nienhaus A. Back disorders and lumbar load in nursing staff in geriatric care: a comparison of home-based care and nursing homes. J Occup Med Toxicol. 2009;4:33.
9. Wendeler D, Dulon M, Nienhaus A. Unfälle und Berufskrankheiten im Jahr 2012 bei der Berufsgenossenschaft für Gesundheitsdienst und Wohlfahrtspflege. In: Nienhaus A, editor. RiRe - Risiken und Ressourcen in Gesundheitsdienst und Wohlfahrtspflege. Landsberg: Ecomed Medizin; 2014. p. 9–26.
10. Jordan C, Luttmann A, Theilmeier A, Kuhn S, Wortmann N, Jager M. Characteristic values of the lumbar load of manual patient handling for the application in workers' compensation procedures. J Occup Med Toxicol. 2011;6:17.
11. Jäger M, Jordan C, Theilmeier A, Wortmann N, Kuhn S, Nienhaus A, et al. Lumbar-load analysis of manual patient-handling activities for biomechanical overload prevention among healthcare workers. Ann Occup Hyg. 2013;57:528–44.
12. Freitag S, Fincke-Junod I, Seddouki R, Dulon M, Hermanns I, Kersten JF, et al. Frequent Bending - An Underestimated Burden in Nursing Professions. Ann Occup Hyg. 2012;56:697–707.
13. Freitag S, Seddouki R, Dulon M, Kersten JF, Larsson TJ, Nienhaus A. The effect of working position on trunk posture and exertion for routine nursing tasks: an experimental study. Ann Occup Hyg. 2014;58:317–25.
14. Nienhaus A, Kesavachandran C, Wendeler D, Haamann F, Dulon M. Infectious diseases in healthcare workers - an analysis of the standardised data set of a German compensation board. J Occup Med Toxicol. 2012;7:8.
15. Haamann F, Dulon M, Nienhaus A. Occupationally acquired MRSA infections in the healthcare sector [Berufliche MRSA-Infektionen bei Beschäftigten im Gesundheitsdienst]. Arbeitsmed Sozialmed Umweltmed. 2011;46:585–9.
16. Schablon A, Nienhaus A, Ringshausen FC, Preisser AM, Peters C. Occupational Screening for Tuberculosis and the Use of a Borderline Zone for Interpretation of the IGRA in German Healthcare Workers. PLoS ONE. 2014;9:e115322.
17. Dulon M, Peters C, Schablon A, Nienhaus A. MRSA carriage among healthcare workers in non-outbreak settings in Europe and the United States: a systematic review. BMC Infect Dis. 2014;14:363.
18. Nienhaus A, Rojahn K, Skudlik C, Wulfhorst B, Dulon M, Brandenburg S. Sekundäre Individualprävention bei FriseurInnen mit arbeitsbedingten Hauterkrankungen [Secondary individual prevention and rehabilitation in female hairdressers suffering from skin diseases]. Gesundheitswesen. 2004;66:759–64.
19. Dulon M, Pohrt U, Skudlik C, Nienhaus A. Prevention of occupational skin disease: a workplace intervention study in geriatric nurses. Br J Dermatol. 2009;161:337–44.

20. Verordnung zur arbeitsmedizinischen Vorsorge (ArbMedVV) vom 18. Dezember 2008 (BGBl. I S. 2768), die zuletzt durch Artikel 1 der Verordnung vom 23. Oktober 2013 (BGBl. I S. 3882) geändert worden ist'. Bundesgesetzblatt. 2013;Teil I:3882–3888.
21. KRINKO. Infektionsprävention in Heimen - Empfehlung der Kommission für Krankenhaushygiene und Infektionsprävention beim Robert-Koch-Institut (RKI). Bundesgesundheitsblatt Gesundheitsforschung Gesundheitsschutz. 2005;48:1061–80.
22. Pocket Leaflet. Clean Care is Safer Care. How to handrub? How to handwash? Five moments for hand hygiene? [http://www.who.int/gpsc/tools/Pocket-Leaflet.pdf?ua=1&bcsi_scan_ce299946edb5e163=1].
23. Kromark K, Dulon M, Nienhaus A. Gesundheitsindikatoren und Präventionsverhalten bei älteren Beschäftigten in der Altenpflege. In: Nienhaus A, editor. Gefährdungsprofile - Unfälle und arbeitsbedingte Erkrankungen in Gesundheitsdienst und Wohlfahrtspflege. 2nd ed. Landsberg, Lech: Ecomed; 2010. p. 180–96.
24. Freitag S, Fincke-Junos I, Nienhaus A. Messtechnische Analyse von belastenden Körperhaltungen bei Pflegekräften - Vergleich zwischen einer geriatrischen Station und anderen Krankenhausstationen. In: Nienhaus A, editor. Gefährdungsprofile - Unfälle und arbeitsbedingte Erkrankungen in Gesundheitsdienst und Wohlfahrtspflege. 2nd ed. Landsberg, Lech: Ecomed; 2010. p. 160–79.
25. Dulon M, Kromark K, Skudlik C, Nienhaus A. Prevalence of skin and back diseases in geriatric care nurses. Int Arch Occup Environ Health. 2008;81:983–92.
26. Andersen LL, Clausen T, Mortensen OS, Burr H, Holtermann A. A prospective cohort study on musculoskeletal risk factors for long-term sickness absence among healthcare workers in eldercare. Int Arch Occup Environ Health. 2012;85:615–22.
27. Peters C, Schablon A, Bollongino K, Maass M, Kass D, Dulon M, et al. Multiresistant pathogens in geriatric nursing - infection control in residential facilities for geriatric nursing in Germany. GMS Hyg Infect Control. 2014;9:Doc22.
28. Aiello AE, Malinis M, Knapp JK, Mody L. The influence of knowledge, perceptions, and beliefs, on hand hygiene practices in nursing homes. Am J Infect Control. 2009;37:164–7.
29. Ashraf MS, Hussain SW, Agarwal N, Ashraf S, El-Kass G, Hussain R, et al. Hand hygiene in long-term care facilities: a multicenter study of knowledge, attitudes, practices, and barriers. Infect Control Hosp Epidemiol. 2010;31:758–62.
30. Larson EL, Bryan JL, Adler LM, Blane C. A multifaceted approach to changing handwashing behavior. Am J Infect Control. 1997;25:3–10.
31. Tai JW, Mok ES, Ching PT, Seto WH, Pittet D. Nurses and physicians' perceptions of the importance and impact of healthcare-associated infections and hand hygiene: a multi-center exploratory study in Hong Kong. Infection. 2009;37:320–33.
32. Alvaran MS, Butz A, Larson E. Opinions, knowledge, and self-reported practices related to infection control among nursing personnel in long-term care settings. Am J Infect Control. 1994;22:367–70.
33. Parmeggiani C, Abbate R, Marinelli P, Angelillo IF. Healthcare workers and health care-associated infections: knowledge, attitudes, and behavior in emergency departments in Italy. BMC Infect Dis. 2010;10:35.
34. Sowirka O, Carron A, Perri M, Zervos M, Hyde K, Maddens M. Prevalence of Staphylococcus aureus carriage among asymptomatic nursing home personnel: a pilot study. J Am Med Dir Assoc. 2000;1:159–63.
35. Olsen K, Sangvik M, Simonsen GS, Sollid JU, Sundsfjord A, Thune I, et al. Prevalence and population structure of Staphylococcus aureus nasal carriage in healthcare workers in a general population. The Tromso Staph and Skin Study. Epidemiol Infect. 2013;141:143–52.
36. Gaspard P, Eschbach E, Gunther D, Gayet S, Bertrand X, Talon D. Meticillin-resistant Staphylococcus aureus contamination of healthcare workers' uniforms in long-term care facilities. J Hosp Infect. 2009;71:170–5.
37. Furuno JP, Krein S, Lansing B, Mody L. Health care worker opinions on use of isolation precautions in long-term care facilities. Am J Infect Control. 2012;40:263–6.
38. Abad C, Fearday A, Safdar N. Adverse effects of isolation in hospitalised patients: a systematic review. J Hosp Infect. 2010;76:97–102.

7

Silicosis: geographic changes in research - an analysis employing density-equalizing mapping

Alexander Gerber*, Doris Klingelhoefer, David A Groneberg and Matthias Bundschuh

Abstract

Background: A critical evaluation of scientific efforts is needed in times of modified evaluation criteria for academic personnel and institutions.

Methods: Using scientometric benchmark procedures and density-equalizing mapping, we analysed the global scientific efforts on "silicosis" of the last 92 years focusing on geographical changes within the last 30 years, specifying the most productive authors, institutions, countries and the most successful cooperations.

Results: The USA as the most productive supplier have established their position as center of international cooperation, followed in considerable distance by the United Kingdom, Germany and China. Asian countries, particularly China, catch up and are expected to excel the USA still in this decade.

Conclusion: The combination of scientometric procedures with density-equalizing mapping reveals a distinct global pattern of research productivity and citation activity. Modified h-index, citationrate and impact factor have to be discussed critically due to distortion by bias of self-citation, language and co-authorship.

Keywords: Silicosis, Scientometria, Density-equalizing mapping, H-Index, Citationrate

Introduction

Silicosis is a fibrotic lung disease caused by inhalation of crystalline silica (Silicon dioxide, SiO2). Universalized insufficient technical protection measures in the past to this day, result in exposition of countless workers over considerable spans of their lives and have made silicosis one of the most important occupational diseases worldwide [1]. The highly fibrogenic crystalline silica is the most abundant mineral worldwide. Of the several crystalline forms quartz, tridymite and cristobalite are the most important ones. Quartz occurs naturally in rocks such as granite, slate and sandstone, as well as in desert sand, which is practically pure silica. Tridymite and cristobalite are even more fibrogenic than quartz and occur naturally as high temperature polymorphs of silica, for example in lava [2]. For occupational purpose, silica is commonly used in the ceramic- and glass-industry, in foundries, chemical industry, electrical industry, natural stone industry, jewellery industry and for working methods such as sand jet polishing, abrasive technics with sand and many more [3]. Although protective measures have resulted in a declining in death rate due to silicosis in developed countries over the past decades, new outbreaks still occur in emerging nations [4,5]. Upon inhalation of respirable silica dusts, the crystals are deposited in the distal airways, and reactive oxygen species are produced on both the particle surfaces and via phagocytic cells. Phagocytosis of crystalline silica causes damage of the phagolysosomal membranes and induces apoptosis. Activation of the NALP3-Inflammasome triggers the inflammatory cascade by production of inflammatory cytocines, subsequently leading to fibrosis [6-8]. Diagnosis of silicosis generally requires a substantial occupational or environmental exposure of respirable cristalline silica and compatible radiologic abnormalities. Other competing diagnoses like infections, carcinomas, idiopathic interstitial pneumonia or interstitial lung diseases associated with a rheumatic disease have to be excluded. Chronic silicosis, the most common form of this disease, is distinguished from the accelerated silicosis and the acute silicosis by its low severity and rapidity of progression and usually develops after 10 to 30 years of low concentrated exposure to silica dust [5,9,10]. Patients may initially be asymptomatic and show shortness of

* Correspondence: gerber@med.uni-frankfurt.de
Institute of Occupational, Social and Environmental Medicine, Goethe-University, Theodor-Stern-Kai 7, Haus 9b, Frankfurt am Main 60590, Germany

breath at later stages. Chest radiography usually shows small round opacities, especially in the upper lung zones, and occasionally diffuse interstitial pattern of fibrosis which may be progressive over years, even after cessation of exposition. With retraction of the lung tissue, compensatory emphysema arises. The hilar and mediastinal lymph nodes often enlarge and frequently calcify in an eggshell pattern. Pulmonary function testing may be without pathological findings or reveals airflow limitation, restrictive defects and reduced diffusion capacity [9]. Accelerated silicosis develops 5–10 years after initial exposure to higher concentrations of crystalline silica dust. Clinical symptoms and radiologic imaging are similar to chronic silicosis but tend to progress more rapidly [11]. Acute silicosis, also known as silicoproteinosis, develops after exposure to high concentrations of respirable crystalline silica dust for a fiew weeks to 5 years. Most affected by acute silicosis are sandblasters and quartzite millers [5,12]. Radiographicaly a ground-glass appearance and air-bronchogramm is described. Dry cough, fever, fatigue, weight loss, respiratory insufficiency, and even death within months occur. Silicosis has been associated with several disorders, of which tuberculosis, COPD and lung cancer are the most important [13,14]. A curative treatment for silicosis does not exist, treatment options focus on preventing complications. In recent years, enormous efforts have been made to improve the understanding of pathogenetic mechanisms in silicosis. Particularly the finding of the NALP3-Inflammasome as major trigger of the inflammatory cascade appears to be an important step to break down into immunologic aspects of the disease and could explain the frequently observed incidence of rheumatic diseases e.g. rheumatoid arthritis or systemic lupus erythematodes as a consequence of breaking the immunologic tolerance [15-18]. Nevertheless, a scientometric approach to the topic "silicosis" has not been available despite an increased need to evaluate quality and quantity of scientific accomplishments. The aim of the present study is to evaluate the scientific effort in silicosis, considering geographical aspects, using large scale data analysis, scientometric approaches and density-equalizing procedures.

Methods

Scientometrics

Scientometrics is the science of measuring and analyzing research. It uses computational approaches and bibliometric methods such as citation analysis, impact factor or h-index.

Data source

Data was retrieved from the database Web of Science (WoS) by Thomson Reuters and from the Medline database (PubMed) by the U.S. National Library of Medicine.

Search strategy

Using PubMed and the MeSH search tags, MeSH heading related to "silicosis" were created, combined with the Boolean operator OR and entered as follows into the WoS search field to approximate the overall number of published items: "Silicosis" OR "Anthracoses" OR "Coal Worker's Pneumoconiosis" OR "Coal Worker Pneumoconiosis" OR "Coal Worker's Pneumoconioses" OR "Coal Workers Pneumoconiosis" OR "Pneumoconioses, Coal Worker's" OR "Pneumoconiosis, Coal Worker's" OR "Pneumoconiosis, Coal Worker" OR "Pneumoconiosis, Coal Workers" OR "Black Lung" OR "Black Lungs" OR "Lung, Black" OR "Lungs, Black" OR "Coal Miner's Lung" OR "Coal Miner Lung" OR "Coal Miner's Lungs" OR "Coal Miners Lung" OR "Miner's Lung, Coal" OR "Miner's Lungs, Coal" OR "Black Lung Disease" OR "Black Lung Diseases" OR "Coalworker's Pneumoconiosis" OR "Coalworker Pneumoconiosis" OR "Coalworker's Pneumoconioses" OR "Coalworkers Pneumoconiosis" OR "Pneumoconioses, Coalworker's" OR "Pneumoconiosis, Coalworker's". Further investigations used the "Analyse Results" function and the "Citation Report" provide by the WoS database.

Timeframe

The analysed timeframe covers the years from 1920 to 2012. Results from 2013 were not considered due to incomplete data acquisition at the time of analysis.

Data analysis and categorization

Citation analysis is used as a tool to estimate quantitative and qualitative research productivity for the scientific community. All publications in the space of time referring to silicosis were analysed with the "citation report" method. Total number of citations and the average citation per item (citation rate) were calculated. Publication date, country of origin, source title, author and institution were other aspects of analysis. Findings were transferred to excel charts and illustrated in diagrams. Density-equalizing mapping procedures based on Gastner`s and Newman`s algorithm were used to visualize the distribution of the total number of published items and the average citation rate in a country-specific manner [19]. Using this approach, territories (countries) were resized in proportion to selected variables (for our purpose the number of published items and average citation rate). For methodical reasons, we decided to attribute any special administrative or autonomous region worldwide to its related country based on the present governmental status in the year 2013. E.g. Hong Kong was grouped to Mainland China despite its being a British colony until its reversion to China in 1997, and its medical system as well as the publications still being independent from Mainland China. Northern Ireland, Wales and Scotland were grouped to the UK and the former

"German Democratic Republic" and the "Federal Republic of Germany" were grouped to Germany. This expectedly caused some distortion in each case for the benefit of the incorporating country and must therefore be regarded as a methodological bias.

H-index

The h-index is a bibliometric device, developed by Hirsch in 2005, to measure productivity and impact of scientists, institutions or countries at a point of time. It is calculated from the set of most cited publications and

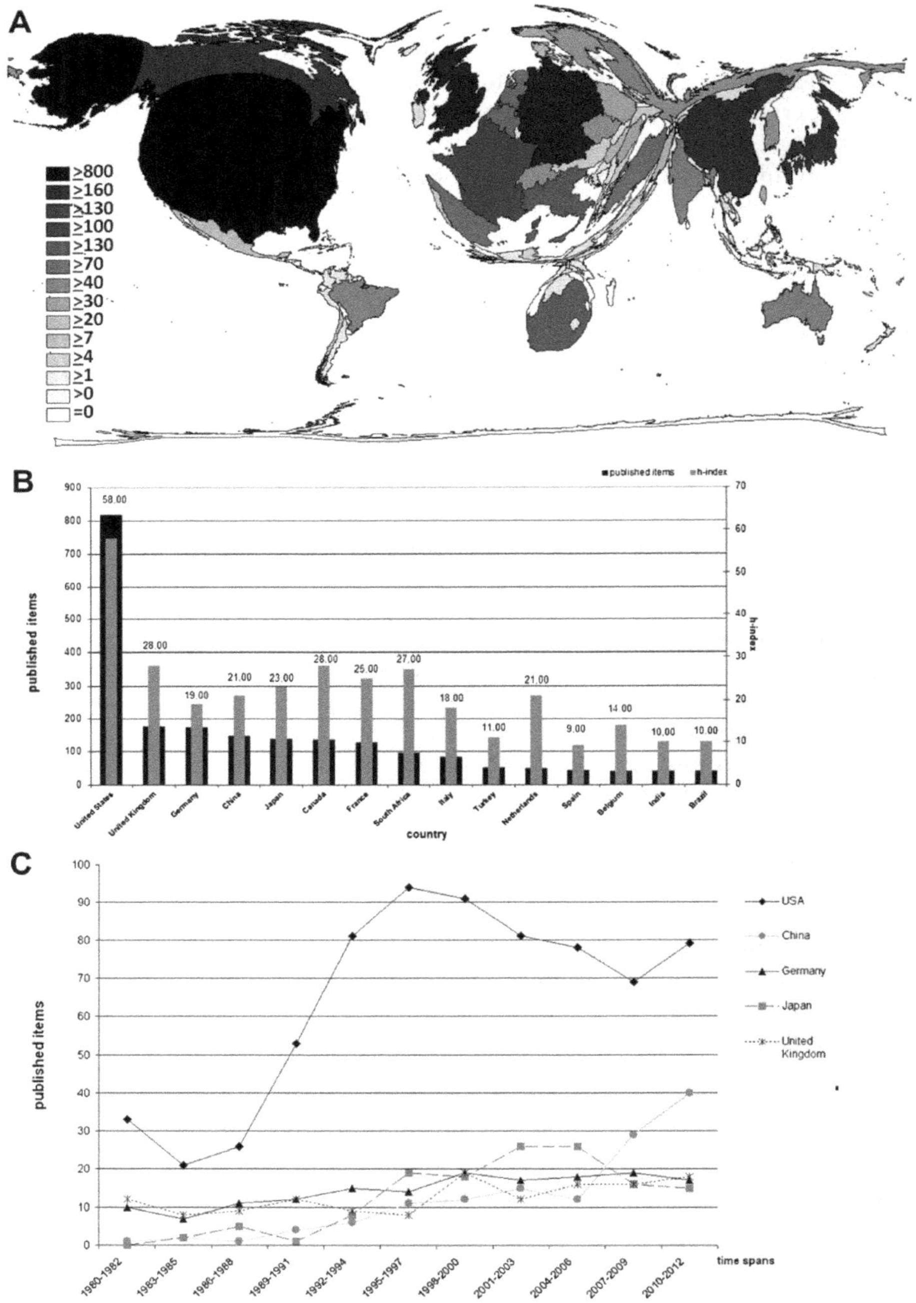

Figure 1 Published items regarding "silicosis". A: Density-equalizing map illustrating the number of publications in each particular country (the area of each country and its colour were scaled in proportion to its total number of publications regarding "silicosis" as illustrated in the panel). **B:** Ranking of country total number of published items an h-index related to "silicosis". **C:** Trend of the scientific productivity of the five most productive countries.

the number of received citations. The height of the h-index suggests the influence of the author in his scientific field [20,21]. For this study we used a modified h-index, generated on the basis of the authors work in the analyzed timeframe referring to silicosis. Only publications listed in the WoS in peer-reviewed journals with an impact factor were considered. Book articles were not considered as well as publications, when referring not explicitly to silicosis.

Impact factor

The impact factor was devised by Eugene Garfield, the founder of the Institute for Scientific Information, to estimate a journals relative importance in its scientific

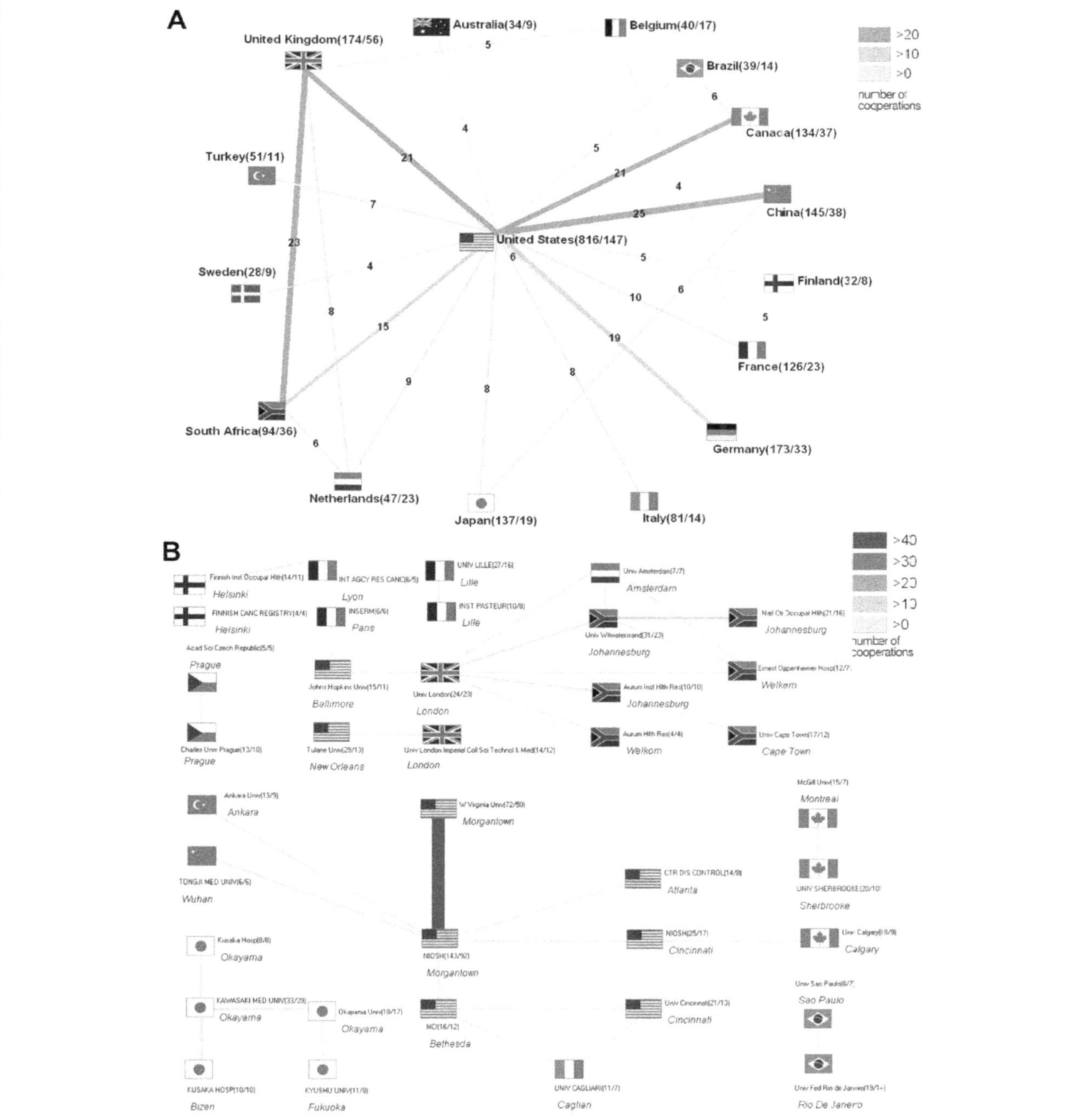

Figure 2 Cooperating articles. A: Analysis of the international cooperations. **B:** Analysis of the interinstitutional cooperations.

field. It reflects the average number of citations per annum, published articles received during the two preceding years [22].

Analysis of cooperation

To investigate cooperation between countries and institutions, data of references were gained from WoS as plain text files and analysed. If at least two authors, coming from different institutions or countries, contributed to a publication, this relationship was defined as a cooperation. To visualize the productivity of cooperation for each pair of institutions or countries, a vector was calculated, proportional to the number of cooperation in thickness and shade of grey.

Results

Total number of published items, analysis of origin and cooperation

The WoS database provided a total of 2,805 published items with a reference to silicosis in the research timeframe. The publications originate from 74 countries with the USA being the most productive supplier (Figure 1A). Overall, US-American scientists participated in 29% of all publications, followed by researchers from the United Kingdom, Germany, China and Japan respectively (Figure 1A + B). Only the USA published more than 500 items hence their dominating the cartogram. Major parts of South America (except for Brazil), Africa (except for South Africa) and East-Asia (except for Japan and China) are minimized. An analysis of developments in the country-specific scientific productivity since 1980 detects remarkable changes in geographic foci. While China started contributing measurably to the worldwide scientific output related to silicosis as late as only in 1980, it has since developed into the currently second most productive country with a tendency to rise (Figure 1C). Most of the scientific efforts are concentrated in the USA. According to this, the USA were placed in the middle of the diagram (Figure 2A). The cooperations between the USA and China, the USA and the United Kingdom, the United Kingdom and South Africa, the USA and Canada, and between the USA and Germany have been identified as the most productive ones. The closest inter-institutional collaboration worldwide exists between the West Virginia University Hospital in Morgantown (USA) and the National Institute for Occupational Safety and Health (NIOSH) in Morgantown (USA) (Figure 2B).

Citation parameters

The United States of America (58), hold the highest h-index in a country-specific manner, followed by the United Kingdom and Canada (both 28), and South Africa (27) (Figure 1B + Figure 3). The highest number of research institutions engaged with the topic "silicosis" is agglomerated in the USA, followed by Germany, Canada, China and Japan (Figure 4A). The USA also receive the highest total amount of citations, followed with considerable distance by Canada and the UK (Figure 4B). As for the citation rate (CR, average citation per publication), the Netherlands attract attention (Figure 4C) with a CR of 23 (47 published items, 1,092 received citations) outnumbering even the most productive and frequently cited countries such as South Africa (CR: 19), the USA (CR:18), Canada (CR: 17) and the UK (CR:16).

Analysis of publishing journals and the most productive authors concerned with silicosis

Identified as the most productive journal dealing with silicosis (Figure 5A), "Occupational and Environmental

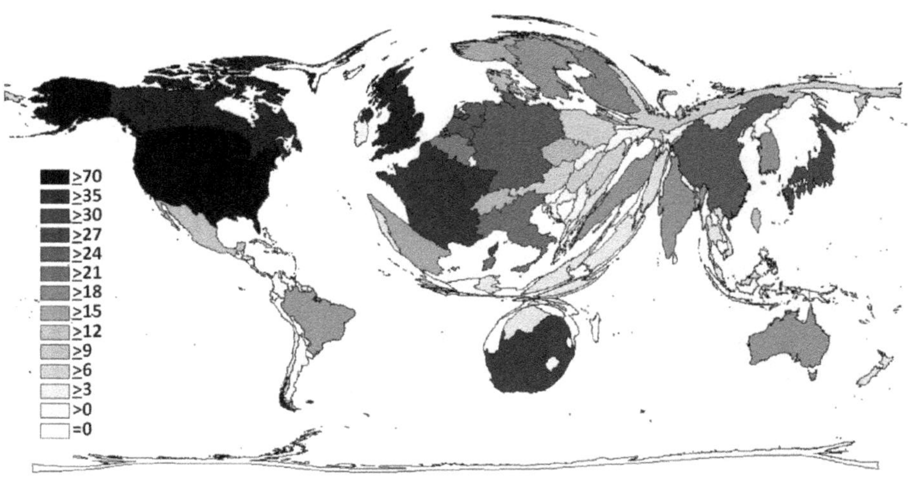

Figure 3 Density-equalizing map showing the h-index of each particular country. The area of each country was scaled in proportion to its h-index regarding "silicosis".

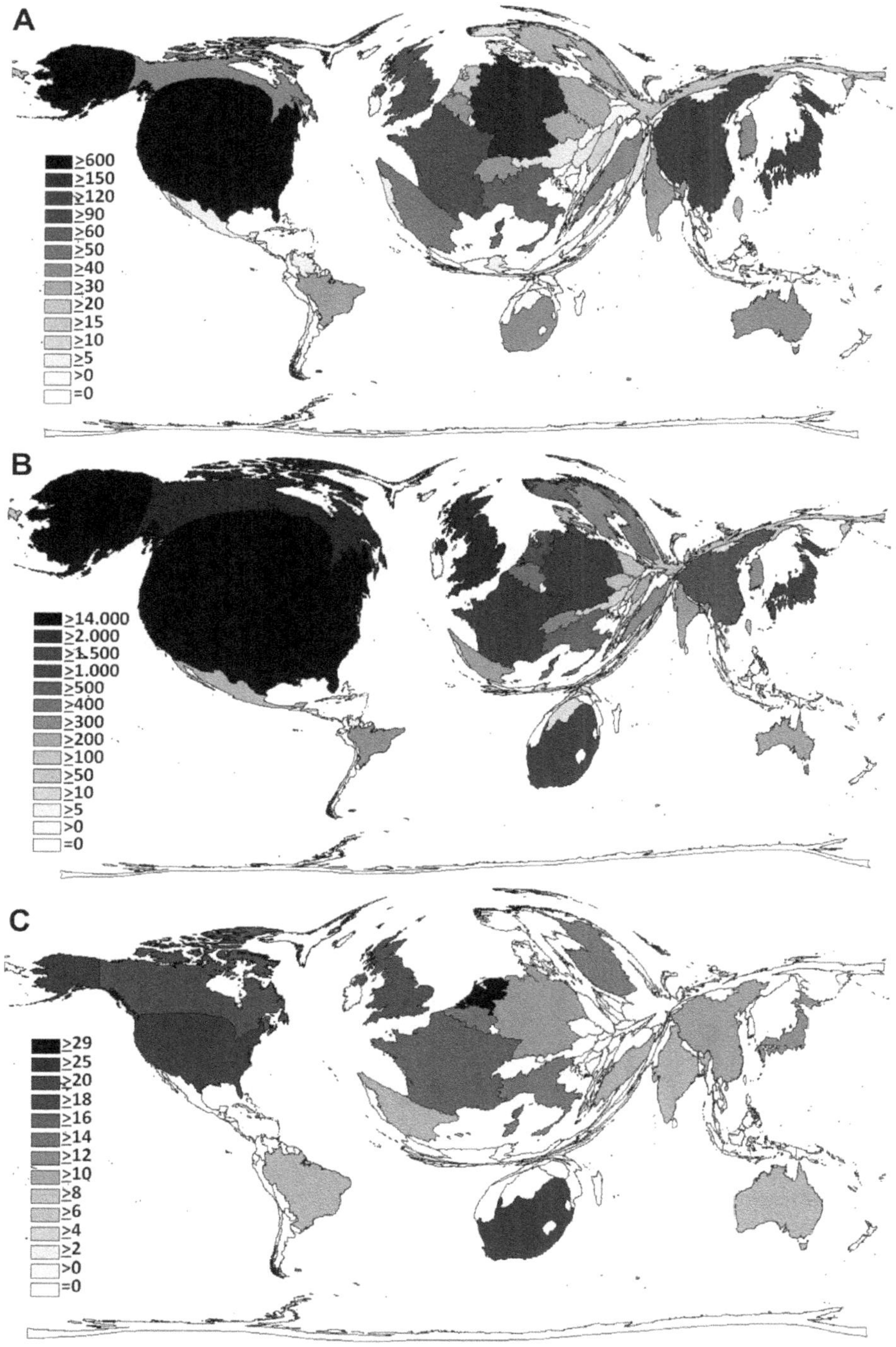

Figure 4 Number of scientific institutions engaged with "silicosis" (A), number of citations received concerning "silicosis" (B) and citations rate (C) of each particular country. A: Density-equalizing map showing the number of scientific institutionsconcerned with the topic "silicosis" of each particular country. The area of each country was scaled in proportion to its number of institutions. **B:** Density-equalizing map illustrating the total number of citations each country received concerning "silicosis". The area of each country was scaled in proportion to its number of received citations. **C:** Density-equalizing map illustrating the citation rate (average citation per publication) of each particular country. The area of each country was scaled in proportion to its citation rate. Threshold > 30 published items.

Medicine", established in 1944 as the "British Journal of Industrial Medicine" leads with 144 published items and an impact factor of 3.02, followed by the "American Journal of Industrial Medicine" with 138 items (impact factor 1.97) and the "British Medical Journal" (impact factor 17.22), publishing 100 items. Furthermore, the ten most productive authors

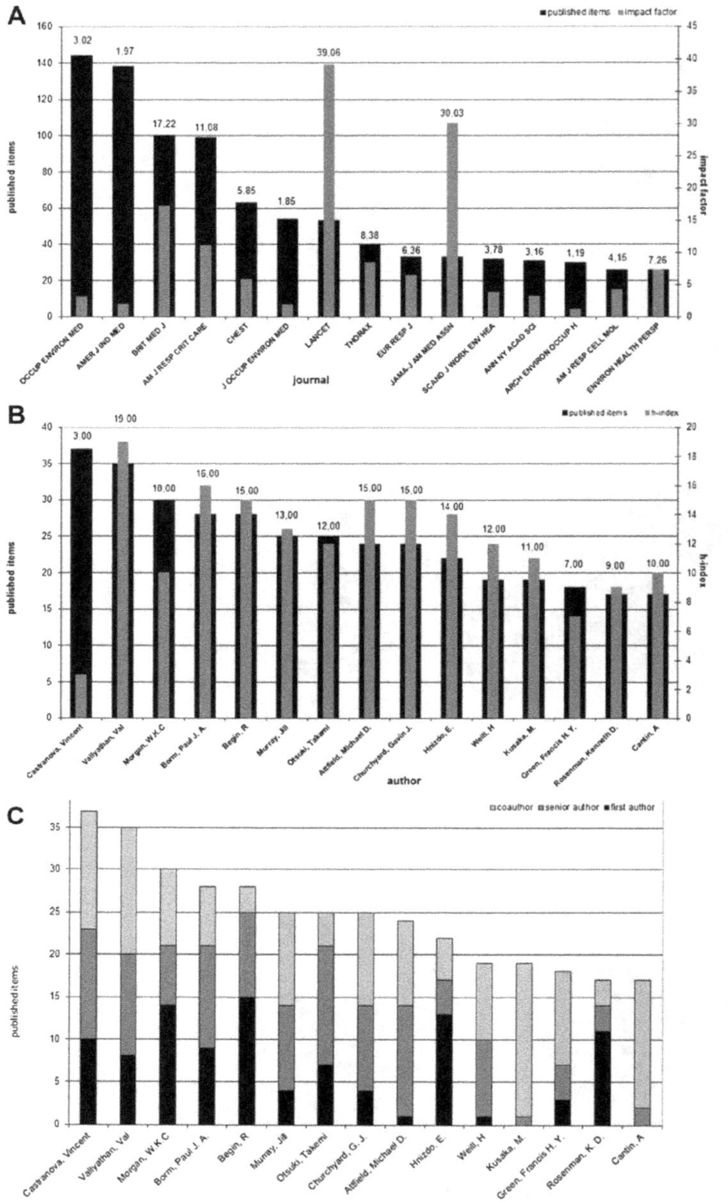

Figure 5 Top 15 journals (A), most productive authors (B) and their proportion of first- authorship and senior-authorship to co-authorship. A: Top 15 ranking of journals by the number of published items and their impact factor items during the period 1920–2012 **B:** 15 most productive authors and their h-index in the period 1920-2012 **C:** 15 most productive authors considering the proportion of first-authorships and senior-authorships to co-authorships.

and their h-index were determined (Figure 5B + C). "Castranova, Vincent" (NIOSH, Morgantown, USA) is the most productive author with 37 published items in the analysed time span, followed by "Vallyathan, V." (NIOSH, Morgantown, USA) with 35 items, "Morgan, W.K.C" (Canada) with 30 items and Borm, Paul JA (Netherlands) with 28 items. The h-index shows a slightly different distribution, as "Vallyathan, V." holds the highest h-index (19), followed by "Borm PJA" (16). Regarding first- and senior-authorship, "Begin, R" with 14 first- and 10 senior-authorships leads by far and shows the best ratio of first- and senior- authorships to co-authorships. To get valid results for all parameters, we checked and corrected each author, institution and country, mentioned in the WoS, for misspelling, variations in name spelling, affiliations and fusions, renaming or unification, usually by making inquiries via world wide web.

Discussion

In the present study, bibliometric tools and density-equalizing procedures were used to evaluate quantitative and qualitative aspects of the scientific output in the field of "silicosis". After a decrease of worldwide research productivity for about ten years beginning in the late 1990ies, new findings in recent years about the NALP 3-Inflammasome and immunologic aspects of silicosis seem to have caused an increase of scientific activity. The USA maintain their predominant position as illustrated in Figure 1A, but Asian countries, particularly China, catch up and are expected to excel the USA still in this decade. The presently outstanding productivity of the USA does not surprise as they dispose the highest agglomeration of research institutions and provide an exemplary scientific infrastructure (Figure 4A). As expected, the USA show the most intensive collaboration behaviour on a national as well as on an international level (Figure 2A + B), of which the most productive notably proved to be the one with China. As international projects tend to have more influence on the scientific community, an intensive collaboration behaviour on an international level increases the likelihood to produce research of higher international relevance, usually leading to higher numbers of received citations in comparison with a collaboration on a lower international or only national level [23,24]. This might explain the dominating position of the Netherlands even compared to the USA and the other most productive countries, when considering only the citation rate but not the h-index or the total number of citations which both are limited by the total amount of publications (Figure 4C). In comparison with their overall scientific output, the Netherlands cooperate intensively on an international level, predominantly with the USA, the UK and South Africa (Figure 2A). Also the forth most productive author worldwide with the second highest h-index is Dutch. To avoid overestimation of a few articles that may have been cited often, we used a threshold of 30 publications for the calculation of the citationrate. In times of growing competition in the scientific community, modified evaluation criteria for academic personnel and a rising need to publish, a subsequent tendency to co-authorship and author self-citation is seen which can artificially inflate an authors productivity and disproportionately affect impact factor and h-index. Several studies and simulations recently have proven that particularly studies with more authors published in lower profile journals are most vulnerable to this effect [25-27]. A recent correspondence in "The Lancet" discussed this problem with regards to the evaluation-practice of medical doctors in China [28,29]. However, after analysing the ratio of first- and senior-authorship to co-authorship of the most productive authors, as well as analysis of self-citations, using the WoS citation report for the most productive countries, biases of co- authorship or self-citation have not turned out to be the reason for the success of the ten most productive authors and countries. To estimate a journals relevance in its scientific field, the impact factor was used as a parameter for the scientific quality of a publishing journal. In this regard, the "British Medical Journal" and the "American Journal of Respiratory and Critical Care Medicine" have the best results (Figure 5A). Apparently, journals explicitly focusing on the field of occupational and environmental medicine as "Occupational and Environmental Medicine" and the "American Journal of Industrial Medicine" are inferior to clinical journals in publishing the most relevant items. It should be mentioned that the subsequent rise of the impact factor among English-language journals results in more citations leading to a language bias [30]. This is supported by the fact that all 15 most productive journals publishing on the subject "silicosis" are in English language. However, scientometric indicators such as h-index, citationrate and impact factor, commonly used for assessment of scientific quality, have to be seen critically due to distortion by self-citation, co-authorship and language-bias. To exclude these biases automatically from calculations of h-index, productivity and impact factor, a further scientometric approach is needed.

Competing interests

The authors declare that they have no competing interests.

Authors' contributions

DAG and MB made substantial contributions to the conception and design of the study, acquisition of the data data and have been involved in drafting and revising the manuscript. DK contributed to creating the figures. All authors have read and approved the final manuscript.

References

1. Greenberg MI, Waksman J, Curtis J: **Silicosis: a review.** *Dis Mon* 2007, **53**(8):394–416.
2. Corrin B, Nicholson AG: *Pathology of the Lungs.* 3rd edition. London, UK: Churchill Livingstone; 2011:778.
3. Kraus T: *Arbeitsmedizin.* 3rd edition. Stuttgart, Germany: Gerhard Triebig, Michael Kentner, Rainer Schiele; 2011:970.
4. Bang KM, Attfield MD, Wood JM, Syamlal G: **National trends in silicosis mortality in the United States, 1981–2004.** *Am J Ind Med* 2008, **51**(9):633–639.
5. Leung CC, Yu IT, Chen W: **Silicosis.** *Lancet* 2012, **379**(9830):2008–2018.
6. Hamilton RF Jr, Thakur SA, Holian A: **Silica binding and toxicity in alveolar macrophages.** *Free Radic Biol Med* 2008 **44**(7):1246–1258.
7. Hornung V, Bauernfeind F, Halle A, Samstad EO, Kono H, Rock KL, Fitzgerald KA, Latz E: **Silica crystals and aluminum salts activate the NALP3 inflammasome through phagosomal destabilization.** *Nat Immunol* 2008, **9**(8):847–856.
8. Huaux F: **New developments in the understanding of immunology in silicosis.** *Curr Opin Allergy Clin Immunol* 2007, **7**(2):168–173.
9. (NIOSH), N I f O S a H: **Health effects of occupational exposure to respirable crystalline silica.** In *Services.* Edited by D o h a h. Cincinnati, OH: Department of Health and Human Services Centers for Disease Control and Prevention National Institute for Occupational Safety and Health; 2002:51–59.
10. Weisman D, Banks D: *Interstitial Lung Disease.* 4th edition. London, UK: BC Decker Inc; 2003.
11. Health, A T S C o t S A o E a O: **Adverse effects of crystalline silica exposure. American Thoracic Society Committee of the Scientific Assembly on Environmental and Occupational Health.** *Am J Respir Crit Care Med* 1997, **155**(2):761–763.

12. Marchiori E, Souza CA, Barbassa TG, Escuissato DL, Gasparetto EL, Souza AS Jr: **Silicoproteinosis: high-resolution CT findings in 13 patients.** *AJR Am J Roentgenol* 2007, **189**(6):1402–1406.
13. Ehrlich RI, Myers JE, te Water Naude JM, Thompson ML, Churchyard GJ: **Lung function loss in relation to silica dust exposure in South African gold miners.** *Occup Environ Med* 2011, **68**(2):96–101.
14. Rees D, Murray J: **Silica, silicosis and tuberculosis.** *Int J Tuberc Lung Dis* 2007, **11**(5):474–484.
15. Vega Miranda J, Pinto Penaranda LF, Marquez Hernandez JD, Velasquez Franco CJ: **Microscopic polyangiitis secondary to silica exposure.** *Reumatol Clin* 2013 [Epub ahead of print].
16. Gomez-Puerta JA, Gedmintas L, Costenbader KH: **The association between silica exposure and development of ANCA-associated vasculitis: systematic review and meta-analysis.** *Autoimmun Rev* 2013 [Epub ahead of print].
17. Lee S, Hayashi H, Maeda M, Chen Y, Matsuzaki H, Takei-Kumagai N, Nishimura Y, Fujimoto W, Otsuki T: **Environmental factors producing autoimmune dysregulation–chronic activation of T cells caused by silica exposure.** *Immunobiology* 2012, **217**(7):743–748.
18. Speck-Hernandez CA, Montoya-Ortiz G: **Silicon, a possible link between environmental exposure and autoimmune diseases: the case of rheumatoid arthritis.** *Arthritis* 2012, **2012**:604187.
19. Gastner MT, Newman ME: **From the cover: diffusion-based method for producing density-equalizing maps.** *Proc Natl Acad Sci USA* 2004, **101**(20):7499–7504.
20. Hirsch JE: **An index to quantify an individual's scientific research output.** *Proc Natl Acad Sci USA* 2005, **102**(46):16569–16572.
21. Hirsch JE: **Does the H index have predictive power?** *Proc Natl Acad Sci USA* 2007, **104**(49):19193–19198.
22. Garfield E: **Which medical journals have the greatest impact?** *Ann Intern Med* 1986, **105**(2):313–320.
23. Andersen J, Belmont J, Cho CT: **Journal impact factor in the era of expanding literature.** *J Microbiol Immunol Infect* 2006, **39**(6):436–443.
24. Mohebbi MR: **The impact of "Impact Factor" on medical journalism in the developing world!** *Indian Pediatr* 2008, **45**(7):604.
25. Bartneck C, Kokkelmans S: **Detecting h-index manipulation through self-citation analysis.** *Scientometrics* 2011, **87**(1):85–98.
26. Haug C: **Authorship and co-authorship.** *Tidsskr Nor Laegeforen* 2006, **126**(4):429.
27. Kulkarni AV, Aziz B, Shams I, Busse JW: **Author self-citation in the general medicine literature.** *PLoS One* 2011, **6**(6):e20885.
28. Qiu J: **Publish or perish in China.** *Nature* 2010, **463**(7278):142–143.
29. Ye B, Liu AH: **Inadequate evaluation of medical doctors in China.** *Lancet* 2013, **381**(9882):1984.
30. Mueller PS, Murali NS, Cha SS, Erwin PF, Ghosh AK: **The association between impact factors and language of general internal medicine journals.** *Swiss Med Wkly* 2006, **136**(27–28):441–443.

8

Cut-off values for the applied version of the Beck Depression Inventory in a general working population

Uwe Rose[1*], Stefanie March[2], Melanie Ebener[3] and Jean-Baptist du Prel[3]

Abstract

Background: The Beck Depression Inventory (BDI) for the assessment of depressive symptoms is well established in clinical settings. An applied version (BDI-V) was previously developed in German for use within epidemiologic studies. The current study analyses the association between this applied version of the BDI and different measures of functioning. The aim is to determine BDI-V cut-off values when used in a population of employees.

Methods: The study included 6339 employees of the first wave of a German cohort study on work, age, health and work participation. Depressive symptoms were assessed by an applied version of the BDI-V. Data on functioning were obtained from personal interviews. The determination of cut-off values is achieved with the min-max principle for classification applied to receiver operating characteristic (ROC) curves.

Results: The min-max principle points to a BDI-V cut-off between 20 and 24 for male and between 23 and 28 for female respondents. The corresponding sensitivities range between 0.64 and 0.75 for males and between 0.59 and 0.74 for females. Specificities range between 0.64 and 0.75 for males and between 0.60 and 0.74 for females. Female respondents have higher BDI-V cut-offs for all criteria.

Conclusions: The range of values is lower than a recommendation in a former study. In addition to this, the values differ for gender. The current analyses focus on an easier-to-use version of the BDI formerly applied for epidemiologic studies. The determination of cut-off values is based on criteria which are indicators for impairment in (work) functioning in a population of employees. Therefore, grouping of individuals according to the reported cut-off values is guided by the relevance of these scores for occupational functioning.

Keywords: Depressive symptoms, Beck Depression Inventory, BDI, Functioning, Employees, Cut-off values, Receiver operating characteristics, Work, Work ability

Background

Depressive symptoms are highly relevant outcomes in population based research fields such as occupational epidemiology. They are associated with a high loss of productivity and working time due to sickness absence and early retirement [1, 2]. Therefore instruments which measure depressive symptoms and have been validated in the setting of a general working population are of high value for research, but unfortunately seldom available.

When applying such instruments to epidemiological studies, there are typically constraints on the length of the interview. Therefore, a questionnaire for depressive symptoms is required to be fairly short. With these aspects in mind we investigated the validity of the applied version of the Beck Depression Inventory (BDI-V) which we used in the context of the lidA (leben in der Arbeit; English: living at work)-study: a German cohort study on work, age, health and work participation [3].

The assessment of depressive symptoms by means of a questionnaire is different than the assessment of clinical depression based on a standardised interview. According to the standards of classification systems such as the fourth and fifth editions of the Diagnostic and Statistical

* Correspondence: rose.uwe@baua.bund.de
[1]Federal Institute of Occupational Safety and Health (FIOSH), Nöldnerstrasse 40-42, 10317 Berlin, Germany
Full list of author information is available at the end of the article

Manual of Mental Disorders (DSM) of the American Psychiatric Association [4, 5] a major depressive episode is diagnosed by a standardised interview. The diagnosis is based on a set of diagnostic criteria, and the application of a rule for classification. Starting with depressed mood and loss of interest or pleasure, the patient is asked about a pattern of symptoms (i.e. changes in appetite, sleep disturbances etc.). A further criterion for an episode is met when the symptoms cause clinically significant distress or impairment in important areas of functioning.

In contrast to the assessment by a clinician using specific criteria there is a long-standing tradition of self-reported measures of depressive symptoms. One example is the BDI. Respondents have to choose one statement from a list of four which best describes how they have been feeling during the past week up to and including the date of assessment. The aggregation of item responses to a score allows for an assessment of depression symptoms severity. A higher score might be an indication for a greater impairment in different areas of life. But this association is only an assumption and is not based on the direct assessment of "an impairment in social, occupational, or other important areas of functioning" in the DSM-V (p.161, [5]).

This DSM criterion is very similar to "activity limitations" as described in the International Classification of Functioning, Disability, and Health (ICF) coordinated by the WHO [6]. The classification system of the ICF goes beyond the diagnosis of particular patterns of symptoms and signs: It focuses on the effects of a health condition on the person and her functioning [7–9]. These effects are classified by performance in daily activities and by participation in life situations, while considering the environmental and personal factors that affect psychological health [7–9]. In this sense, self-report measures are narrowed in their assessment to symptomatology and do not provide a direct link to consequences for a person's daily functioning. Such reduction to symptomatology as found in typical self-reporting instruments is not a hidden fault or shortcoming. It is rather a prerequisite for establishing the validity of scores in depression inventories by appraising the evidence with regards to their relation to other relevant criteria. This procedure for a validation is in line with "The Standards for Educational and Psychological Testing" [10], which describe several sources of evidence to illuminate different aspects of validity even in the absence of a gold standard for testing.

The starting point for the current study is an applied version of the original BDI [11, 12]. This instrument is well established in clinical settings. It has been modified for applications in survey research. Criterion-referenced validity of this applied version of the BDI (German BDI-V) was investigated [13] using correlations between the BDI-V and similar or convergent self-rating scales of depression. Moreover, Schmitt et al. [13] compared the scores between different clinical and nonclinical samples. This kind of evidence supports the assumption that all these instruments are similar representations of the same concept (depression). But the relationship between BDI-V and other external criteria like general functioning in relevant areas of life remains unclear, whereas both aspects are part of standardised clinical interviews. Therefore, the current analysis will examine these aspects of general functioning and work ability, including their association with the BDI-V scores, in a sample of middle-aged employees. The main aim is the determination of BDI-V cut-off values with reference to functioning.

Methods

Design

lidA is a German prospective cohort study in which individuals will be followed up in three year intervals. The study investigates the associations of work, health and employment in an ageing work force. The current validation study is based on respondents from the first wave. The focus was on the association between depressive symptoms and functioning. The responses regarding functioning were obtained by a computer assisted personal interview (CAPI). Depressive symptoms were assessed by the BDI-V (see below). The BDI-V used was a paper and pencil version returned to the interviewer in a closed envelope.

Sample

Employees were recruited in the frame of the first wave of the German lidA-cohort study, which targets work, age, health and work participation in employees born in 1959 and 1965. Forming part of the German baby-boom generation, these employees are highly relevant for lidA's primary research goal [3]. The response rate was 27.3 percent. The sample was selected in a two stage random process: First 222 sample points from all over Germany were randomly chosen. Second, 6585 study participants were randomly selected from the database of the Institute for Employment Research (IAB) of the Federal Employment Agency on the reference date 31th December 2009. This data, also referred to as Integrated Employment Biographies (IEB), includes all German employees subject to social insurance contributions. Persons who are unemployed, self-employed, freelancers as well as civil servants are excluded by definition [3].

Following the International Labour Organization (ILO), an employee is defined as a person who works at least one hour a week [14]. Thus 6339 employees were available for this analysis.

In Germany, there are extensive legal requirements for data protection. Therefore, an application process in accordance with German social legislation was required to carry out the sampling procedure [15]. The approval was issued by the ethics commitee of the University of Wuppertal.

Measurements

Depressive symptoms

In the original version of the BDI depressive symptoms are assessed by 21 typical symptoms, each with four statements ranked according their severity level and resulting in 84 statements. The wording of items and comprehensiveness of the questionnaire's structure might be well suited for a clinical setting, but the applicability of the BDI in epidemiological studies is limited by the length of the instrument. This was part of the motivation behind constructing an applied version of the BDI in German by Schmitt et al. [13]. For this reason, only 20 items from the original BDI were selected. One item about weight loss was dropped. Instead of the original BDI consisting of four statements for each symptom, only one statement is used in the simplified version. This sole statement serves as a reference point when participants are asked to rate their frequency of experience by using a simple six-level scale. The range of the sum scores goes from 0 to 100. Schmitt et al. [13] compared the reliability of the original BDI and their simplified version: Cronbach's alpha of the original version was lower ($\alpha = 0.84$) than that of the simplified version ($\alpha = 0.94$). The simplified BDI and the original version correlated with $r = 0.83$. This high degree of convergence supported by the results of a confirmatory factor analysis showed only a slight deviation from perfect measurement equivalence, in spite of the higher efficiency of the applied BDI-V. Moreover, norm values are provided by Schmitt et al. [16] based on a sample from the general population in Germany. Criterion-referenced validity was investigated [13] by correlations between BDI-V and similar or convergent self-rating scales of depression and by comparing the score of BDI-V between different clinical and nonclinical samples. This kind of evidence supports the assumption that all these instruments are similar representations of the same concept (depression).

Functioning

Two items of the Work Ability Index [17] were selected in order to define dichotomous criteria for functioning at work:

- The respondents are asked "How do you rate your current work ability with respect to the physical demands of your work?" (Work ability - physical), and
- "How do you rate your current work ability with respect to the mental demands of your work?" (Work ability - mental)

The response categories for both items are "very good", "rather good", "moderate", "rather poor", "very poor". The cut-off is made between "moderate" and "rather poor".

Three items of the CAPI were extracted from the modified German version of the SF-12 [18]. They are related to mental health, emotional problems and social limitations: "During the last four weeks, how often did you feel that due to ..."

- "mental health or emotional problems you achieved less than you wanted to at work or in everyday activities?" (SF-12 role emotional 1),
- "mental health or emotional problems you carried out your work or everyday tasks less thoroughly than usual?" (SF-12 role emotional 2),
- "physical or mental health problems you were limited socially, that is, in contact with friends, acquaintances, or relatives?" (SF-12 social functioning).

The response categories for these three items are "always", "often", "sometimes", "almost never", and "never". The cut-off was made between "sometimes" and "almost never".

Statistical analysis

Criterion referenced validity of the BDI-V was assessed by the rank correlation between BDI-V score and the values of five indicators of functioning. Receiver operating characteristic (ROC) analysis was used to define cut-off values for the BDI-V (Figs. 1 and 2). ROC curves originate from signal detection theory and were later introduced in medicine to validate and improve diagnostic measures [19]. In the classical paradigm for evaluating test performance, the result of an index test is compared with a reference test, typically an instrument widely accepted as a gold standard. An example is liver biopsy as the standard for evaluating liver fibrosis. Such a gold standard as this is to date not available for depressive symptoms. There are however in the field of psychometrics other strategies to evaluate the validity of an index test [10]. An important source for interpretations and inferences of validity is evidence based on relations to other variables. The current analysis focusses on the relationship of the BDI-V to other variables relevant to the participants' daily functioning and ability to work. ROC curve analysis is then carried out on the basis of these other variables serving as external criteria. BDI-V values were chosen for optimally distinguishing cases with impaired functioning in different areas of life. Participants who have a sum-score above a given cut-off value are cases with impairment. Those below are non-cases. Within a range from 0 to 100

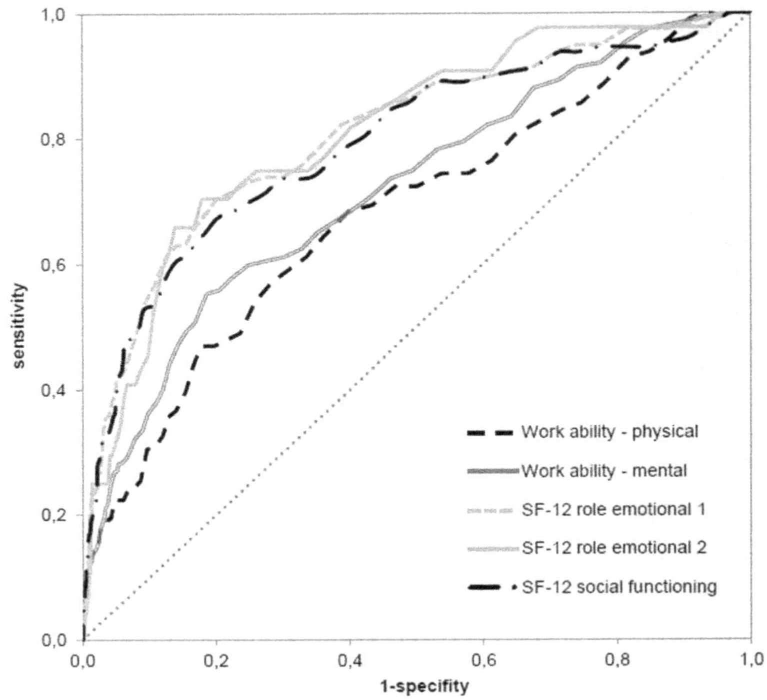

Fig. 1 Area Under the Curve for male; sensitivity and 1-Specificity for all BDI-V scores

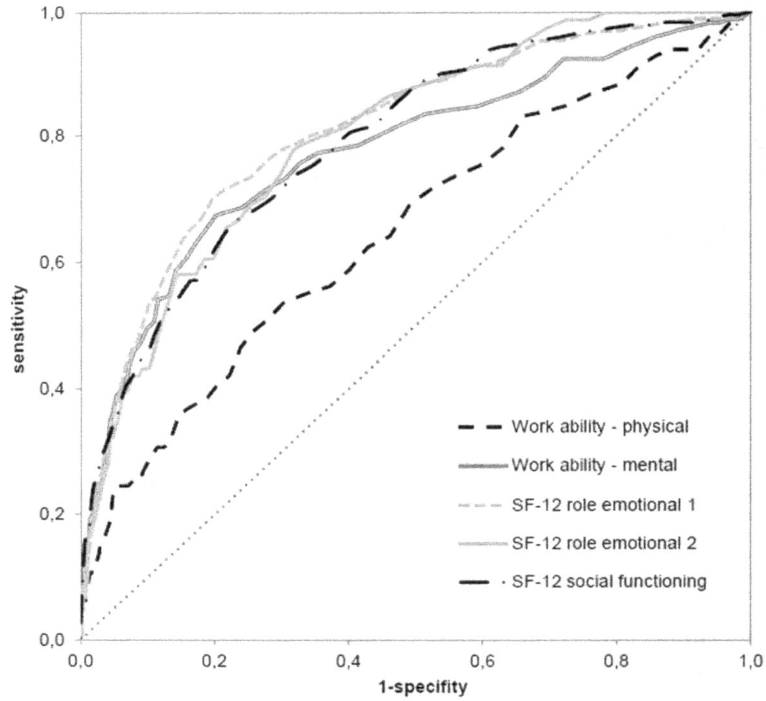

Fig. 2 Area Under the Curve for female; sensitivity and 1-Specificity for all BDI-V scores

there are 100 possible cut-off values each corresponding to a cumulative percentage. This cumulative distribution is used for the computation of sensitivity (SENS) and specificity (SPEC). The misclassification of cases and non-cases is given by 1 – sensitivity (1 – SENS) and 1 – specificity (1 – SPEC). The area under the curve (AUC) indicates the accuracy of the instrument to detect impairment. It is generated by plotting 1 – SPEC against SENS (see e.g. [19]). There are different strategies and rules to determine the optimal cut-off and to reduce the risk for misclassification (1 – SENS, 1 – SPEC). One common approach is the computation of the Youden-Index (Y): Y = SENS + SPEC – 1 for each possible cut-off. The optimal cut-off is then indicated by the highest Y-value. This rule however allows low values of SENS to be compensated by high values of SPEC and vice versa. Such a compensation is avoided by computing the maximum of both errors in classification. The subsequent selection of a cut-off is based on a minimization of these maximum errors (min-max principle) [20].

Results

Sample characteristics

All participants were born in either 1959 or 1965. The predominant employment status among men in these birth cohorts is full time employment (94.7 %), only 3.3 % of the male employees worked part-time (Table 1). The latter is more frequent among women (45.8 %) while 43.4 % were in full-time work. Changes in the employment status (unemployment etc.) are possible due to the time lag between the sampling of addresses and the date of interview in the field. On the other hand, the percentages for the remaining categories (including less than part-time work) are 2.0 % for male and 10.8 % for female respondents. The most prevalent category for the highest school leaving qualification is intermediate qualification with a higher percentage among female (48.0 %) than male respondents (34.7 %). Civil servants, self-employed, and freelancers were excluded from the sampling process. The distribution for net income on this background is characterized by low (male 4.3 %, female 38.1 %) and middle income (male 37.5 %, female 43.8 %).

The median value for BDI-V among males is 16 (central 95 %: 0–50) and among females 20 (central 95 %: 1–56). Both age cohorts are represented by the same median value (18). The lowest value within the central 95 % of the BDI-V distribution for both age cohorts is 1, whereas the highest values are 52 and 55 for 1959 and 1965 cohorts, respectively.

Analysis of the BDI-V scores

Among male participants the correlation of the BDI-V scores with five criteria was computed using Kendall Tau_b. Higher values for this rank correlation were found for three criteria: -0.37 for impairment of everyday activities (SF-12 role emotional 1), -0.35 for impairment of everyday tasks (SF-12 role emotional 2), -0.35 for impairment of social functioning (SF-12 social functioning). Smaller (positive) correlations were found for the physical dimension of work ability (Work ability - physical) (0.21) and the mental dimension (Work ability - mental) (0.30).

The correlations among female participants were -0.39 (SF-12 role emotional 1), -0.34 (SF-12 role emotional 2), -0.38 (SF-12 social functioning), with physical dimension of work ability at 0.22 and mental dimension

Table 1 Sample characteristics

Variable		Males		Females	
	n	2,552	47.2 %	2,360	52.8 %
Highest school leaving graduation	Low graduation	781	30.6 %	544	19.0 %
	Middle graduation	886	34.7 %	1,374	48.0 %
	High graduation	837	32.8 %	899	31.4 %
	Other/w.o. graduation	51	2.0 %	309	10.8 %
Employment status	Full time	2,417	94.7 %	1,242	43.4 %
	Part time	84	3.3 %	1,309	45.8 %
	Other	51	2.0 %	309	10.8 %
Personal net income	<1000 Euro	109	4.3 %	1,091	38.1 %
	1000 - <2000 Euro	958	37.5 %	1,254	43.8 %
	2000 - <3000 Euro	838	32.8 %	312	10.9 %
	3000 - <4000 Euro	287	11.2 %	49	1.7 %
	≥4000 Euro	242	9.5 %	25	0.9 %
	Missing data	118	4.6 %	129	4.5 %

of work ability at 0.27 (Table 2). These associations are mirrored in the values of AUC in Tables 3 and 4.

The min-max principle points to a BDI-V-cut-off between 20 and 24 for male and between 23 and 28 for female respondents. The resulting cut-offs depend on the criteria and the corresponding sensitivities ranges: They are between 0.64 and 0.75 for males and between 0.59 and 0.74 for females (Tables 3, 4). Specificity ranges between 0.64 and 0.75 for males and between 0.60 and 0.74 for females. Female respondents have higher BDI-V cut-offs for all criteria.

Discussion

The BDI was primarily constructed as an instrument for use in clinical settings. By contrast, the applied version BDI-V was tested within a general population [16]. To the best of our knowledge this is the first time that the validity of the instrument has been investigated within a general working population.

The sample of the current study comprises workers who – despite possible impairments to health and functioning – are still employed. This is an important difference to those studies which include clinical samples of participants who are not at work for health reasons. Moreover, the selected sampling frame also had an influence on the decision to use work ability and functioning as relevant criteria for a validation. Our strict focus on employees is a major difference to the studies of Schmidt et al. [13, 16].

The distribution of BDI values differs between a clinical setting and a general working population. In a clinical setting there is mainly a need to differentiate between moderate and severe types of depressive episodes. In contrast, high depression scores are less common among employees. Furthermore, there is some evidence that the BDI provides more detailed information about higher severity levels than other depression scales [21].

Beyond the distributional aspects, there is an important difference between the application of the BDI and an assessment of major depression by a clinical interview. The latter addresses depressive symptoms along with questions towards impairment or functioning. Hence, the association between depressive symptoms and impairment is part of the diagnosis. This association is not known for the BDI-V, it is rather an assumption which formed a focus of the current study. Evidence for this association is given by rank correlations with five indicators and their corresponding AUC values, confirming the criterion referenced validity of the BDI-V. However, these results give no indication on how to classify persons as impaired or not impaired on the basis of a particular cut-off. A cut-off value given for a revised form of the original BDI is a score of 18 [22]. But a direct comparison of scores between the BDI and the BDI-V is not possible due to the different ranges of the two instruments. The revised BDI contains the 21 items of the original BDI and the sum scores cover a range from 0 to 63. The BDI-V contains 20 items and the range for scores goes from 0 to 100. In both cases the relevant cut-off value is contained within about the first third of the range, which indicates a clinically relevant depression in the framework of a validation of the revised BDI (BDI-II [23]). The selection of an appropriate cut-off value for depressive symptoms as assessed by the BDI-V depends firstly on their relation to general functioning and work ability and secondly, on the negative consequences of low sensitivity or specificity. If sensitivity is too low, there is a higher risk for misclassification by overlooking relevant impairments in the general functioning and work ability of employees. Otherwise, low specificity would result in employees with moderate depressive symptoms being classified as impaired even though they are not. Thus we are aware that methods used to determine a cut-off value for a

Table 3 BDI cut-off score, sensitivity, 1 – specificity, min-max, AUC for different criteria for male ($n = 2,552$)

Criterium	BDI-V Score	SENS	1 - SPEC	min- max	AUC
Work ability - physical[a]	≥ 20	0.64	0.36	0.36	0.68
Work ability - mental[a]	≥ 20	0.65	0.35	0.35	0.72
SF-12 role emotional 1	≥ 24	0.73	0.25	0.27	0.81
SF-12 role emotional 2	≥ 24	0.75	0.26	0.26	0.81
SF-12 social functioning	≥ 23	0.71	0.27	0.29	0.79

[a]reversed coding for Work ability

Table 2 Rank Correlations (Kendall Tau b) with BDI-V

Variable	Males ($n = 2,552$)	Females ($n = 2,860$)
Work ability - physical[a]	0.21*	0.22*
Work ability - mental[a]	0.30*	0.27*
SF-12 role emotional 1	-0.37*	-0.39*
SF-12 role emotional 2	-0.35*	-0.34*
SF-12 social functioning	-0.35*	-0.38*

[a]reversed coding for Work ability, *$p < .01$

Table 4 BDI cut-off score, sensitivity, 1 – specificity, min-max, AUC for different criteria for female ($n = 2,860$)

Criterium	BDI-V Score	SENS	1 - SPEC	min- max	AUC
Work ability - physical[a]	≥ 23	0.59	0.40	0.40	0.65
Work ability - mental[a]	≥ 27	0.72	0.29	0.29	0.78
SF-12 role emotional 1	≥ 28	0.74	0.26	0.26	0.81
SF-12 role emotional 2	≥ 28	0.70	0.28	0.30	0.80
SF-12 social functioning	≥ 26	0.71	0.30	0.30	0.79

[a]reversed coding for Work ability

meaningful dichotomy in reference to the association of depressive symptoms with general functioning and work ability should be both sensitive as well as specific. We chose the min-max principle as an appropriate method for finding an optimal cut-off value by minimizing both types of misclassification [20].

One of the most striking results of our study was the difference in the cut-off-values between women and men, with higher values for women. This might be related to the observation of Schmitt et al. [16] that women in general have a higher average level of BDI-V scores than men. Higher levels of depression in women have also been reported in several other studies using different instruments to measure depressive symptoms (e.g., [24–26]). The higher threshold for women could be the result of a tendency for symptom aggravation in women or a tendency for underreporting of depressive symptoms in men. An alternative explanation could be that women and men did report their depressive symptoms accurately but the coping strategies for depressive symptoms are more efficient in women than in men. In this case, similar levels of depressive symptoms in women and men would result in less impairment for women. A third explanation could be that women and men reported differently on the scales of general functioning and work ability. Then women would have a tendency to overestimate or men to underestimate their general functioning and work ability at a given level of depressiveness. All these explanations would lead to higher cut-off values in women than in men and have to be studied further in future investigations.

The overall response rate of our investigation was quite low at 27.3 %. However, a selectivity analysis of our study sample was carried out to investigate possible sources of bias. In comparison to the sampling frame of all employees subject to social security contributions, only minor differences were found in 16 crucial sociodemographic variables [27]. It is therefore likely that our responders are highly representative of all participants in the sampling frame selected for this study. Some limitations to the external validity of our investigation should be mentioned. One serious limitation is that only two age groups (1959, 1965) were included in our validation study. Therefore our results regarding cut-off values may be restricted to these middle-aged employees, meaning that these cut-off values might be not comparable to those of other age groups. This assumption, however, should be investigated by future studies. Another limitation is that our working population includes only employees subject to social security contributions. Although this applies to the vast majority of German employees, we can only hypothesize about the situation of civil servants, self-employed persons and freelancers. Furthermore, missing values could have introduced some sort of bias in our results. As the percentage of missing values, especially in the BDI-V, was not negligible in our data set, selection bias cannot be excluded. This is due to the possibility that the percentage of non-responders is either positively or negatively associated with the amount of depressive symptoms. Last but not least this is an exploratory data analysis. These considerations should be addressed in future investigations.

Conclusion

It is our view that the question of whether higher BDI-V values indicate a reduction in general functioning and work ability as a consequence of a depressive mood is highly relevant in a work setting: When exceeding a certain threshold, the impairment of general functioning in the daily lives and work ability of employees may lead to a loss of productivity, higher absenteeism and higher retirement rates. This is especially a challenge for ageing societies as is the case in Germany [28]. Moreover, the use of cut-off values in the BDI-V for indicating relevant impairments in functioning and work ability is also interesting at an individual level, e.g. within the context of examinations by occupational physicians. Lastly, a more efficient assessment of depressive symptoms by means of validated instruments and the availability of cut-off values would have great practical value in the fields of occupational research and public health.

The current study focussed on a subset of indicators for functioning and work ability. The selection was predetermined by the availability of adequate instruments and variables. However, there are other options in the choice of instruments and variables beyond those realised in this study. This leads to the question of how these associations and cut-off values would be related when other indicators are simultaneously considered. The use of other indicators in further replication studies for the purpose of establishing consistency would be an important additional step in the validation of the BDI-V.

Competing interests

The authors declare that they have no competing interests.

Authors' contributions

All authors contributed to the design and concept of the study. UR introduced the decision criterion. ME and SM performed the statistical analysis. All authors contributed to the interpretation of the results. UR and JP drafted main parts of the manuscript. All authors revised the manuscript critically. All authors read and approved the final manuscript.

Acknowledgement

The authors would like to thank the participants of the study. The authors would also like to thank Jon Scouten and Enno Swart for critical review of the text, Inna Friedland for assistance in the preparation of the text and would like to thank the Pearson Assessment & Information GmbH for permission to use the BDI-V-questionnaire.

Primary financial support was provided for SM and JP by the German Federal Ministry of Education and Research [grant numbers 01ER0825, 01ER0826, 01ER0827 and 01ER0806], for ME by the University of Wuppertal, and additional support was provided by the Federal Institute of Occupational Safety and Health.

Author details
[1]Federal Institute of Occupational Safety and Health (FIOSH), Nöldnerstrasse 40-42, 10317 Berlin, Germany. [2]Institute of Social Medicine and Health Economics, Otto-von-Guericke-University of Magdeburg, Leipziger Str. 44, 39120 Magdeburg, Germany. [3]Institute for Safety Engineering, University of Wuppertal, Gaußstr. 20, 42119 Wuppertal, Germany.

References

1. Jacobi F, Hoyer J, Wittchen HU. Seelische Gesundheit in Ost und West: Analysen auf der Grundlage des Bundesgesundheitssurveys. Z Klin Psychol Psychother. 2004;33:251–60.
2. Henderson M, Harvey SB, Overland S, Mykletun A, Hotopf M. Work and common psychiatric disorders. J R Soc Med. 2011;104:198–207.
3. Hasselhorn HM, Peter R, Rauch A, Schröder H, Swart E, Bender S, et al. Cohort profile: The lidA Cohort Study - a German Cohort Study on Work, Age, Health and Work Participation. Int J Epidemiol. 2014;43:1736–49.
4. American Psychiatric Association. Diagnostic and Statistical Manual of Mental Disorders. 4th ed. Washington, DC: American Psychiatric Association; 2000.
5. American Psychiatric Association. Diagnostic and Statistical Manual of Mental Disorders. 5th ed. Arlington: American Psychiatric Publishing; 2013.
6. World Health Organization. International Classification of Functioning, Disability, and Health (ICF). Geneva: World Health Organization; 2001.
7. Baron S, Linden M. The role of the "International Classification of Functioning, Disability and Health, ICF" in the description and classification of mental disorders. Eur Arch Psychiatry Clin Neurosci. 2008;258:81–5.
8. Baron S, Linden M. Disorders of functions and disorders of capacity in relation to sick leave in mental disorders. Int J Soc Psychiatry. 2009;55:57–63.
9. Peterson DB. Psychological Aspects of Functioning, Disability, and Health. New York: Springer Publishing Company; 2011.
10. Joint Committee on Standards for Educational and Psychological Testing of the American Educational Research Association, the American Psychological Association, and the National Council on Measurement in Education. Standards for Educational and Psychological Testing. Washington: American Educational Research Association; 1999.
11. Beck AT, Steer RA. Beck Depression Inventory - Manual. San Antonio: The Psychological Corporation; 1987.
12. Beck AT, Steer RA. Beck Depression Inventory (BDI). In Handbook of psychiatric measures. Edited by Association AP. Washington, DC: American Psychiatric Association; 2000: 519-523
13. Schmitt M, Beckmann M, Dusi D, Maes J, Schiller A, Schonauer K. Messgüte des vereinfachten Beck- Depressions-Inventars (BDI-V). Diagnostica. 2003;49:147–56.
14. ILO labour market statistics. [https://www.destatis.de/EN/Publications/STATmagazin/LabourMarket/2012_01/Explanations.html]
15. March S, Rauch A, Thomas D, Bender S, Swart E. [Procedures according to data protection laws for coupling primary and secondary data in a cohort study: the lidA study]. Gesundheitswesen. 2012;74:e122–129.
16. Schmitt M, Altstötter-Gleich C, Hinz A, Maes J, Brähler E. Normwerte für das vereinfachte Beck-Depressions-Inventar (BDI-V) in der Allgemeinbevölkerung. Diagnostica. 2006;52:51–9.
17. Tuomi K, Ilmarinen J, Jahkola M, Karajarinne L, Tulkki A. Work Ability Index. First reprint of the 2nd revised edition. Helsinki: Finnish Institute of Occupational Health; 2006.
18. Nübling M, AH H, Mühlbacher A. Data documentation 16. Entwicklung eines Verfahrens zur Berechnung der körperlichen und psychischen Summenskalen auf Basis der SOEP – Version des SF 12 (Algorithmus). Berlin: DIW; 2006.
19. Du Prel JB, Muttray A. Validität von Diagnostik- und Screeningstudien. In: Porzsolt F, editor. Grundlagen der Klinischen Ökonomik. 1st ed. Berlin: PVS Schriftenreihe; 2011. p. 43–56.
20. Smith RD, Slenning BD. Decision analysis: dealing with uncertainty in diagnostic testing. Prev Vet Med. 2000;45:139–62.
21. Olino TM, Yu L, Klein DN, Rohde P, Seeley JR, Pilkonis PA, et al. Measuring depression using item response theory: An examination of three measures of depressive symptomatology. Int J Methods Psychiatr Res. 2012;21:76–85.
22. Hautzinger M, Bailer M, Worall H, Keller F. Beck-DepressionsInventar (BDI). Testhandbuch. 1995.
23. Hautzinger M, Keller F, Kühner C. BDI-II. Beck-Depressions-Inventar. Revision. 2nd ed. Frankfurt: Pearson Assessment; 2009.
24. Immerman RS, Mackey WC. The depression gender gap: a view through a biocultural filter. Genet Soc Gen Psychol Monogr. 2003;129:5–39.
25. Kessler RC. Epidemiology of women and depression. J Affect Disord. 2003;74:5–13.
26. Buber I, Engelhardt H. The Association between Age and Depressive Symptoms among Older Men and Women in Europe. Findings from SHARE. Comp Popul Stud. 2011;36:103–26.
27. Schröder H, Kersting A, Steinwede J. Methodenbericht zur Haupterhebung lidA – leben in der Arbeit. Nürnberg: FDZ; 2013.
28. Germany's Population by 2060: Results of the 12th coordinated population projection. [https://www.destatis.de/EN/Publications/Specialized/Population/GermanyPopulation2060.pdf?__blob=publicationFile]

9

Subjective stress, objective heart rate variability-based stress, and recovery on workdays among overweight and psychologically distressed individuals

Tiina Föhr[1*], Asko Tolvanen[2], Tero Myllymäki[3], Elina Järvelä-Reijonen[4], Sanni Rantala[5], Riitta Korpela[5], Katri Peuhkuri[5], Marjukka Kolehmainen[4], Sampsa Puttonen[6,7], Raimo Lappalainen[3], Heikki Rusko[8] and Urho M. Kujala[1]

Abstract

Background: The present study aimed to investigate how subjective self-reported stress is associated with objective heart rate variability (HRV)-based stress and recovery on workdays. Another aim was to investigate how physical activity (PA), body composition, and age are associated with subjective stress, objective stress, and recovery.

Methods: Working-age participants ($n = 221$; 185 women, 36 men) in this cross-sectional study were overweight (body mass index, 25.3–40.1 kg/m^2) and psychologically distressed (≥3/12 points on the General Health Questionnaire). Objective stress and recovery were based on HRV recordings over 1–3 workdays. Subjective stress was assessed by the Perceived Stress Scale. PA level was determined by questionnaire, and body fat percentage was assessed by bioelectrical impedance analysis.

Results: Subjective stress was directly associated with objective stress ($P = 0.047$) and inversely with objective recovery ($P = 0.046$). These associations persisted after adjustments for sex, age, PA, and body fat percentage. Higher PA was associated with lower subjective stress ($P = 0.037$). Older age was associated with higher objective stress ($P < 0.001$). After further adjustment for alcohol consumption and regular medication, older age was associated with lower subjective stress ($P = 0.043$).

Conclusions: The present results suggest that subjective self-reported stress is associated with objective physiological stress, but they are also apparently affected by different factors. However, some of the found associations among these overweight and psychologically distressed participants with low inter-individual variation in PA are rather weak and the clinical value of the present findings should be studied further among participants with greater heterogeneity of stress, PA and body composition. However, these findings suggest that objective stress assessment provides an additional aspect to stress evaluation. Furthermore, the results provide valuable information for developing stress assessment methods.

Keywords: Heart rate variability, Objective stress, Perceived stress scale, Physiological stress, Physical activity, Psychological stress, Recovery, Stress assessment, Subjective stress, Work-related stress

* Correspondence: tiina.fohr@jyu.fi
[1]Department of Health Sciences, University of Jyväskylä, P.O. Box 35, FIN-40014 Jyväskylä, Finland
Full list of author information is available at the end of the article

Background

Stress at work can be considered a major public health risk. In many theories and definitions, stress is determined as a psychological or physiological response of the organism to an external load [1]. Stress is associated with psychological disturbances, as well as physiological changes, such as lowered heart rate variability (HRV) [2]. It may even lead to cardiovascular diseases if prolonged [3, 4]. Recovery from stress is an important issue, as incomplete recovery is also suggested to be a risk factor for cardiovascular diseases [5]. Common to the definitions of recovery is that recovery occurs when the exposure to stress is over. Recovery repairs the negative effects of stress and it is a process during which individual recovers to the specific baseline level and is recovered from the possible previous loads [1]. Furthermore, stress has detrimental economic consequences due to decreased job satisfaction and increased sickness-related absences from work [6].

Most stress assessment methods primarily focus on an individual's subjective perception of stress. However, HRV has been proposed to be a good indicator for investigating the physiological effects of stress and recovery [2, 7]. HRV is the beat-to-beat (R–R interval) variation in times between the consecutive heartbeats expressed in normal sinus rhythm on an electrocardiogram (ECG) recording [8, 9]. HRV is very individual and it is modulated by both parasympathetic and sympathetic activity of the autonomic nervous system (ANS). Stress is associated with increased activation level of the body when sympathetic activity dominates the ANS whereas recovery is associated with reduced activation level of the body when parasympathetic activation dominates the ANS over sympathetic activity [10–12]. Studies investigating the association between self-reported, psychological stress and HRV in real-life settings have found controversial results (e.g. [7, 13–16]). Most of these studies have used traditional time- or frequency-domain measures of HRV. However, it is also possible to describe the state of stress and recovery using HRV-derived variables that include information that is difficult to obtain from traditional measures of HRV [7]. These novel variables take into account factors such as HRV-derived respiratory variables and individual resting heart rate (HR) and HRV values. Due to very high inter- and intra-individuality of HRV, new approaches which take into account individuality in HRV could provide additional insight into quantification of stress and recovery.

Physical activity (PA) can help the individual to build resources to buffer the negative effects of stress and promote his/her recovery from stress [17]. On the other hand, stress is suggested to be associated with physical inactivity (e.g. [7, 18, 19]) and being overweight [7, 20]. High stress levels could attenuate an individual's willingness or ability to engage in regular exercise and to be physically active [21], resulting in failure to achieve the beneficial effects of PA against stress.

The present study aimed to examine the associations between subjective self-reported psychological stress and objective physiological HRV-based measures of stress and recovery on workdays. The second aim was to investigate how PA, body composition, and age are associated with subjective stress, objective stress, and recovery.

Methods

Participants

The present cross-sectional study included individuals of different occupations with symptoms of metabolic syndrome and psychological distress, who met the inclusion criteria in an initial screening and underwent baseline measurements for a controlled and randomized trial called the Elixir study [22]. The initial purpose of the Elixir study was to investigate the effect of different psychological interventions on psychological and metabolic health. Data collection was carried out in three Finnish study centers at the universities of Helsinki, Jyväskylä, and Kuopio. The inclusion criteria were self-reported body mass index (BMI) of between 27–34.9 kg/m^2, and perceived psychological stress indicated by at least 3/12 points on the General Health Questionnaire [23]. The participants did not have any severe chronic illnesses, and any regularly taken medications were reported. Details of the inclusion and exclusion criteria have been reported previously [22].

Further inclusion criteria specifically for the present secondary cross-sectional baseline analyses were available data regarding objective stress and recovery (HRV recording) and subjective stress (Perceived Stress Scale; PSS). Individuals who used α- or β-adrenergic blocking agents affecting the heart were excluded from the present analysis. However, other regular medication was allowed. The final study group of the present analyses comprised of 221 individuals who also met the additional inclusion and exclusion criteria. Table 1 presents the characteristics of the participants. All participants were informed about the initial study, and they signed written informed consent prior to any measurements. This study was conducted according to the Declaration of Helsinki, and the study protocol was approved by the ethics committee of the Central Finland Health Care District.

Measurements

Objective stress and recovery were determined from recordings of the beat-to-beat R–R interval in real-life settings over 1–3 workdays. R–R interval data were collected using a Firstbeat Bodyguard measurement device (Firstbeat Technologies Ltd, Jyväskylä, Finland). The data were then analyzed using the Firstbeat Analysis Server

Table 1 Characteristics of the participants

	All ($N = 221$)		Female ($N = 185$)		Male ($N = 36$)	
	Mean	Range	Mean	Range	Mean	Range
Age (yrs)	48	26–60	48	26–60	45	31–60
Weight (kg)	87.7	64.0–120.1	85.4	64.0–113.9	99.3	83.8–120.1
Height (cm)	167.8	149.0–195.6	165.4	149.0–184.8	179.7	167.5–195.6
BMI (kg/[m]^2)	31.1	25.3–40.1	31.2	25.3–40.1	30.8	26.3–37.0
Body fat%	38.6	12.8–50.8	40.7	28.4–50.8	28.0	12.8–35.1
Physical activity (MET index[a])	3.2	0.0–18.0	3.0	0.0–15.3	4.3	0.1–18.0
Subjective stress (PSS[b])	26.5	7.0–52.0	26.5	7.0–52.0	26.2	17.0–38.0
Objective stress (stress index)	163.0	88.5–455.8	163.2	88.5–455.8	162.2	89.1–308.3
Objective recovery (stress balance)	0.35	−1.00–1.00	0.34	−1.00–1.00	0.40	−0.98–1.00

[a]MET-h/day, based on retrospective physical activity questionnaire
[b]Perceived Stress Scale

software (version 5.3.0.4), which included a powerful artifact correction feature for irregular ectopic beats, and signal noise. The original R-R interval series were resampled at the rate of 5 Hz by using linear interpolation to obtain equidistantly sampled time series, and second-by-second HRV indices were calculated with the short-time Fourier transform method by using constant duration Hanning window [24, 25]. Thereafter, the software categorizes the data into different physiological states such as stress, recovery, and physical activity of different intensities by taking into account individual characteristics (e.g. the individual levels and scales of HR and HRV, and the individual relationships between HRV and autonomic control e.g. [24]). Stress means sympathetic dominance of the ANS without metabolic requirements caused by physical activity whereas recovery means parasympathetic dominance of the ANS. In this categorization, second-by-second HRV indices, HRV-derived respiration rate, oxygen consumption calculated by HR, HRV-derived respiration rate, and on-off kinetics, and parameter describing excess-post exercise oxygen consumption are used with neural network data modeling [25–27] (for more details, see the white papers by Firstbeat Technologies Ltd [28]). The intensity of stress reaction is calculated from the HR, high frequency (0.15–0.4 Hz), and low frequency (0.04–0.15 Hz) components of HRV and respiratory variables. The intensity of stress is high when HR is elevated, HRV is reduced, and the frequency distribution of HRV is inconsistent because of changes in respiratory period. The intensity of recovery is calculated from the HR and high frequency component of HRV, and it is high when HR is low and high frequency component of HRV is high and regular. From the Firstbeat Analysis Server, the stress index was used as an indicator of objective stress and the stress balance value as an indicator of objective recovery. The stress index characterizes the magnitude of stress processes during the whole day. This index describes the mean intensity of the recognized stress reactions (theoretically ranging from 0 to ∞, ranging in our material 88.5 – 455.8). The stress balance value (ranging from −1 to 1) indicates the proportion of time of stress and recovery reactions during self-reported sleep periods during the measurement period. Values from 0.5 to 1 indicate good recovery, values from 0 to 0.5 indicate moderate recovery, and values from 0 to −1 indicate weak recovery [7].

The HRV data consisted of successfully recorded workdays, with an allowed maximum of 15 % regarding the grade of detected and corrected artifacts in R–R intervals. The values of the HRV-based variables of stress and recovery were the mean values of the workdays. Data from two workdays were included for 191 participants, from one workday for 20 participants, and from three workdays for 10 participants. For each monitored day, the participants reported their working hours, sleeping hours, and alcohol consumption in measurement diaries. Alcohol consumption was reported in standard units of approximately 12 g of ethanol (one unit: 33 centiliter [cl] beer, 12 cl red or white wine, 8 cl fortified wine, or 4 cl liquor).

Subjective stress during the preceding month was assessed using the 14-item PSS, which measures the degree to which situations in one's life are stressful on a 5-point scale ranging from 0 (never) to 4 (very often) [29]. PSS total scores are generally calculated by reversing the scores of the seven positive items and then summarizing the scores of all 14 items. Internal reliability (Cronbach's α) for the PSS was 0.86. To reduce the measurement error of the PSS sum score, we used a factor that included all 14 questions in the present analysis instead of the sum score.

PA was assessed using a questionnaire with items regarding present activity and changes within the last two months. The questionnaire included structured questions covering leisure-time PA and commuting activity [30, 31]. A multiple of the resting metabolic rate (MET) was assigned for each activity to describe the intensity of the form of PA. The MET indices for each form of PA were calculated by multiplying the intensity (MET), duration (h), and frequency of the activity, and the MET index was expressed as the sum score of different activities (MET-h/d).

Body composition was evaluated using bioelectrical impedance analysis (InBody720; Jyväskylä, Kuopio/Tanita BC-418 MA; Helsinki) in the morning after 10–12 h of fasting. This device provides information about the whole body fat percentage. Body weight and height were also measured during the same laboratory visit.

Statistical analysis

Statistical analyses were performed using Mplus version 5.21 [32]. Within this program, we used the MLR estimator, which comprises maximum likelihood with robust standard errors and with scale-corrected chi-square test values correcting for the effect of non-normality. To analyze the measurement structure of the PSS score, we used confirmatory factor analysis (CFA). Based on the results of the CFA the latent factor model was used in the estimation of the correlations and in structural equation modeling analysis to investigate the associations of objective stress and recovery with subjective stress, as well as to investigate the associations of PA, body composition, and age with objective and subjective stress. The significance level of the study was set at 0.05. The model fit was evaluated using the χ^2 test, comparative fit index (CFI), Tucker Lewis index (TLI), root mean square error of approximation (RMSEA), and standardized root mean square residual (SRMR). For a good-fitting model, the χ^2 test is non-significant, CFI and TLI are at least 0.95, RMSEA is no more than 0.06, and SRMR no more than 0.08 [33].

Results

The one-factor solution for the PSS did not sufficiently fit the data (χ^2 (77) = 345.12, $P < 0.001$; CFI = 0.786; TLI = 0.747; RMSEA = 0.126; SRMR = 0.084); therefore, the factor structure was altered based on modification indices. The factor subjective stress was merged to contain two specific factors, as covariance existed between the residuals of questions 2, 3, 8, 12, 13, and 14 (related to perception of uncontrollable life) and the questions 1, 3, 6, and 11 (related to perception of overload) (Fig. 1). This estimated model fit the data well (χ^2 (66) = 109.25, $P < 0.001$; CFI = 0.966; TLI = 0.952; RMSEA = 0.054; SRMR = 0.044). All of the modification indices were lower than 4, indicating that there were no additional parameters that would have increased the fit of the model for the analysis.

Table 2 presents the results of the associations of subjective stress with objective stress and recovery. Subjective stress correlated with objective stress ($r = 0.139$, 95 % CI 0.002 to 0.276, $P = 0.047$) and with objective recovery ($r = -0.140$, 95 % CI −0.277 to −0.003, $P = 0.046$) without any adjustments (Model 1). In Model 2, the associations of subjective stress with objective stress and recovery were adjusted for sex and age. Subjective stress was associated with objective stress (residual $r = 0.209$, 95 % CI 0.075 to 0.343, $P = 0.002$) and with objective recovery (residual $r = -0.137$, 95 % CI −0.275 to 0.000, $P = 0.050$). Age was positively associated with objective stress (β = 0.435, 95 % CI 0.327 to 0.543, $P < 0.001$). Sex was not associated with subjective stress, objective stress, or recovery. The associations of subjective stress with objective stress and recovery were not influenced by further adjustment for alcohol consumption or for regular medication.

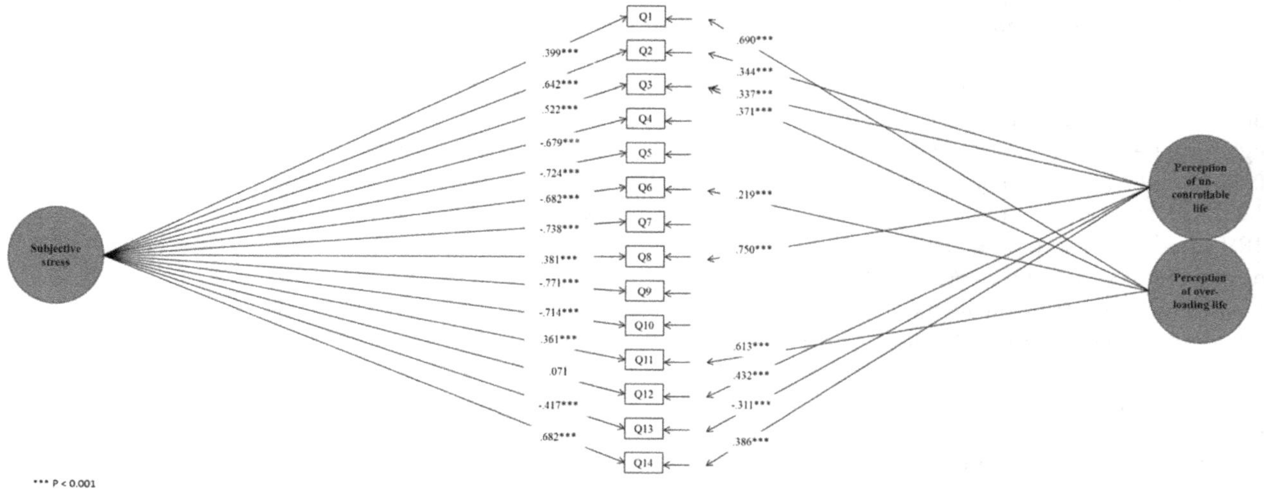

Fig. 1 The structure of the factor constructed of the questions of the Perceived Stress Scale (PSS). Factor loadings (standardized estimates) for the 14 questions, and loadings of the two specific factors for residual variances

Table 2 Correlations of subjective stress with objective stress and recovery

	Subjective stress							
	Model 1				Model 2			
	r	S.E.	95 % CI	*P*	r_e	S.E.	95 % CI	*P*
Objective stress (Stress index)	0.139	0.070	0.002 to 0.276	0.047	0.209	0.068	0.075 to 0.343	0.002
Objective recovery (Stress balance)	−0.140	0.070	−0.277 to −0.003	0.046	−0.137	0.070	−0.275 to 0.000	0.050

Standardized model results: correlation (r), residual correlation (r_e), standard error (S.E.), 95 % confidence interval (95 % CI), and *P* value
Model 1: no adjustments Model 2: age- and sex adjusted

Figure 2 presents the association of subjective stress with objective stress and recovery after adjustment for sex, age, PA, and body fat percentage. Subjective stress was associated with objective stress (residual $r = 0.217$, 95 % CI 0.084 to 0.351, $P = 0.001$) and recovery (residual $r = -0.146$, 95 % CI −0.283 to −0.009, $P = 0.037$). PA was negatively associated with subjective stress ($\beta = -0.149$, 95 % CI −0.289 to −0.009, $P = 0.037$). The negative association of subjective stress with body fat percentage was non-significant ($\beta = -0.187$, 95 % CI −0.384 to 0.011, $P = 0.064$). Objective stress and recovery were not associated with PA or body fat percentage. Sex was not associated with subjective stress, objective stress, or recovery. Age was positively associated with objective stress ($\beta = 0.439$, 95 % CI 0.330 to 0.547, $P < 0.001$). The results were not influenced by further adjustment for alcohol consumption or regular medication, except that age was negatively associated with subjective stress ($\beta = -0.143$, 95 % CI −0.282 to −0.004, $P = 0.043$).

Discussion

The present findings suggest that the higher the subjective self-reported stress the higher the objective HRV-based stress and the lower the objective HRV-based recovery on workdays. We also found that within our psychologically distressed and overweight study group, higher level of PA was associated with lower subjective stress.

Our results showed that higher subjective stress was associated with higher objective stress when adjusted for the effects of age and sex. This rather weak but statistically significant association strengthened after accounting for PA and body fat percentage. This finding is in line with those of previous studies. Uusitalo et al. [34] found that daily emotions at work and chronic work-related stress were associated with cardiac autonomic function. They used the same HRV-based measurement method as we did, and reported that the associations of HRV-based measures and the traditional HRV measures with subjective stress were alike. Other previous studies have reported similar findings using traditional time or frequency domain measures of HRV (e.g. [14, 16]). Collins et al. [14] observed that job strain and low decision latitude were associated with reduced cardiac vagal control, and that job strain was associated with elevated sympathetic control during working hours. These results of Collins et al. [14] were obtained from 24-h ECG recordings. Additionally, other study results obtained from both short-time [35, 36] and 24-h ECG

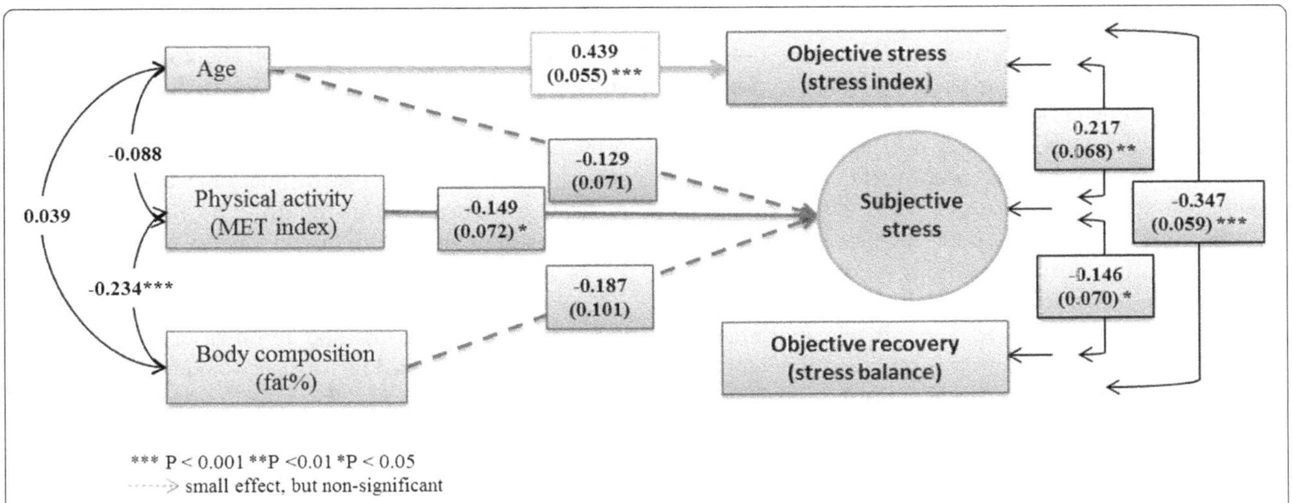

Fig. 2 Sex-adjusted associations of age, physical activity, and body composition with subjective stress, with objective stress, and with recovery. The presented values are standardized model results (estimate and standard error). Residual correlation and standard error between subjective stress and objective stress and recovery, and correlations between age, physical activity, and body composition are also presented

recordings (e.g. [37]) have observed the association between subjective stress and HRV with larger populations.

We also found that higher subjective stress was associated with lower objective recovery during sleep. This rather weak but statistically significant association strengthened after taken into account sex, age, PA and body fat percentage. This finding supports the previous study, which found that daily emotions at work were associated with night time traditional HRV measures [34]. In contrast, Hynynen et al. [13] found that low- and high-stress groups exhibited no differences in nocturnal traditional measures of HRV. Further studies are needed to investigate the association between subjective stress and HRV-based recovery during sleep. Recovery is an important factor in preventing the detrimental effects of stress, as good recovery during sleep has been suggested to confer protection from cardiovascular disease risk factors [2, 38]. An effort-recovery model shows that in cases of incomplete recovery, an employee must expend extra effort to perform properly at work [1].

The present results showed that higher level of PA was weakly but statistically significantly associated with lower levels of subjective stress among our overweight participants with low inter-individual variability in PA. Within our study group, PA was not associated with objective stress or objective recovery. The present study design does not enable us to draw any broader conclusions about the association between PA and subjective stress, and it remains unclear whether stress or inactivity is a cause or a consequence in this relationship. However, our finding of a negative association between PA and subjective stress supports the conclusions of previous studies. Hamer [39] suggests that regular exercise may have stress-buffering benefits largely because exercisers are more often in the post-exercise window when they encounter daily stressors. In line with our present cross-sectional finding, Kouvonen et al. [18] found that increased work-related stress was weakly associated with decreased PA during 6–8 year follow-up. In contrast to our present results, we found in our previous study [7] that a higher level of PA was associated with lower objective stress and higher objective recovery among participants with great inter-individual variability in their PA levels.

Within our study group, body fat percentage was not associated with objective stress or recovery. According to magnitude-based inference with confidence intervals [40, 41] our results showed a small negative effect of body fat percentage on subjective stress. In line with this, previous findings in large study groups suggest that a higher obesity level may confer protection from burnout (e.g. [42]). Whereas, our previous study found that a more favorable body composition was associated with lower objective stress and higher objective recovery [7] and obesity is known to cause stress to the body, as visceral obesity is a key factor in metabolic syndrome [43].

Here we also found that older age was associated with higher objective stress, but not with objective recovery. Additionally, the results showed an unclear negative non-significant association between age and subjective stress. Our inference is that any effect of age on subjective stress is at most small. HRV is individual, and is known to decrease with age [11]. The objective method presently used recognizes stress and recovery reactions and determines different physiological states of the body based on individual scaling of HR and HRV data. The presently used stress index as an indicator of magnitude of the objective stress reactions is, however, calculated from HR, HRV and respiratory variables during the recognized stress states on the whole day. Therefore, the aging-related decrease in HRV likely explains this finding to some extent and inhibits us to conclude that older employees were more sensitive to physiological stress. Whereas, the presently used stress balance value as an indicator of objective recovery was calculated from the recognized stress and recovery states during sleep, and this value takes into account all individuality in HRV. In the present study, age did not affect objective recovery during sleep. However, older persons seemed to perceive less stress than their younger counterparts. Further research on the association between age and objective stress, including the effect of PA, would be interesting and warranted.

In the present study, subjective stress was assessed by PSS. This scale has been found to be a reliable and valid measure of perceived stress. To analyze the measurement structure of the PSS score, we further used CFA to test whether the 14 questions of the PSS were consistent with the factor consisting of these 14 questions. We found that the fit factor solution included two specific factors. Based on the results of the CFA and to get more reliable results we used this factor solution as a variable of subjective stress in the present analysis. PSS assesses subjective stress during the preceding month. So, it is important to take into account that the present results provide information about the association of perceived stress over one month with the objective stress and recovery at the end of this month.

Subjective methods were used to assess both the level of stress and the level of PA. Even though, it is known that subjective assessment may include some reporting bias, it is a commonly used method for measuring stress. The most frequently utilized instrument is a questionnaire that has been widely criticized because it relies on individual self-reporting. In contrast, physiological measures represent objective data, which are considered to be more reliable as they are not affected by an individual's cognition, social context, or emotions [44]. Therefore, it is reasonable and important to develop objective measures of stress that acknowledge the physiological burden of stress. The assessment of PA was based on a questionnaire. However, this questionnaire took into account a long-term level of PA and may give more trustful information about individual's PA than an objective measurement from a short period.

HRV assessment is a promising clinical tool for assessing health and identifying health impairments [10, 24, 45]. However, due to a limited applicability of the traditional measures of HRV into changing and uncontrollable real-life setting, it is important to develop methods that apply HRV data and are able to provide valuable information on stress and recovery in individuals' everyday life. By utilizing both HRV and additional HRV-derived information it is possible to produce knowledge of physiological states, such as stress and recovery that is not available from the basic HRV measures which represent the average level of the autonomic activity over a period of the time. This kind of information can also be utilized in supporting lifestyle change. Previous findings also support the validity and reliability of the HRV-based method used in the present study [7, 34]. In addition to subjective assessment of stress, the method has been validated against neuroendocrine responses to stress. The indicators of stress and recovery during sleep have been found to be associated with free salivary cortisol after awakening [46]. As HRV measurement is dependent on the duration of the R – R interval recording [47], it is a strength of the present study that HR and HRV data were recorded in real-life settings over a rather long time period, usually two workdays. Secondly, the method produced stress- and recovery-related variables based on the HR, HRV, and respiratory variables. These variables are more informative for both health-care professionals and patients/clients than traditional measures of HRV and they are suitable for application in general health care.

Although, HRV assessment is a promising clinical tool for assessing health and identifying health impairments, several points must be considered regarding the HR- and HRV-based measurement of stress. HR and HRV are very individual, and are dependent on age and sex [10, 11, 24]. HRV decreases with age, and the variation is greater among female population. Therefore, it is important to account for age and gender, as well as PA, when investigating the associations of objective stress and recovery with subjective stress. The present study excluded subjects who used α- or β-blockers, as these drugs have substantial effects on HR and HRV. However, our participants included individuals using regular medication such as other cardiac medications or psychopharmacological, metabolic or analgesic medication. This could also potentially affect HR and HRV since many medications directly or indirectly act on the ANS [11]. Therefore, we also accounted for regular medication and alcohol consumption in our present analysis. These adjustments did not affect the associations of objective stress and recovery with subjective stress. However, it is important to acknowledge that the measurement was accomplished in real-life settings and it takes participant's word for confounding factors, such as medication and alcohol consumption.

The present study participants were psychologically distressed and overweight composing an ideal study group for investigating the association of subjective stress with objective stress and recovery. Furthermore, they represent a group of Finnish workers of different occupations, mainly trade and office workers. However, there were limited variations in the levels of psychological stress, fat percentage and PA within our participants. Therefore, these presently found associations should be studied further among more heterogeneous study group and the present results can thus be generalized to overweight individuals with psychological distress. It would have been interesting to further study the possible gender differences; however, such analyses were not reasonable within the present group due to the low number of men. Data collection was carried out in three study centers. However, adjustment for study center did not affect the results.

There is a recognized need for further research about the reliability of HRV measurement. The results of Cipryan & Litschmannova [48] suggest that researchers should be very cautious when drawing conclusions based only on short-term HRV analysis. Such methods as presently described and evaluated HRV-based method for assessing objective stress and recovery in real-life settings mainly over two workdays, are necessary to improve the reliability of HRV analysis and to provide informative and suitable variables for application in general health care and lifestyle counselling. This kind of individual counselling would be the optimal way to utilize HRV-based method in stress assessment. Real-life setting includes several uncontrollable confounding factors complicating the group-level analyzing of the data. This fact together with the participants' low inter-individual variation in the main variables of the present study result to the fact that the found associations are rather weak. From the perspective of magnitude-based inference with confidence intervals [40] there is a possibility that some of our findings are somewhat trivial. On the whole, there is a limited number of studies that have utilized long-term HRV monitoring and it is difficult to compare the present findings with the previous findings obtained from short-term ECG recordings and with studies that have used different measures than we did. Nevertheless, based on previous evidence, we assume that similar findings to our present findings and overall conclusion would have been reached by using traditional measures of HRV. More research with larger study populations and further follow-up studies are needed.

Conclusions

The present results suggest that subjective self-reported stress is associated with objective HRV-based stress and recovery. Subjective psychological and objective physiological stress are apparently affected by different factors, such as PA. However, some of the found associations among the overweight and psychologically distressed participants with low inter-individual variation in PA are rather weak and the clinical value of the present findings should be studied further among participants with greater heterogeneity of stress, PA and body composition. However, these findings suggest that the presently described method for objective stress assessment provides an additional and important aspect to stress assessment. Furthermore, the results provide valuable information for the development of stress assessment methods.

Abbreviations

ANS: Autonomic nervous system; BMI: Body mass index; CFA: Confirmatory factor analyses; CFI: Comparative fit index; ECG: Electrocardiogram; HR: Heart rate; HRV: Heart rate variability; MET: Multiple of the resting metabolic rate; PA: Physical activity; PSS: Perceived stress scale; RMSEA: Root mean square error of approximation; SRMR: Standardized root mean square residual; TLI: Tucker Lewis index.

Competing interests

T. Myllymäki is an employee of and H. Rusko is a stockowner in Firstbeat Technologies Ltd. They did not contribute to writing the conclusions of the study. The authors declare that they have no competing interests.

Authors' contributions

Study conception and design: TF, AT, RK, MK, RL, UK. Data acquisition: TF, TM, EJ-R, SR, KP, UK. Data analysis and interpretation: TF, AT, TM, EJ-R, SR, RK, KP, MK, SP, RL, HR, UK. Statistical analysis: TF, AT. Drafting the manuscript: TF. Critical revision of the manuscript for important intellectual content: TF, AT, TM, EJ-R, SR, RK, KP, MK, SP, RL, HR, UK. Final approval of the version to be published: TF, AT, TM, EJ-R, SR, RK, KP, MK, SP, RL, HR, UK. Obtained funding: TF, RK, MK, RL, UK. Administrative, technical, or material support: AT, RK, MK, SP, RL, UK.

Acknowledgements

This study was supported by the SalWe Research Program for Mind and Body (Tekes - the Finnish Funding Agency for Technology and Innovation grant 1104/10). T. Föhr's work was supported by a personal grant from the Juho Vainio Foundation.

Author details

[1]Department of Health Sciences, University of Jyväskylä, P.O. Box 35, FIN-40014 Jyväskylä, Finland. [2]Methodology Centre for Human Sciences, Faculty of Social Sciences, University of Jyväskylä, P.O. Box 35 (Y 33), FIN-40014 Jyväskylä, Finland. [3]Department of Psychology, University of Jyväskylä, P.O. Box 35, FIN-40014 Jyväskylä, Finland. [4]Institute of Public Health and Clinical Nutrition, University of Eastern Finland, Kuopio Campus, P.O. Box 1627, FIN-70211 Kuopio, Finland. [5]Medical Faculty, Pharmacology, Medical nutrition physiology, University of Helsinki, P.O. Box 63, FIN-00014 Helsinki, Finland. [6]Finnish Institute of Occupational Health, Topeliuksenkatu 41 a A, FIN-00250 Helsinki, Finland. [7]Institute of Behavioral Sciences, University of Helsinki, P.O. Box 9, FIN-00014 Helsinki, Finland. [8]Department of Biology of Physical Activity, University of Jyväskylä, P.O. Box 35, FIN-40014 Jyväskylä, Finland.

References

1. Meijman TF, Mulder G. Psychological aspects of workload. In: Handbook of work and organizational psychology: Work psychology. 2nd ed. United Kingdom: Redwood Books Ltd; 1998. p. 5–33.
2. Van Amelsvoort LGPM, Schouten EG, Maan AC, Swenne CA, Kok FJ. Occupational determinants of heart rate variability. Intern Arch Occup Environ Health. 2000;73 Suppl 4:255–62.
3. Chandola T, Heraclides A, Kumari M. Psychophysiological biomarkers of workplace stressors. Neurosci Biobehav Rev. 2010;35 Suppl 1:51–7.
4. Kivimäki M, Nyberg ST, Batty GD, Fransson EI, Heikkilä K, Alfredsson L, et al. Job strain as a risk factor for coronary heart disease: a collaborative meta-analysis of individual participant data. Lancet. 2012;380 Suppl 9852:1491–7.
5. Kivimäki M, Leino-Arjas P, Kaila-Kangas L, Luukkonen R, Vahtera J, Elovainio M, et al. Is incomplete recovery from work a risk marker of cardiovascular death? Prospective evidence from industrial employees. Psychosom Med. 2006;68 Suppl 3:402–7.
6. Duijts SF, Kant I, Swaen GM, van den Brandt PA, Zeegers M. A meta-analysis of observational studies identifies predictors of sickness absence. J Clin Epidemiol. 2007;60 Suppl 11:1105–15.
7. Teisala T, Mutikainen S, Tolvanen A, Rottensteiner M, Leskinen T, Kaprio J, et al. Associations of physical activity, fitness, and body composition with heart rate variability–based indicators of stress and recovery on workdays: a cross-sectional study. J Occup Med Toxicol. 2014;9:16.
8. Reed MJ, Robertson CE, Addison PS. Heart rate variability measurements and the prediction of ventricular arrhythmias. QJM. 2005;98 Suppl 2:87–95.
9. McMillan DE. Interpreting heart rate variability sleep/wake patterns in cardiac patients. J Cardiovasc Nurs. 2002;17 Suppl 1:69–81.
10. Acharya UR, Joseph KP, Kannathal N, Lim CM, Suri JS. Heart rate variability: a review. Med Bio Eng Comput. 2006;44:1031–51.
11. Task Force of the European Society of Cardiology and the North American Society of Pacing and Electrophysiology. Heart rate variability: standards of measurement, physiological interpretation and clinical use. Circulation. 1996;93 Suppl 5:1043–65.
12. Malliani A, Pagani M, Lombardi F, Gerutti S. Cardiovascular neural regulation explored in the frequency domain. Circulation. 1991;84 Suppl 2:482–92.
13. Hynynen E, Konttinen N, Kinnunen U, Kyröläinen H, Rusko H. The incidence of stress symptoms and heart rate variability during sleep and orthostatic test. Eur J Appl Physiol. 2011;111 Suppl 5:733–41.
14. Collins SM, Karasek RA, Costas K. Job strain and autonomic indices of cardiovascular disease risk. Am J Ind Med. 2005;48 Suppl 3:182–93.
15. Riese H, Van Doornen LJ, Houtman IL, De Geus EJ. Job strain in relation to ambulatory blood pressure, heart rate, and heart rate variability among female nurses. Scand J Work Environ Health. 2004;30 Suppl 6:477–85.
16. Hanson EKS, Godaert GLR, Maas CJM, Meijman TF. Vagal cardiac control throughout the day: the relative importance of effort–reward imbalance and within-day measurements of mood, demand and satisfaction. Biol Psychol. 2001;56 Suppl 1:23–44.
17. Gerber M, Pühse U. Do exercise and fitness protect against stress-induced health complaints? A review of the literature. Scand J Publ Health. 2009;37 Suppl 8:801–19.
18. Kouvonen A, Vahtera J, Oksanen T, Pentti J, Väänänen AK, Heponiemi T, et al. Chronic workplace stress and insufficient physical activity: a cohort study. Occup Environ Med. 2013;70 Suppl 1:3–8.
19. Ahola K, Pulkki-Råback L, Kouvonen A, Rossi H, Aromaa A, Lönnqvist J. Burnout and behavior-related health risk factors: results from the population-based finnish health 2000 study. J Occup Env Med. 2012;54 Suppl 1:17–22.
20. Iversen LB, Strandberg-Larsen K, Prescott E, Schnohr P, Rod NH. Psychosocial risk factors, weight changes and risk of obesity: the Copenhagen City heart study. Eur J Epidemiol. 2012;27 Suppl 2:119–30.
21. Sonnentag S, Jelden S. Job stressors and the pursuit of sport activities: a day-level perspective. J Occup Health Psychol. 2009;14 Suppl 2:165–81.
22. Lappalainen R, Sairanen E, Järvelä E, Rantala S, Korpela R, Puttonen S, et al. The effectiveness and applicability of different lifestyle interventions for enhancing wellbeing: the study design for a randomized controlled trial for persons with metabolic syndrome risk factors and psychological distress. BMC Publ Health. 2014;14 Suppl 1:310.
23. Makowska Z, Merecz D, Moscicka A, Kolasa W. The validity of general health questionnaires, GHQ-12 and GHQ-28, in mental health studies of working people. Int J Occup Med Environ Health. 2002;15 Suppl 4:353–62.

24. Martinmäki K, Rusko H, Kooistra L, Kettunen J, Saalasti S. Intraindividual validation of heart rate variability indexes to measure vagal effects on hearts. Am J Physiol Heart Circ Physiol. 2006;290:640–7.
25. Saalasti S. Neural networks for heart rate time series analysis. In: PhD Thesis. Finland, Jyväskylä Studies in Computing 33. Jyväskylä: Department of Mathematical Information Technology, University of Jyväskylä; 2003.
26. Kettunen J, Saalasti S, inventors; Firstbeat Technologies Ltd, assignee. Procedure for deriving reliable information on respiratory activity from heart period measurement. United States: patent US 20050209521A1; 2005.
27. Kettunen J, Saalasti S, inventors; Firstbeat Technologies Ltd, assignee. Procedure for detection of stress by segmentation and analyzing heart beat signal. United States: patent US 007330752B2; 2008.
28. White papers [http://www.firstbeat.com/physiology/white-papers]
29. Cohen S, Kamarck T, Mermelstein R. A global measure of perceived stress. J Health Soc Behav. 1983;24 Suppl 4:385–96.
30. Kujala UM, Kaprio J, Sarna S, Koskenvuo M. Relationship of leisure-time physical activity and mortality: The finnish twin cohort. JAMA. 1998;279 Suppl 6:440–4.
31. Waller K, Kaprio J, Kujala UM. Associations between long-term physical activity, waist circumference and weight gain: a 30-year longitudinal twin study. Int J Obes. 2007;32 Suppl 2:353–61.
32. Muthén LK, Muthén BO. Mplus user's guide. 7th ed. Muthén & Muthén: Los Angeles: CA; 1998.
33. Hu LT, Bentler PM. Cutoff criteria for fit indexes in covariance structure analysis: conventional criteria versus new alternatives. Struct Equ Model. 1999;6 Suppl 1:1–55.
34. Uusitalo A, Mets T, Martinmäki K, Mauno S, Kinnunen U, Rusko H. Heart rate variability related to effort at work. Appl Ergon. 2011;42 Suppl 6:830–8.
35. Hintsanen M, Elovainio M, Puttonen S, Kivimäki M, Koskinen T, Raitakari OT, et al. Effort—reward imbalance, heart rate, and heart rate variability: the cardiovascular risk in young finns study. Int J Behav Med. 2007;14 Suppl 4:202–12.
36. Zanstra YJ, Schellekens JM, Schaap C, Kooistra L. Vagal and sympathetic activity in burnouts during a mentally demanding workday. Psychosom Med. 2006;68 Suppl 4:583–90.
37. Vrijkotte TG, van Doornen LJ, de Geus EJ. Effects of work stress on ambulatory blood pressure, heart rate, and heart rate variability. Hypertension. 2000;35 Suppl 4:880–6.
38. Steptoe A, Marmot M. Impaired cardiovascular recovery following stress predicts 3-year increases in blood pressure. J Hypertens. 2005;23 Suppl 3:529–36.
39. Hamer M. Psychosocial stress and cardiovascular disease risk: the role of physical activity. Psychosom Med. 2012;74 Suppl 9:896–903.
40. Batterham AM, Hopkins WG. Making meaningful inferences about magnitudes. Sportscience. 2005;9:6–13.
41. Cohen J. A power primer. Psychol Bull. 1992;112 Suppl 1:155–9.
42. Armon G, Shirom A, Berliner S, Shapira I, Melamed S. A prospective study of the association between obesity and burnout among apparently healthy men and women. J Occup Health Psychol. 2008;13 Suppl 1:43–57.
43. Rosmond R. Role of stress in the pathogenesis of the metabolic syndrome. Psychoneuroendocrinology. 2005;30 Suppl 1:1–10.
44. Kompier M. Assessing the psychosocial work environment-"subjective" versus"objective" measurement. Scand J Work Environ Health. 2005;31 Suppl 6:405–8.
45. Vanderlei LCM, Pastre CM, Hoshi RA, Carvalho TD, Godoy MF. Basic notions of heart rate variability and its clinical applicability. Rev Bras Cir Cardiovasc. 2009;24 Suppl 2:205–17.
46. Rusko H, Rönkä T, Uusitalo A, Kinnunen U, Mauno S, Feldt T, et al. Stress and relaxation during sleep and awake time, and their associations with free salivary cortisol after awakening. Nordic Ergonomics Society congress 2006 [http://www.firstbeat.com/userData/firstbeat/download/rusko_et_al_nes_2006_congress.pdf]
47. Pinna G, Maestri R, Torunski A, Danilowicz-Szymanowicz L, Szwoch M, La Rovere M, et al. Heart rate variability measures: a fresh look at reliability. Clin Sci. 2007;113:131–40.
48. Cipryan L, Litschmannova M. Intra-day and inter-day reliability of heart rate variability measurement. J Sports Sci. 2013;31 Suppl 2:150–8.

10

Stonefish envenomation of hand with impending compartment syndrome

Terence Khai Wei Tay*, Han Zhe Chan, Tunku Sara Tunku Ahmad, Kok Kheng Teh, Tze Hau Low and Nuraliza Ab Wahab

Abstract

Background: Marine stings and envenomation are fairly common in Malaysia. Possible contact to various marine life occurs during diving, fishing and food handling. Even though majority of fish stings are benign, there are several venomous species such as puffer fish, scorpion fish, lionfish, stingray and stonefish that require urgent medical treatment. Stonefish is one of the most venomous fish in the world with potential fatal local and systemic toxicity effects to human.

Case Presentation: We reported a case of stonefish sting complicated with impending compartment syndrome.

Conclusions: Medical staff should be alert about the possibility of this potential emergency in standard management of stonefish stings.

Keywords: Stonefish, Synanceia, Bites and stings, Marine toxins, Impending compartment syndrome

Background

Synanceia spp. is a genus of fish from the family Synanceiidae, the Stonefish, whose members are dangerous and even fatal to human. It is one of the most venomous fish currently known in the world [1]. They are found in the coastal regions of Indo-Pacific oceans as well as off the coast of Florida and in the Caribbean.

Stonefish has potent neurotoxins secreted from glands at the base of their needle-like dorsal fin spines, which stick up when disturbed or threatened. The name, "Stonefish", derives from its ability to camouflage with a grey and mottled color similar to the color of a stone. They are often covered by a coat of slime to which algae adhere. This excellent camouflage and their habit of partially burying themselves in the sand, makes them difficult to detect and avoid. Many small fishes easily fall prey to its superior camouflage ability. Human too, may not notice them most of the time, and thus inadvertently touch or step on them, triggering a sting. When disturbed, the stonefish injects an amount of venom proportional to the amount of pressure applied to it. They have earned labels such as 'the master of deceit' and 'devil-fish' due to their unaesthetic appearance and toxic venom. Like other venomous animal venoms, stonefish venom exhibits hemorrhagic, hemolytic, and proteolytic enzymatic activity [2]. The stings will lead to excruciating pain and gross oedema of the affected limb.

In Malaysia and Singapore, stonefish stings are rare. There were only eight cases reported within year 2001 and 2003 [3].

Case report

Our patient is a thirty-year-old Burmese aquarium cleaner in Aquaria KLCC, who was accidentally stung on his right index finger by a stonefish during a cleaning work. He immediately suffered from intense burning pain over radial aspect of his right index finger. The sharp pain soon spread to his ipsilateral axilla. Rapid-onset gross swelling developed in the affected finger and within two hours, his entire right index finger and radial half of the hand were swollen and erythematous. There was no stonefish spine retained in the wound. Despite receiving regular analgesia in the form of fentanyl and morphine, he still suffered from intense pain over his index finger. Anti-tetanus injection, antihistamine and steroid were administered and the limb elevated in attempt to reduce the swelling. Intravenous antibiotics (amoxicillin/clavulanic acid and metronidazole) were also given.

Twelve hours later, the pain had progressively worsened again and swelling had spread to involve the

* Correspondence: terencetkw99@yahoo.com
Department of Orthopaedic Surgery, Faculty of Medicine, University of Malaya, 50603 Kuala Lumpur, Malaysia

dorsum and radial half of his right hand (Fig. 1). Blisters appeared on his right index finger and he had paraesthesia over the median nerve distribution over the affected hand. Sensation reduced over the tip of right index finger and oxygen saturation on pulse oximeter dropped to 89 %, which raised the fear of impending compartment syndrome associated with symptoms of acute carpal tunnel syndrome. Clinically, patient was afebrile with stable vital signs. Laboratory results, including a white blood cell count, haemoglobin level, clotting profile; renal (electrolytes) and liver function tests were all normal. No gas shadow was seen in the right hand plain radiograph. All Gram stains and subsequent cultures were negative. There was no specific anti-venom for stonefish available in National Poison Centre. Patient was treated with warm water immersion and elevation in between immersion. Swelling gradually subsided. Fasciotomy was not required as the patient had responded well with the conservative management. His right hand swelling and circulation improved gradually. There was no local skin necrosis. Patient was discharged well with good recovery from pain and numbness after 4 days of hospital stay. There was no associated neurogenic or vascular sequelae noted during subsequent follow up. He had a full motion in his fingers and wrists joints at six weeks follow up.

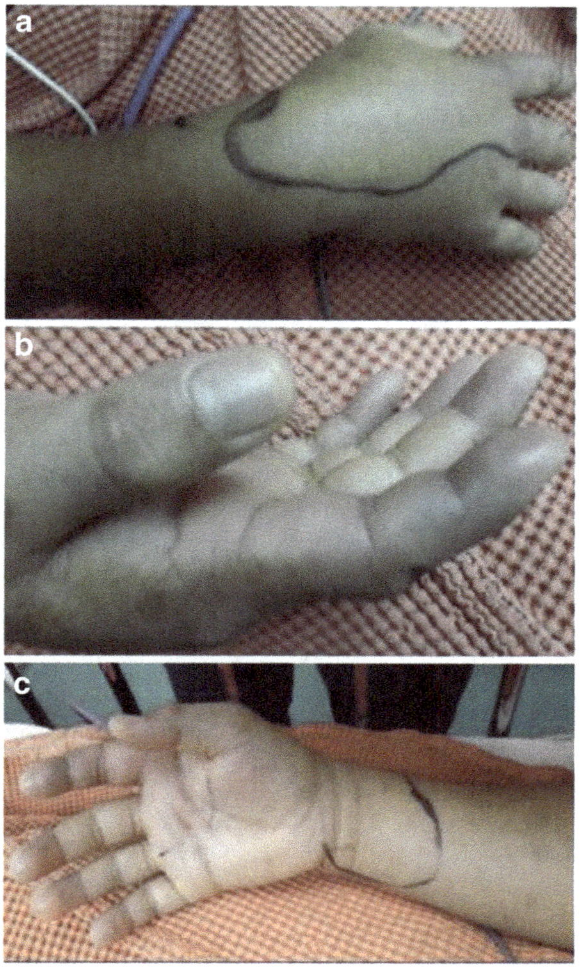

Fig. 1 Extensive erythema, gross swelling up to the entire index finger, dorsum, and distal third forearm

Discussion

Bio-toxicity

To date, there has been a tremendous effort to identify the specific bioactive venomous properties of stonefish toxin. The lethal effect of these venoms seems to reside in a signature protein unique to individual species within each family. Within the stonefish family, stonustoxin is the lethal protein from *Synanceja horrida*, trachynilysin from *Synanceja trachynis* and verrucotoxin from *Synanceja verrucosa* [4]. However, exact relationships of the toxin are still inconclusive. The most commonly accepted bioactive agents include the enzyme hyaluronidase, stonustoxin, and trachynilysin. Stonefish **hyaluronidase** has potency many times higher than the enzyme from snake venom [5]. Hyaluronidase, through its ability to break down connective tissue, accounts for the significant necrosis associated with stonefish envenomation [6]. It is believed to be responsible for the rapid spread. **Stonustoxin**, the lethal fraction is another bioactive element of the venom reported to be haemolytic and vasorelaxant. It contributes to extensive oedema after envenomation. Stonutoxin is also a potent hypotensive agent, which has myotoxic and neurotoxic activity as well. Marked hypotension appears to be the primary cause of death in animals in vivo studies [7]. **Trachynilysin** is a neurotoxin that depletes neurotransmitter levels at the synapses resulting in hyperstimulatory neuroblockade. As yet, these findings are largely experimental and further investigations are required before definite conclusions can be drawn.

Research shows that the venom is an unstable protein, with a pH of 6.0 and a molecular weight of 150,000. In vitro, it may be denatured by heat (2 min at 50 °C), acid and alkalis (pH > 9,pH < 4), potassium permanganate and Congo red [8]. Its heat labile nature is the basis for the stonefish sting treatment.

Management of stonefish injury by Hot Water Immersion (HWI)

Generally, standard stonefish envenomation management protocols include initial resuscitation, symptomatic relief with heat immersion therapy, anti-venom administration for systemic or severe local symptoms, and surgical removal of spines or foreign bodies. The evidence for the treatment of puncture-type stings by this method comes from one small experimental study [9] and a total of 99 reports of its effective use in 110 cases from several papers [10, 11]. This evidence has led to recommendation of this treatment method by organizations such as the International Life Saving Federation and the British Marine Life Study Society. The use of HWI is advised in toxicology guidelines such as Toxbase and the BNF and is supported in all five published review articles on marine envenomation. On the other hand, Tang et al [12] have advised caution with heat immersion, because the warmth may create an optimal environment for the development of vibrio necrotising fasciitis, most guidelines and studies still suggest that hot water immersion therapy is an effective treatment.

Two theories have been proposed on how HWI works. Marine venoms consist of multiple proteins and enzymes, and there is evidence that these become deactivated when heated to temperatures above 50 C [13]. A long-held view is that deactivation of these heat labile proteins by direct heat application leads to inactivation of the venom. They showed that venom lost its lethality more rapidly at temperatures over 43 C. However, no significant loss of lethality was seen after exposure to temperatures less than 39 C. The theory of deactivation has been questioned by authors who feel that such direct inactivation would require temperatures so high as to result in burns and tissue necrosis in the patient. Despite the concern of burn injury, there is only a single recorded case of significant thermal burn from over 200 cases of the use of HWI [14]. It is an inexpensive, and as there is reasonable evidence that it can relieve pain after a variety of types of fish sting. An alternative theory is that HWI causes modulation of pain receptors in the nervous system leading to a reduction in pain. Established pain hypotheses such as the gate control theory and the diffuse noxious inhibitory control theories have been proposed as possible mechanisms of action for HWI [15].

The most common methods of application are thermal packs, basins with hot water, and hot showers. Application of hot, but not scalding, water (40–42 C) for 30 min or until the pain resolves is the standard advice. American Journal of Public Health concluded that an exposure to water with maximum temperature of 49° Celcius for 8 min can cause burn injuries. Their studies also showed that prolong exposure to water with temperature about 45° Celcius for 2 h or more will cause scalded injuries. Immersion in water heated to the warmest bearable temperature (40–42 °C) is a relatively safe, easily accessible, and effective first-line management for stonefish injuries.

Stonefish Anti-venom

Most studies support the use of injected anti-venom as a potent tool in the management of stonefish envenomation [16, 17]. Due to its equine origin the anti-venom could theoretically cause serum sickness or precipitate anaphylactic reactions but there is little documented evidence that these adverse effects occur in practice. Indications for the use of stonefish anti-venom include systemic symptoms, severe pain, paralysis or multiple punctures are present. While the intramuscular (IM) route is well established, intravenous administration remains controversial. In general, one ampule (2000U) of Australia Commonwealth Serum Laboratories (CSL) of Melbourne Stonefish Anti-venom is given intramuscularly for puncture wounds from one or two spines. For three to four spine envenomation two vials are administered.

Compartment syndrome

Current international stonefish management guidelines mainly focused on heat immersion and anti-venom administration. Surgery has been reserved for removal of foreign bodies, especially the fish spines. Stonefish venom is believed to have hemolytic and proteolytic effect to skin and underlying soft tissue including neurovascular bundles. The vicious cycle of vascular permeability and soft tissue oedema can impinge on peripheral nerves and vessels, which can worsen over time, resembling compartment syndrome. In our case, patient presented with impending compartment syndrome that may have required a fasciotomy surgery. Fortunately, his swelling resolved with the elevation and hot water immersion therapy. If the swelling progresses, fasciotomy would have been warranted.

Conclusions

The stonefish is an environmental hazard to the unwary swimmer, angler, aquarium cleaner, and chefs. Their unparalleled camouflage ability makes them virtually undetectable and unavoidable. Envenomation can lead to unwanted local morbidity, excruciating pain, gross oedema of the affected limb, and severe systemic reactions have been reported. In majority, most of the cases do not result in protracted morbidity and it only requires prompt recognition, early pre-hospital care, and supportive management for symptomatic relief. We figured out that conservative management with short period of hot water immersion at temperature below 45° is generally safe and it helps to prevent unnecessary surgical intervention.

Consent

Appropriate written informed consent was obtained for publication of this case report. A copy of the written consent is available by the Editor-in-Chief of this journal.

Competing interests
The authors declare that they have no competing interests.

Authors' contributions
TTKW, CHZ and TKK were involved in conception, design and acquisition of data. LTH, NAW and ATS made the analysis, interpretation and editing data. All authors read and approved the final manuscript.

Author's information
Ahmad TS is Hand Consultant at Department of Orthopaedic Surgery, University Malaya. Terence TKW, Teh KK and Low TH are senior lecturer at Department of Orthopaedic Surgery, University of Malaya. Chan HZ is a medical officer at University Malaya Medical Centre (UMMC). Nuraliza AW work as Research Assistant at Department of Orthopaedic, University of Malaya.

References

1. Smith MM, Heemstra PC. Smith's sea fishes. Berlin–Heidelberg–New York: Springer Verlag; 1986. p. 1047.
2. Wiener S. Observations on the venom of the stone fish (Synanceja trachynis). Med J Aust. 1959;46(19):620–7.
3. Lee JY, Teoh LC, Leo SP. Stonefish envenomations of the hand–a local marine hazard: a series of 8 cases and review of the literature. Ann Acad Medicine Spore. 2004;33(4):515–20.
4. Khoo HE. Bioactive proteins from stonefish venom. Clin exp pharm & physiol. 2002;29(9):802–6.
5. Poh CH, Yuen R, Chung MC, Khoo HE. Purification and partial characterization of hyaluronidase from stonefish (Synanceja horrida) venom. Comp Biochem Physiol B. 1992;101(1–2):159–63.
6. Poh CH, Yuen R, Khoo HE, Chung M, Gwee M, Gopalakrishnakone P. Purification and partial characterization of stonustoxin (lethal factor) from Synanceja horrida venom. Comp Biochem Physiol B. 1991;99(4):793–8.
7. Low KS, Gwee MC, Yuen R, Gopalakrishnakone P, Khoo HE. Stonustoxin: effects on neuromuscular function in vitro and in vivo. Toxicon. 1994;32(5):573–81.
8. Edmonds C, Lowry C, Pennefather J. Diving and subaquatic medicine: Butterworth-Heinemann; 1992
9. Auerbach PS. Marine envenomations. N Engl J Med. 1991;325(7):486–93.
10. Halpern P, Sorkine P, Raskin Y. Envenomation by Trachinus draco in the eastern Mediterranean. Eur J Emerg Med. 2002;9(3):274–7.
11. Isbister GK. Venomous fish stings in tropical northern Australia. Am J Emerg Med. 2001;19(7):561–5.
12. Tang WM, Fung KK, Cheng VC, Lucke L. Rapidly progressive necrotising fasciitis following a stonefish sting: a report of two cases. J Orthop Surg (Hong Kong). 2006;14(1):67–70.
13. Carrette TJ, Cullen P, Little M, Peiera PL, Seymour JE. Temperature effects on box jellyfish venom: a possible treatment for envenomed patients? Med Aust. 2002;177(11–12):654–5.
14. Muirhead D. Applying pain theory in fish spine envenomation. Med Soc J. 2002;32:150–3.
15. Kizer KW, McKinney HE, Auerbach PS. Scorpaenidae envenomation. A five-year poison center experience. JAMA. 1985;253(6):807–10.
16. Lau FL. Emergency management of poisoning in Hong Kong. Hong Kong Med J. 2000;6(3):288–92.
17. Lehmann DF, Hardy JC. Stonefish envenomation. N Engl J Med. 1993;329(7): 510–1.

Evaluation of Darkroom disease's symptoms among radiographers in the West Bank hospitals

Hamzeh Al Zabadi[1,2*] and Yaser Nazzal[2]

Abstract

Background: Radiographers report many unexplained work related symptoms attributed to "darkroom disease symptoms" such as headache, skin rash, mouth sores, blurred vision, palpitation, and chemical taste. The aim of the present study was to assess the prevalence of occupationally-related darkroom disease symptoms among male radiographers in the West Bank hospitals.

Methods: A cross sectional study was conducted on a non-random purposive sample of male radiographers (study group) and nurses (control group) using a previously validated and standardized questionnaire.

Results: We were able to recruit 330 radiographers and 242 nurses. Data analysis showed that the majority of both groups aged between (36–43) years. Furthermore, the differences in the reported prevalence of symptoms among radiographers showed a statistically significant higher percentage for each reported symptom compared to nurses (P-values <0.001). In multivariate linear regression, staying more than 30 minutes in the darkroom per shift was associated with a significant increase in the mean number of reported symptoms (P-value < 0.001). However, the availability of a ventilating machine in the darkroom showed a strong negative association with the mean number of reported symptoms (P-value < 0.001).

Conclusions: Our findings could help overcome the limitations usually encountered in such complex occupational exposure. However, trying to interpret our finding directly to chemicals exposure in the radiographers' occupational setting should be done with caution due to the absence of active or passive monitoring for the suspected chemicals.

Background

In many occupational settings, some chemicals could adversely affect health and contaminate the environment [1]. Extensive use of x-ray processing chemistry on a world-wide basis has raised professional concerns regarding darkroom disease which is a term used to describe unexpected multiple symptoms attributed by radiographer to their work environment when being exposed to film processing chemicals [2-6]. These symptoms include: headaches, skin rashes, shortness of breath, mouth ulcers, unusual heart rhythms, painful joints, runny/stuffy nose and nausea.

* Correspondence: halzabadi@gmail.com
[1]Public Health Department, Faculty of Medicine and Health Sciences, An-Najah National University, PO.Box 7, West Bank, Nablus, Palestine
[2]Master of Public Health Program, Faculty of Graduate studies, An-Najah National University, Nablus, Palestine

X-rays could create a latent image on the film surface by reducing the silver halide crystals to elemental silver then the image is amplified and stabilized during the development process using agents such as hydroquinone. The image is fixed by agents, which dissolve and remove the unused silver halides [7]. Automated x-ray film processing machines achieve short development times by using elevated temperatures (28-35°C), by including glutaraldehyde as a hardening agent within the developer solution, and by actively drying the fixed and washed film with heated air [8]. This process of radiographic film development might therefore induce potential exposures to hydroquinone, glutaraldehyde, formaldehyde, glycols (diethylene, triethylene), acetic acid, sodium sulphite, sulfur dioxide, ammonium chloride, silver compounds, 5-nitroindazole, Thiosulphate, 1-phenyl-3-pyramzolidone and other chemicals [9-12].

Radiography departments could have poor structural designs together with operational deficiencies of ventilation system and closed/dark workplace [13]. During manual film processing, cleaning of the internal components of the film processor or during the normal processing procedures, radiographers might be exposed to the above mentioned chemicals through either direct or indirect skin contact, fumes inhalation or via ingestion. Therefore, this exposure in such an occupational setting is complex and implies multiple chemicals. Consequently, it is not appropriate to assess the exposure to a single chemical as the outcomes could be related to the overall synergistic and pharmacokinetics interactions between these chemicals in the human body. Worldwide, few studies have been conducted on the radiographers in order to clarify the link between their exposures and the workplace related symptoms [14]. As an expected outcome, this study will assess the prevalence of occupationally-related darkroom disease symptoms among the radiographers (exposed group) compared to the nurses (non-exposed group) in the West Bank hospitals in order to implement preventive and effective protocols for the control of this occupationally-related disease. The results of this study will improve our understanding in a way that might help overcome the limitations of environmental exposure assessment in such a very complex occupational setting.

Methods

Study design and population

A cross sectional study was conducted. The study population involved subjects recruited from the two professional health team members; the radiographers (exposed group) and the hospital's nurses (non-exposed group) selected from the chosen Palestinian governmental and non-governmental hospitals listed in Table 1. As most of the radiographers personnel were males, only male nurses were included in the study to avoid bias from gender differences. Both study populations were selected from the same occupational setting, from similar demographic category, had worked in the field since at least one year and agreed to participate. However, those with physician diagnosed asthma before their current occupation were excluded, as asthma symptoms could interfere with the study outcomes (i.e. darkroom disease symptoms). Although random sampling would have been more appropriate, our method of recruitment could have limited our selection and classification biases to the minimum as well.

Study settings

The study was conducted in the x-ray departments in the governmental and non-governmental hospitals in the West Bank over 3 months period (1st January-1st April 2012). The selected hospitals were chosen primarily because they have large numbers of radiographers and therefore are representative of the most Palestinian hospitals in the West Bank.

Sample size

There were nearly (518) radiographers who currently (at the time of study) work in the x-ray departments all over the Palestinian hospitals in the West bank. Out of them, 471 are males. About 330 radiographers were selected of all those met the selection criteria and agreed to participate using non-random purposive sampling technique. Similarly, the male nurses (n = 242) responded by the same sampling method from the same hospitals assuring that the selection criteria are fit. Based on the study type I error (α) that has been estimated up to 5% for the study and a power expectation of 80%, a sample size of 250 in each group was found to be sufficiently large enough to highlight the expected differences (10%) between the two study groups.

Ethical considerations

The study protocol was approved by the Institutional Review Board (IRB) and the scientific research committee of the Public Health Department as well as the

Table 1 The study selected hospitals stratified by governorate, and sector (governmental and non-governmental)

Governorate	Governmental hospitals	Non-governmental hospitals
Ramallah	Al-Mujamaa' Al-Tibi	Red Crescent society; Arab Medical Care; Al-Mustaqbal
Jenin	Martyer Dr. Khalil Suleiman	Al-Razi; Patient Friend Society
Tulkarm	Thabit Thabit	Al-Zakat; Red Crescent Society
Nablus	Rafedia; Al-Watani	Al-Injili; Al-Ittihad; Al-Arabi Al-Takhasussi
Qalqilya	Darwish Nazzal	Al-Aqsa
Salfit	Salfit	*None
Jericho	Jericho	*None
Bethlehm	Alhussein	*None
Hebron	A'alia	Alahli

*None: No non-governmental hospitals in these Governorates.

Faculty of Graduate Studies Scientific Research Board at An-Najah National University. Permissions to conduct the study in the hospitals' x-ray departments were obtained from the Palestinian Ministry of Health (MoH) for the governmental hospitals and from the hospital's managers for the non-governmental hospitals. A written and signed informed consent was obtained from each participant who met the selection criteria and agreed to participate voluntary.

Data collection

Data were collected by using a standardized and a previously-validated face-to-face administered questionnaire adapted with permission from Damases, (2006) [15]. In each hospital, male radiographers available at that time who met the inclusion criteria and where able to sign the consent form voluntary were interviewed. The interview was in private with each radiographer and in a face-to-face assuring that every question in the questionnaire was answered and clear. After conducting x-ray departmental questionnaires, face-to-face interviews with the available male nurses in the nursing wards at that time were conducted in the same manner taking into consideration equal numbers with radiographers (although this was not always the case).

The questionnaire included questions dealing with the study independent and dependant variables. It included; (1) Socio-demographic factors and exposure to some factors that might influence health such as smoking status and habits, (2) Exposure to external factors such as living near to industrial areas and sharing home with people who smoke, (3) A self-reported list of symptoms of darkroom disease such as; headache, nausea, irritation of throat, sneezing or nose itchy (not including common cold), heart beating abnormally and others, (4) Questions for radiology workers only covered the availability and conditions of services such as; performing daily radiographic images and duration time spent in the darkroom per working shift; availability of windows and more than one door, availability of ventilating machine and exhaust to transmit the fumes outside the darkroom.

Pilot testing of the questionnaire

The questionnaire was piloted before using in the field and on the Palestinian population. Indeed, ten radiographers and ten nurses (who work in the male wards in Jenin hospitals) were asked to fill in the questionnaires in order to examine its clarity and comprehensiveness for the Palestinian population. As a result of this pre-test (pilot testing), no major changes were found to be necessary. However, minor modifications were judged necessary to improve the questionnaire clarity and presentation of questions for the local Palestinian conditions. The data gathered from the pilot testing was not included in the main study.

Data analysis

All data were analyzed using the statistical software 16 package SPSS (Statistical Package for the Social Sciences) [16]. Chi-square test for trends was carried out to analyze the differences between the dependant variable and the qualitative independent variables and in regard to the percentages of the reported symptoms. Students-t test and ANOVA were used to test the mean differences of the continuous dependant variable (number of symptoms) among different categorical independent variables. Multivariate linear regression analysis adjusted for possible confounders was developed to assess the associated occupational factors with the mean number of symptoms among radiographers (out of 20 studied symptoms). *P*-value less than 0.05 was always considered significant. In the questionnaire, there were 20 questions about symptoms, and the answers' categories for each question were (yes, no). These questions were used to develop new variables with scorings. Each score was the sum answer "yes" for each of the 20 symptoms' questions. Therefore, the score ranged from 0–20. This new variable was then analyzed as continuous variable in the analysis.

We have conducted a one-Way ANOVA analysis for all questionnaire variables (those with two and those with more than two categories. However, variables that where more than two categories and showed significant associations in this stage of analysis with the mean number of symptoms (out of 20 total symptoms) were categorized again into two categories and re-tested for significance using the same ANOVA analysis. Indeed, all that were significant on more than two categories remained also significant after re-categorization into two categories (data available upon request).This process of re-categorization of some variables where done due to the large number of variables that showed a significant association with the mean number of symptoms in the bivariate analysis. Therefore, and for the purpose of developing not an overloaded multivariate linear regression model, we have categorized the variables with more than two categories into two categories. Then, we have calculated the mean number of symptoms (out of 20 total symptoms) among each variable category in the radiographers' subjects in order to predict the variables that could be associated with the mean number of symptoms among those subjects (radiographers).

Variables entered in the final multivariate regression model were those with a significant P value of less than or equal 0.05. However, the variables "number of working hours-less than or equal 8 hrs/more than 8 hrs; is there a window in the darkroom-no/yes; and is there an exhaust in the darkroom-no/yes" were also entered in the final model although they were not significant in the first stage of analysis due to their possible effects and associations with the model dependant variable "number of symptoms among radiographers" after adjusting for other variables.

Results

Characteristics of the study population

In this study, we were able to recruit 572 participants from both groups (radiographers and male nurses). The radiographers were 330 subjects who represent nearly 57.7% of all population. However, the male nurses were 242 participants representing nearly 42.3% of all population in both groups. The distribution of the study population is shown in Table 2 below.

As shown in the Table 2, the largest number of respondents among radiographers and nurses indicated their age as between "36-43" years (n = 92 and 27.9%; n = 68; 28.1%; respectively). No statistically significant differences were found between the study groups regarding the age and the marital status. However, a significant relationship was found between the study groups in regard to the educational level where nearly 65.5% and only 41.3% of radiographers and nurses (respectively) reported having a Bachelor degree. The other remaining factors showed statistically significant differences between the two study groups (for more details, see Table 2).

Exposure to internal and external factors

As shown in the Table 2 below, participants were also asked to offer information concerning their neighborhood residence. Nearly only 20% of radiographers (n = 66) reported that they reside in an industrial area, while about only 7.4% of nurses (n = 18) reported that they live in such areas with a statistically significant relationship between current occupation and neighborhood locality. On the other hand, there were no statistically significant relationship between current occupation and sharing home with people who smoke neither there was in regard to smoking status (for more details, see Table 2).

Evaluation of darkroom disease's symptoms

We have evaluated the darkroom disease's symptoms as the main study objective. Table 3 below shows the self-reported frequency (percent) of darkroom disease's symptoms among the two study groups (radiographers and nurses). As shown in the Table 3, the differences in the reported percentage of symptoms among radiographers showed a statistically significant higher percentage for each reported symptom compared to the nurses (P-values <0.001; see Table 3 for the remaining symptoms).

Table 2 Description of the study subjects

Variable	Total	Current occupation n (%)*		*P*-Value
	N (%)* = 572	Radiographers n (%)*	Nurses n (%)*	
Age				
20-27years	106 (18.5)	60 (18.2)	46 (19)	
28-35 years	154 (26.9)	88 (26.7)	66 (27.3)	
36-43 years	160 (28)	92 (27.9)	68 (28.1)	0.092
44-51 years	124 (21.7)	80 (24.2)	44 (18.2)	
>51 years	28 (4.9)	10 (3)	18 (7.4)	
Marital status				
Single	152 (25.6)	86 (26.1)	66 (27.3)	
Married	410 (71.7)	238 (72.1)	172 (71.1)	0.942
Widower	10 (1.7)	6 (1.8)	4 (1.6)	
Educational level				
Diploma	236 (41.3)	104 (31.5)	132 (54.5)	
Bachelor	316 (55.2)	216 (65.5)	100 (41.3)	0.000**
Master	14 (2.4)	8 (2.4)	6 (2.5)	
PhD	6 (1[illegible]	2 (0.6)	4 (1.7)	
Monthly net income				
1500-2000NIS	84 (14.7)	36 (10.9)	48 (19.8)	
2001-2500NIS	382 (66.8)	236 (71.5)	146 (60.3)	0.005**
2501-3000NIS	106 (18.5)	58 (17.6)	48 (19.8)	
Residence place				
City	210 (36.7)	124 (37.6)	86 (35.5)	
Village	268 (46.9)	164 (49.7)	104 (43)	0.018**
Refugee camp	94 (16.4)	42 ([illegible]2.7)	52 (21.5)	
Type of hospital				
Non-Governmental	302 (52.8)	160 (48.5)	142 (58.7)	0.016**
Governmental	270 (47.2)	170 (51.5)	100 (41.3)	
Duration in current occupation				
1-5years	218 (38.1)	126 (38.2)	92 (38)	
6-10years	126 (22)	64 (19.4)	62 (25.6)	0.001**
11-15years	128 (22.4)	74 (22.4)	54 (22.3)	
>15 years	100 (17.5)	66 (20)	34 (14)	
Daily working hours				
<8hours	120 (2[illegible])	88 (26.7)	32 (13.2)	
8hours	394 (68.9)	222 (67.3)	172 (71.1)	0.001**
> 8hours	58 (10.1)	20 (6)	38 (15.7)	
Do you live in an industrial area?				
Yes	84 (14.7)	66 (20)	18 (7.4)	0.001**
No	488 (85.3)	264 (80)	224 (92.6)	
Do you share your home with people who smoke?				
Yes	118 (20.6)	72 (21.8)	46 (19)	0.412
No	454 (79.3)	258 (78.2)	196 (81)	

Table 2 Description of the study subjects *(Continued)*

Smoking status				
Current smoker	166 (29)	86 (26.1)	80 (33.1)	0.176
Ex-smoker	38 (6.6)	24 (7.3)	14 (5.8)	
Non-smoker	368 (64.4)	220 (66.7)	148 (61.2)	

*Data are expressed as number (percent) of each group. **Statistically significant (p <0.05).

The specific health symptoms of the radiographers and nurses are mentioned in Table 3. The most predominant health symptoms in descending order of frequency, addressed by radiographers were: headache (75.8%), sneezing/nose itchy (70.9%), irritation of throat (69.1%), unexpected fatigue (65.5%), runny nose (63%), chemical taste (61.2%), skin rash (59.4%), ringing in the ears (55.8%), nausea (51.5%), unusual numb arms and legs (49.1%), abdominal pain (48.5%), dizziness (46.7%), runny eyes (44.2%), mouth sores (43%), lip sores (41.2%), blurred vision (41.2%), heart beating abnormally (35.2%), urination pain (32.1%), palpitation (30.9%) and finally night sweat (29.7%).

Table 3 The self-reported frequency (percent) of darkroom disease's symptoms among radiographers and nurses in the past six months

Symptom	Radiographers n (%)*	Nurses n (%)*	Chi-square *P*-value
Headache	250 (75.8)	142 (58.7)	< 0.001**
Nausea	170 (51.5)	36 (14.9)	< 0.001**
Runny nose	208 (63)	38 (15.7)	< 0.001**
Irritation of throat	228 (69.1)	50 (20.7)	< 0.001**
Unexpected fatigue	216 (65.5)	88 (36.4)	< 0.001**
Ringing in the ears	184 (55.8)	38 (15.7)	< 0.001**
Lip sores	136 (41.2)	42 (17.4)	< 0.001**
Mouth sores	142 (43)	26 (10.7)	< 0.001**
Heart beating abnormally	116 (35.2)	38 (15.7)	< 0.001**
Unusual numb arms and legs	162 (49.1)	60 (24.8)	< 0.001**
Skin rash	196 (59.4)	26 (10.7)	< 0.001**
Abdominal pain	160 (48.5)	64 (26.4)	< 0.001**
Blurred vision	136 (41.2)	42 (17.4)	< 0.001**
Dizziness	154 (46.7)	52 (21.5)	< 0.001**
Runny eyes	146 (44.2)	34 (14)	< 0.001**
Night sweat	98 (29.7)	18 (7.4)	< 0.001**
Palpitation	102 (30.9)	28 (11.6)	< 0.001**
Urination pain	106 (32.1)	34 (14)	< 0.001**
Chemical taste	202 (61.2)	0 (0)	< 0.001**
Sneezing/nose itchy	234 (70.9)	40 (16.5)	< 0.001**

*Data are expressed as number (percent) of each positive answer (yes) to each symptom. The non presented data equals the negative answer (No).
**Statistically significant (p <0.05).

Evaluation of occupational conditions for radiographers

Table 4 below shows some of the occupational conditions for the radiographers. The frequency of radiographers and the number of symptoms among each different category of an occupational condition are shown below. As shown in the table, the majority (63%) of the radiographers reported performing more than 15 images per day and the higher number of performed images per day the higher number of symptoms reported as well. On the other hand, nearly 104 (31.5%) gave an account of spending (1–30) minutes in the darkroom during the working shift, while the minority (16.4%) stated of spending more than 90 minutes per working shift. The vast majority of radiographers (n = 292; 88.5%) reported not having windows in the darkrooms. Moreover, most of the radiographers (n = 254; 77%) indicated not having alternative/additional door in the darkroom and about 47.3% of them reported not having ventilating machines in the darkrooms, whilst 74.5% notified not having an exhaust to transmit the fumes and odors outside the darkroom. Clearly and as shown in Table 4, the radiographers were more likely to report symptom clusters associated with working factors expected to reflect greater workplace chemical exposures and symptoms; less local exhaust of machines, less frequent adequate ventilation in the processing area, intense load of images done daily, elongated time spent in the darkroom, low accessibility of a window and an extra door in the darkroom.

Multivariate analysis of the mean number of symptoms

The final multivariate linear regression model with all possible predictors is shown in the Table 5. As shown in Table 5, the monthly income was a significant predictor for the mean number of symptoms with a positive association. However, living in a village, reporting living in an industrial area (yes), reporting sharing home with people who smoke (yes), the years of experience (more than 10 years) showed a significantly positive association with the mean number of reported symptoms.

Regarding some occupational factors, the period of stay in the darkroom per shift showed a strong significant association with the mean number of reported symptoms (i.e., reporting staying more than 30 minutes in the darkroom per shift was associated with a significant increase in the mean number of reported symptoms). However, the availability of a ventilating machine in the darkroom showed a strong negative association with the mean number of reported symptoms (i.e., reporting having a ventilating machine in the darkroom was associated with a significant decrease in the mean number of reported

Table 4 Occupational condition variables by number (percent) of subjects and number (percent) of total reported symptoms (3346) among radiographers (n = 330)

Working condition variables	Radiographers n (%)*	Number of symptoms among radiographers No. (%)[!]
How many radiographic images do you perform every day?		
1-5 images	28 (8.5)	290 (8.7)
6-10 images	10 (3)	30 (0.9)
11-15 images	84 (25.5)	756 (22.6)
>15 images	208 (63)	2270 (67.8)
The time spent in the darkroom during the working shift?		
1-30 minutes	104 (31.5)	1002 (29.9)
31-60 minutes	72 (21.8)	660 (19.7)
61-90 minutes	100 (30.3)	1048 (31.3)
> 90 minutes	54 (16.4)	636 (19)
Is there a window in the darkroom?		
Yes	38 (11.5)	444 (13.3)
No	292 (88.5)	2902 (86.7)
Does the darkroom have more than one door where you work?		
Yes	76 (23)	444 (13.3)
No	254 (77)	2902 (86.7)
Is there a ventilating machine in the dark room where you work?		
Yes	174 (52.7)	1566 (46.8)
No	156 (47.3)	1780 (53.2)
Is there an exhaust to transmit the fumes outside the darkroom?		
Yes	84 (25.5)	898 (26.8)
No	246 (74.5)	2448 (73.2)

*Data is expressed as number (percent) for each variable's category. [!]Number of symptoms (percent from the total number of symptoms reported among radiographers; 3346).

Table 5 Multivariate linear regression model* for the association of the mean number of symptoms with some possible predictors among radiographers (N = 330)

Independent variables	B	SE	Beta	*P*-value	95% CI for B
Age (20–40 years/>40 years)	0.92	0.66	0.07	0.16	(−0.37-2.22)
Monthly net income (≤2500/>2500) NIS	2.35	0.70	0.14	0.001	(0.96-3.74)*
Residence place (city and refugee camp/village)	1.15	0.52	0.09	0.03	(0.12-2.19)*
Years of experience (1–10 years/>10 years)	1.31	0.59	0.10	0.03	(0.15-2.47)*
Daily working hours (≤8 hours/>8 hours)	0.51	1.11	0.02	0.65	(−1.68-2.69)
Living in industrial area (no/yes)	5.63	1.13	0.37	0.001	(3.39-7.86)*
Sharing home with people who smoke (no/yes)	3.79	1.12	0.25	0.001	(1.57-6.004)*
Daily images performed per working shift (≤15 images/>15 images)	−0.12	0.65	−0.009	0.85	(−1.39-1.16)
Period of stay in darkroom per shift (1–30 minutes />30 minutes)	3.28	0.62	0.27	0.001	(2.06-4.51)*
Availability of a window in the darkroom (no/yes)	1.58	1.11	0.08	0.15	(−0.61-3.77)
Availability of an extra door in the darkroom (no/yes)	1.19	0.80	0.08	0.13	(−0.38-2.77)
Availability of a ventilating machine in the darkroom (no/yes)	−1.98	0.54	−0.16	0.001	(−3.05- -0.91)*
Availability of an exhaust in the darkroom (no/yes)	−0.57	0.64	−0.04	0.37	(−1.83-0.68)

*Variables entered in the model are those with a P-value of <0.05 in One-way ANOVA. Number of worked hours per day, availability of exhaust, availability of window in the darkroom were entered in the model although not significant in the bivariate analysis; NIS, New Israeli Shekels; SE, standard error; B, unstandardized regression coefficient; Beta, standardized regression coefficient; CI, confidence interval. *Statistically significant ($p < 0.05$). Enter regression method was used. R for the model = 0.71; Adjusted R square = 0.46 ($R^2 = 0.477$; P value of the overall significance of regression model <0.001).

symptoms). All other variables did not remain significant after adjusting for other variables in the model.

Discussion

The aim of the present study was to assess the prevalence of occupationally-related darkroom disease symptoms among the radiographers (exposed group) compared to the nurses (non-exposed group) in the Palestinian hospitals in the West Bank. The main study findings was that, the reported prevalence of symptoms among radiographers showed a statistically significant higher percentage for each reported symptom compared to the nurses (P-values <0.001). In multivariate linear regression analysis, the monthly income was a significant predictor for the mean number of symptoms with a positive association among radiographers. However, living in a village, reporting living in an industrial area (yes), reporting sharing home with people who smoke (yes), the years of experience (more than 10 years) showed a significantly positive association with the mean number of reported symptoms among radiographers.

Regarding some occupational factors, the period of stay in the darkroom per shift showed a strong significant association with the mean number of reported symptoms among radiographers (i.e., reporting staying more than 30 minutes in the darkroom per shift was associated with a significant increase in the mean number of reported symptoms). However, the availability of a ventilating machine in the darkroom showed a strong negative association with the mean number of reported symptoms among radiographers.

Participants' socio-demographic factors

The possible reasons which could have contributed to a lower response rate for both groups are scheduling of examinations, vacation leave, sick leave, resignation and scheduling of work shifts. Nurses were chosen as the non-exposed group. There were some significant differences between the exposed and non-exposed group in some aspects like monthly income, educational level, duration in the current occupation and daily working hours (see Table 2 for more details). Due to large number of outcome variables (symptoms) compared between radiographers and nurses (Table 3) and not to overload the data with many adjusted models, we only described the univariate differences in the percentages of symptoms between the two groups. However, when we developed our final multivariate model of the symptoms, we have adjusted for all these possible confounders (see Table 5 for details). Furthermore, no significant differences in age and marital status were noted between the two groups and both groups showed a statistical similarity regarding sharing home with people who smoke and smoking status variables.

Evaluation of darkroom disease's symptoms among radiographers and nurses

In Palestine, data about darkroom disease symptoms among radiographers are lacking. The present study has found that radiographers have a total of 3346 symptoms, while nurses count for about 896 symptoms in cumulative. These symptom clusters were significantly more common among radiographers than among nurses, occurring over four times as often and are consistent with previous studies of darkroom disease symptoms [4,10]. The most significant symptoms measured in the exposed group were headache, sneezing/nose itchy, irritation of throat, unexpected fatigue, runny nose and chemical taste. In addition to these common symptoms, the exposed group also reported chest illness, nausea, painful joints, ringing ears, skin rash, lip sores, mouth sores, abnormal heart beat and numbness of arms and legs.

It is suggested that these darkroom disease symptoms clusters could be related to exposure to high air concentrations of chemicals (this should be mentioned with caution in this study as we didn't perform an air sampling of the workplace). However, the findings of this study are in accordance with those found in other studies [6] on medical radiation technologist which found that sore throat, headache, sore or itchy eyes, abnormal heart beating and runny nose were significant symptoms compared to non-exposed group. The respiratory problems reported in this study are in parallel with other studies findings. For example, a study [17] showed that respiratory problems among radiographers were several times higher than compared group (physiotherapists) with increased respiratory complains within working hours. These increased related symptoms were attributed to the exposures of radiographers to chemical fumes in the darkroom in the mentioned study.

The reported prevalence of the symptom bad chemical taste amongst radiographers was nearly 61.2% of all radiographers, while nurses did not practice such chemical taste at all. Although we didn't assess the exposure quantitatively in this study, it is well-known that sulphur dioxide, a by-product of the fixation process, is known to be responsible for an unpleasant metallic taste and a bad odour within X-ray departments. The obvious differences between the two professions regarding the prevalence of bad taste should encourage active sulfur dioxide monitoring within X-ray departments. It should be reminded that smoking status was not statistically significant between the two study groups which could minimize or diminish interference and confliction of smoking on results.

Association of the mean number of symptoms with possible predictors

Many factors were shown to be associated with the mean number of symptoms among radiographers in multivariate linear regression model (see Table 5 for details). These results suggest that safety defensive measures are however not operative in darkrooms in Palestine. Our results could further demonstrate a lack of information about darkroom disease among the Palestinian radiographers. However, a study in Gaza strip found that persons at high risks of developing darkroom disease symptoms were those who spend long periods in diagnostic imaging departments (>10 hours per week) [13]. This conclusion is in accordance with our results that found a significant positive association of the period of stay in darkroom per shift with the mean number of reported symptoms among radiographers. Indeed, our study results were consistent and concurrent with the study conducted by Teschke et al. 2000 [10], which showed that the number of films processed and the time workers spent near the machines increased exposures to chemicals and eventually this was linked to darkroom disease symptoms.

It is of notion that most of radiographers (67.8%) task more than 15 images a day which was found to be positively associated with the mean number of reported darkroom disease symptoms among radiographers. However, in another study carried out in the year 2004, about 8% of the radiographers who reported darkroom disease symptoms were spending an average of 8.8 hours per week in the darkroom [6].

On the other hand, our results revealed no significant differences in the multivariate linear regression model for the association of the mean number of symptoms with the availability of a window in the darkroom among radiographers (95%CI for B, −0.61-3.77). Also, current study findings showed no significant differences in the multivariate linear regression model for the association of the mean number of symptoms with the availability of an extra door in the darkroom among radiographers (95%CI for B, −0.38-2.77). However, the availability of a ventilating machine in the darkroom showed a strong negative association with the mean number of reported symptoms. This coincides with the study conducted by Al Ajerami and Sirdah, 2008 [13], who attributed mainly the exposure of radiographers to chemical fumes in the darkroom to the closed ill-ventilated processing darkrooms and revealed deficiency of quality control measures for darkroom processing in almost 80% of all studied darkrooms, also the authors found a lack of effective departmental ventilation system in almost 73.7% and lack of special dark room ventilation system in almost 78.9% of all studied darkrooms. Hence, different studies concluded that the poor design together with the operational ventilation deficiencies were the major characteristics that resulted in the increased percentages of reported symptoms in such an occupational complex setting [8,13].

In our study, the health complains and problems of radiographers could be attributed to poor ventilation procedures such as weak structural design and deficiencies in operational materials and equipment. Concur to our study results, the study conducted by Taro et al. 2004 [6], showed significant correlation between the darkroom disease symptoms to radiographers and poor design of the radiographic departments presented by mal-ventilation, thereby presenting occupational hazard of chemical exposure to the radiographic personnel. In fact, automatic processors can generate considerable heat to hasten the film development process, thus, it is essential that the darkroom ventilation systems meet the international guidelines.

Study limitations

This is a recall study where an over or under-estimation of the reported symptoms could have been occurred. Furthermore, our results could have been more consistent if we have performed clinical examinations in parallel to the self-reported symptoms. Furthermore, and although we have used a validated questionnaire, we did not directly ask about the work-relatedness of the participants self-reported symptoms, e.g., "are those symptoms worsened during the working day, working week and/or are they improved during the weekend or during the week absent from work (holidays)". Therefore, this could be considered as one of the weakness and limitations of this study. Other limitation of this study could be the voluntary participation and the low response rate mainly among nurses which could have led to selection bias on health conditions (either sick or healthy are more willing to participate depending on the context). Clearly enough, a more possible limitation of this study might have also been attributed to the healthy-worker bias where sick workers might have been absent or in vacation so underestimation of the reported symptoms could have been occurred. Due to the study design we have performed, we can't generate causal relationships between the symptoms of darkroom disease and exposed chemicals in the darkroom. Furthermore, the resulted symptoms could have been attributed to some other factors (living in an industrial area, sharing home with people who smoke) or other confounders that haven't been studied. One of other shortcomings of this study is that only the radiographers have been asked about the workplace environmental conditions and their effects analysis on symptoms. Therefore, it is possible that the recall bias made symptomatic more prone to answer "yes" also on the worsening factors especially at work.

Conclusions

Radiographers showed an increase in the prevalence of certain symptoms representing the darkroom disease in comparison with the non-exposed group (hospitals' nurses). However, trying to interpret this finding in relation to chemicals exposure in their workplace should be done with caution due to the absence of active or passive monitoring in the workplace for the suspected chemicals. The severity of darkroom disease symptoms illustrates the need for legal compliance in order to minimize the occurrence of these symptoms. We recommend educational and training programs for the radiographers and developing clear diagnostic criteria for the darkroom disease. Adoption of digital imaging processes is also necessary.

Competing interests

The authors declare that they have no competing interests.

Authors' contributions

HA drafted the manuscript and participated in the statistical analysis of the data. YN and HA designed the study. YN collected the data and participated in writing the first draft of the manuscript. Both authors read and approved the final version of the manuscript.

Acknowledgements

The authors would like to thank the Palestinian Ministry of Health for cooperation and permission to conduct the study in the Governmental hospitals. Sincere thanks also to the participated Non-governmental hospitals and mainly the managers for their kind support and cooperation. We are grateful to all participants in this study for the time they devoted and their understanding.
Sincere and duly acknowledgements to the Open Society Institute (OSI) foundation/higher education support program and its academic fellowship program for maintaining regular and on-going interaction with wider academic community on professional development which helped in the motivation to publish this work.

References

1. Kolarzyk E, Stepniewski M, Zapolska I: **Occurrence of pulmonary diseases in steel mill workers.** *Int J Occup Med Environ Health* 2000, **13**:31–301.
2. Spicer J, Hay D, Gordon M: **Workplace exposure and reported health in New Zealand diagnostic radiographers.** *Australas Radiol* 1986, **30**:281–286.
3. Glass B: **Exposure to glutaraldehyde alone or in a fume mix.** *MAG Mem Sem and Shadows* 1997, **40**:2.
4. Genton M: **Shedding light on darkroom disease-progress and challenges in understanding radiology workers' occupational illness.** *Can J Med Radiat Technol* 1998, **29**:60–65.
5. Sanchez T: **When it hurts to breathe: Chemicals and R.T.s.** *ASRT Scanner* 1999, **31**:6–8.
6. Tarlo SM, Liss GM, Greene JM, Purdham J, McCaskell L, Kipen H, Kerr M: **Work-attributed symptom clusters (darkroom disease) among radiographers versus physiotherapists: associations between self-reported exposures and psychosocial stressors.** *Am J Ind Med* 2004, **45**:513–521.
7. Carlton RR, Adler AM: *Principles of Radiographic Imaging.* 3rd edition. Albany, NY: Delmar; 2001.
8. Hewitt PJ: **Occupational health problems in processing of X-ray photographic films.** *Ann Occup Hyg* 1993, **37**:287–295.
9. Johnston JN, Killion JB: **Hazards in the radiology department.** *Radiol Technol* 2006, **6**:417–423.
10. Teschke K, Chow Y, Beauer M, Chessor E, Hirtle B, Kennedy SM, ChanYeung M, DimichWard H: **Exposures and their determinants in radiographic film processing.** *Am Ind Hyg Assoc J* 2002, **63**:11–21.
11. Leacy E, Brennan PC: **The 'Darkroom Disease': a randomized control trial.** *Radiography* 2002, **8**:127–132.
12. NIOSH (National Institute for Occupational Safety and Health): Pocket Guide to Chemical Hazards: *DHHS (NIOSH) 2005 Publication No: 2005–149.* http://www.cdc.gov/niosh/npg/default.html. Last accessed October 2011.
13. Al-Ajerami Y, Sirdah M: **Effects of x-Ray film processing on health status of medical radiographers at gaza strip, Palestine.** *J Al Azhar Univ Gaza (Nat Sci)* 2008, **10**:59–76.
14. Chessor E, Svirchev L: **X-ray processor ventilation: small air flow, big result.** *App Occup Environ Hyg* 1997, **12**:511–516.
15. Damases C: **An evaluation of sulphur dioxide fume levels and the prevalence of darkroom disease symptoms amongst radiology workers in Namibia.** In *Thesis (M.Tech.: Radiography)-Dept. of Radiography, Durban University of Technology 2006 xi*, 86 leaves, Annexures A-Q. http://ir.dut.ac.za/bitstream/handle/10321/40/Damases_2006.pdf?sequence=14. Last accessed December 2013.
16. SPSS Institute Inc: *SPSS for Window-Statistical Package for the Social Sciences, Version 16.* Chicago, USA: SPSS Institute Inc; 2008.
17. Prabhakara PV, Lakshman KV: **Assessment of risk at workplace: A study on radiographers work practices in Vizag Steel.** *OHS & RC* 2005, **9**:26–28.

12

Development of a self-management intervention for employees with complaints of the arm, neck and/or shoulder (CANS): a focus group study with experts

Nathan Hutting[1,2*], Josephine A Engels[2], J Bart Staal[1,2], Yvonne F Heerkens[2] and Maria W G Nijhuis-van der Sanden[1]

Abstract

Background: Many people suffer from complaints of the arm, neck and/or shoulder (CANS). The complaints are persistent and there is a need for intervention programs for those with longstanding CANS. Studies suggest that a behavioural change is needed in employees with CANS. A self-management program with an add-on eHealth module might be an effective option to achieve the behavioural change needed to manage the complaints in employees with CANS. The aim of this study was to determine the content and strategies of the intervention and to gain insight into possible barriers and facilitators for implementation. Therefore, we examined the views of experts on the problems and characteristics associated with employees with CANS as well as their opinion on a self-management program consisting of self-management sessions and an eHealth module.

Methods: A qualitative study was performed consisting of three focus groups involving a total of 17 experts (with experience with CANS, self-management and/or eHealth interventions). Experts were asked their opinion about the content and requirements of a self-management program for employees with CANS, including an eHealth module. Data were analysed using qualitative data analysis. After coding, the emergent themes were used to organise the data into main categories, expressing the ideas and opinions of experts on CANS, self-management and/or eHealth interventions.

Results: The experts pointed out that the intervention should focus on increasing employees' self-efficacy and empowerment, and address topics related to the possible risk factors for CANS, symptoms, work environment, social environment and personal factors. The eHealth module should be self-explanatory and attractive, and the information provided should be brief, clear and concise.

Conclusions: Experts appeared to see a role for a self-management program for employees with CANS. They indicated that the combination of group sessions and eHealth can work well. Experts provided valuable information with regard to the content of the self-management intervention and the design of the eHealth module.

Keywords: Complaints of the arm, Neck and/or shoulder, CANS, Work-related upper extremity disorders, WRUED, Focus group, Self-management

* Correspondence: Nathan.Hutting@han.nl
[1]Radboud Institute for Health Sciences, IQ Healthcare, Radboud University Medical Center, Nijmegen, The Netherlands
[2]Research Group Occupation and Health, HAN University of Applied Sciences, PO Box 6960, Nijmegen 6503 GL, The Netherlands

Background

Many people suffer from complaints of the arm, neck and/or shoulder (CANS). Reported point prevalence for this disorder ranges from 1.6–53% and the 12-month prevalence from 2.3–41% depending on the setting, definition, and classification used [1-3]. In various working populations the reported 12-month prevalence ranges from 22–40% [3].

Although the exact aetiology of nonspecific CANS is unknown, it is reported to be of multifactorial origin in which work-related factors may play a major role [4-7]. Physical characteristics (i.e. awkward working posture, repetitive work), psychosocial characteristics (i.e. lack of social support from colleagues or supervisor), personal factors (i.e. an ineffective approach to stress management) of the individual worker, as well as characteristics of their work environment (i.e. high job demands, lack of control), contribute to the development and persistence of complaints [4-13]. The importance of each factor, and its individual contribution to the risk of provoking symptoms, varies among individuals and work environments [14].

CANS may cause significant work problems, including absenteeism (sickness absence), presenteeism (decreased work productivity) and, ultimately, job loss [15,16]. A recent focus group study showed that employees with CANS have to deal with their complaints in their daily life and at work [17]. That study also showed that participants are not fully aware of the possibilities to influence their complaints, or of their own role in coping with their complaints. Participants generally suffer from pain, are often approaching their individual limits, and fatigue has a major impact on their life; in addition, they also have to deal with hindering physical and social environmental factors, such as misunderstanding from others [17]. Employees with CANS are often confronted with a wide range of problems. Most have taken many steps in an attempt to reduce their complaints, which can vary from workplace adaptations to different types of (physical) therapies [17].

About 19% of the patients report chronic complaints of which 58% report the use of healthcare, such as care given by the general practitioner, medical specialist and physical therapist [1]. Thus, there seems to be a need for intervention programs for people with longstanding CANS [17-19]. Therefore, information on the experiences and needs of employees with CANS can be valuable in developing such interventions. To determine the content of the intervention, and to guarantee that strategies will be adopted and implemented, the perspective of the healthcare professional should also be taken into account, because they refer clients to these programs or give the care themselves. Experts on care for those with CANS can probably provide valuable information that can be used in the development of intervention programs for employees with CANS.

Self-management is an approach increasingly used in chronic disease care to improve self-efficacy and a healthy lifestyle [20]. Self-management interventions focus primarily on encouraging patients to be involved with and in control of their own treatment, as well as improving their understanding of how their condition and treatment affect their lives [21]. Self-management often includes preparing people to manage their health behaviours on a day-to-day basis, participating in treatment or education designed to attain specific results, practicing tasks, and developing attitudes that reduce the emotional or physical impact of illness, with or without assistance from clinicians [22]. There is inconsistent evidence for the effects of self-management programs for patients with chronic musculoskeletal pain [23-25] and there is some evidence that group-delivered short programs (< 8 weeks) with a healthcare professional involved have the best potential [23].

A promising medium for facilitating patient empowerment is the Internet [26]. Many home-based disease-management programs have been developed to improve the health of patients [27]. eHealth interventions have become popular in number and reach [28]. A recent systematic review indicates that web-based interactive interventions have a beneficial effect on patient empowerment and/or physical activity in patients with various chronic conditions [26].

Unfortunately, web-based interventions also have some possible disadvantages. For example, it is common for users who experience difficulties with the program to discontinue program use or drop out of a study before completion [29,30]. Moreover, for the specific group of participants with CANS, who often work with computers at work, more prolonged computer use (by following an eHealth program) could worsen their physical problems [31]. Also, eHealth alone limits the (often very supportive) personal contacts between participants. Therefore, a combination of a self-management program with an add-on eHealth module could be an effective option to achieve behavioural change in the management of complaints in employees with CANS, especially in those suffering from longstanding complaints. CANS has a multifactorial origin and symptoms are diverse; by adding an eHealth module, information can be provided in a more tailored way (in which participants can make their own choices) [17]. In this way, the time during the meetings can be used more effectively, whilst relevant information is available at every moment due to the eHealth module. Our research group plans to adapt the self-management program developed by Detaille et al. [32,33] following the process of intervention mapping [34,35] and add an eHealth module for use in employees with CANS persisting for ≥ 12 weeks.

The aim of the present explorative study is to determine the content and strategies of the self-management program and eHealth module and to gain insight into possible hindrances and facilitators for implementation. Therefore, this study evaluates the experiences and opinions of experts in the field of CANS, self-management and/or eHealth, regarding the problems and characteristics of employees with CANS, as a step towards developing a self-management program consisting of self-management sessions and an eHealth module. Using this information, the existing self-management program developed by Detaille et al. [32,33] can be adapted and designed to fit the needs of the target population in order to make it easier for them to achieve healthy behaviours and management of their symptoms.

Methods

Study design

In March 2012, three focus groups with experts in the field of CANS, self-management and/or eHealth were held. Two focus groups were held at the HAN University of Applied Sciences, Nijmegen, and one focus group was held at a hotel in Utrecht (both in the Netherlands). The Medical Ethical Committee at Radboud university medical center declared (registration number 2013/316) that the study does not fall within the Dutch law on 'Medical Research involving Human Subjects' (the WMO) and that therefore, no approval is required from a medical ethic committee. The research protocol fulfilled the criteria of the Declaration of Helsinki on Ethical Principles for Medical Research Involving Human Subjects.

We used focus groups to investigate the broad range of ideas that experts had about CANS, self-management and eHealth. Focus groups can uncover factors that influence opinions, behaviour or motivation [36] and provide an interactive environment in which ideas can emerge from the group [36]. A group possesses the capacity to become more than the sum of its parts and to exhibit a synergy that individuals alone do not possess [36]. Therefore, focus groups were considered the most suitable tool to address the aim of this study.

Participants

Between January and March 2012, a purposive sampling technique was used to identify potential participants. Experts (defined as persons with a high degree of practice skills or knowledge, i.e. relevant postgraduate professional qualifications, a PhD, and/or experienced clinicians) in the field of CANS, self-management and/or eHealth interventions were identified by the authors, contacted by email or telephone, and asked to participate in the study. The different areas of expertise represented by the experts were distributed over the three focus groups, thereby ensuring that all areas of expertise were represented in all focus groups. Each participant was informed that participation was voluntary and that data would be used anonymously. All participants were asked to fill out a short questionnaire (demographics) prior to the start of the focus group. All participants agreed to audio-recording of the sessions. All participants received a gift of 75 euro for their participation.

A total of 17 experts, divided in three groups of five or six participants each, participated in this focus group study; of these, 12 (70.6%) were female and five (29.4%) were male. The mean age of the participants was 45.3 (range 28–60) years. The demographic profile of the participating experts is presented in Table 1. Experts worked in various professions. All participants had postgraduate qualifications in the field of CANS, eHealth and/or self-management. Five experts (29.4%) had a higher professional education and 12 (70.6%) had an academic higher education. Of the participants, 64.7% was an expert on CANS, 64.7% an expert on self-management, and 58.8% an expert on eHealth (some experts had more than one kind of expertise).

Focus groups

Following the recommendations of Krueger and Casey [36] a semi-structured interview guide with open-ended questions was developed (Appendix) by the authors. The interview guide was based on the expertise of our research group (NH, JE, BS, YH, MN, and SD). The expertises included: guideline development, self-management, work-related disorders, and clinical experience with CANS. The interview guide was pilot-tested in the first focus group and, because no modifications were necessary, we used the same interview guide in all three focus groups. The group members were asked for their opinion and experiences on CANS and/or self-management, including an eHealth module. Moreover, they were asked for their ideas on the content of the self-management intervention, and the requirements to be fulfilled by the eHealth module and the self-management sessions. Moreover, possible barriers and facilitators were explored. The participants had no knowledge about the results of the focus groups held earlier with employees with CANS, described in an earlier article [17] and no other information was provided. Each focus group was moderated by the first author (NH) using a standardized script. All focus groups were audio-recorded and notes were taken by an assistant (LD). In each meeting the pre-developed interview guide was followed. The moderator made sure that every participant was involved in the discussion. The moderator actively generated interaction and discussion between participants. Each of the three sessions lasted about 120 min. After each session, the moderator and the assistant discussed the group dynamics and made a summary of the most striking results [36].

Table 1 Demographic profile of the participating experts

Expert number	Gender	Age (years)	Group	Education level	Education	PhD	Profession	Expertise		
								CANS	SM	EH
1	Female	60	1	AHC	Psychology	Yes	Researcher	No	Yes	No
2	Female	44	1	HPE	Physiotherapy, occupational health physiotherapy	No	Physiotherapist	Yes	Yes	Yes
3	Male	57	1	AHC	Medicine	No	Occupational health physician	Yes	Yes	No
4	Female	31	1	AHC	Occupational therapy, health sciences	No	Occupational therapist, lecturer	Yes	No	No
5	Female	50	1	HPE	Work and Organization	No	Work and Organization expert	Yes	No	No
6	Female	45	1	HPE	Physiotherapy, occupational health physiotherapy	No	(Occupational health) physiotherapist	Yes	Yes	No
7	Female	53	2	HPE	Management	No	Health and Safety Coordinator	Yes	No	No
8	Female	47	2	AHC	Speech therapy, speech and language pathology	PhD.c	Researcher	No	Yes	Yes
9	Female	30	2	AHC	Psychology	PhD.c	Researcher	No	Yes	Yes
10	Male	47	2	AHC	Occupational therapy	PhD.c	Lecturer, researcher	Yes	Yes	No
11	Female	47	2	HPE	Occupational therapy	No	Occupational therapist	Yes	Yes	Yes
12	Female	42	3	AHC	Health sciences	Yes	Researcher	Yes	No	Yes
13	Male	33	3	AHC	Movement sciences, epidemiology	Yes	Product manager eHealth	No	No	Yes
14	Male	56	3	AHC	Physiotherapy, occupational health physiotherapy	No	(Occupational health) physiotherapist	Yes	Yes	Yes
15	Female	42	3	AHC	Health sciences	Yes	Researcher	No	Yes	Yes
16	Female	58	3	AHC	Sociology	Yes	Researcher, development	No	Yes	Yes
17	Male	28	3	AHC	Physiotherapy, health sciences	PhD.c	Researcher	Yes	No	Yes

HPE = Higher professional education, AHC = Academic higher education, CANS = Complaints of arm, neck, and/or shoulder, SM = Self-management, EH = eHealth, PhD = Doctor of Philosophy, PhD.c = Doctor of Philosophy candidate.

Data analysis

The audio-recordings were transcribed by an assistant (LD). The draft version of the Results section was sent to all participants and they were asked to screen the text for misinterpretations and to make additions if necessary. If the participants did not respond to the first email within 10 days, one reminder was sent to them by email. The first author (NH), who was trained in qualitative research methods, performed the data analysis.

After reading each transcript multiple times, the transcripts were analysed using qualitative data analysis with an open-coding system [37]. New codes were added when considered necessary. After that the codes were sorted into themes based on how the different codes are related and linked [37]. Then the emergent themes were used to organise the data into main categories [37], expressing the ideas and opinions of experts on CANS, self-management and/or eHealth interventions. Moreover, the relationship between the categories was explored [37].

The Atlas.ti (version 7.082) program was used for analysis. During data analysis, the emerging themes were discussed in the research group. Moreover, by reading all the transcripts, the research group checked that no main categories were missed. The supporting quotes related to each theme were discussed by the research group.

Results

With regard to the development of the intervention the experts indicated, for example, that insight into the complaints and self-awareness and knowledge about the complaints (e.g. about risk factors) are important. They also stated that self-management starts as a personal problem of the employee and that it is important that the employee him/herself is in control. The attitude of employees towards their complaints and possible social support was also considered important. During data analyses, it appeared that these categories emerging from the data showed similarities with the I-Change model

(2.0) (Figure 1), which consists of three phases of behavioural change [38]. Therefore, the derived categories with regard to the content of the intervention were clustered according to the three phases (Awareness, Motivation and Behaviour) of the I-Change model (2.0) [38]. Moreover, experts gave their opinions on the combination of self-management sessions and an additional eHealth module, and the conditions and requirements concerning the eHealth module.

All data and information presented here are the opinions and statements of the experts.

Awareness

Insight into the complaints

Experts in the focus groups stated that employees with CANS have to work on identifying factors regarding the onset and persistence of their complaints. Experts considered it important that, at the start of the intervention, participants evaluate their individual problem areas, gain insight into their complaints, and develop self-awareness. It was mentioned that identifying risk factors and contextual factors can start in the self-management sessions, because here people feel most at ease and reassured. In addition, the eHealth module can be helpful because it can give additional explanations and background information. According to the experts, it also seems advisable to involve an expert on CANS in the program, to provide information and to answer company-specific questions of the participants.

Some experts indicated that for successful participation in a self-management program participants should have a certain cognitive level and must have a learning capacity. Participants in the program must have the ability to perform self-reflection and to look critically at their work environment, colleagues and at themselves. For awareness and self-reflection a considerable amount of information must be available and appropriate tools must be provided during the intervention. People need to examine their own problems and address them individually. Incorporating a screening tool or test to gain insight into their own situation and contributing factors is also advisable.

Putting priority on the health problem

Listening to the body was considered important. One expert said that if workers have complaints for ≥ 12 weeks, then they have not listened properly to their body. Self-awareness was indicated as one of the most important items; in addition, employees must be able to manage their own workload and complaints. One expert said:

> *It's striking that most of the employees who I see are under a lot of pressure at work and take almost no breaks... and then they also have difficulty in being able to self-manage. Because they think that they have to finish their work, there is no time for a break. Then you come into a type of conflict situation.* (Expert 4)

Experts stated that many employees have a high workload and take almost no breaks, leading to a type of conflict, because they feel they cannot take the time to take these breaks. Therefore, it is difficult to manage their own health problems and the workload. Especially for this group of workers, awareness and behavioural change were considered important. Complaints do not always go away, but a self-management program could offer support to these employees. One expert stated:

> *At the time that someone personally achieves insight into the causality of the story and can thereby also take control into his/her own hands, then you retain someone in the work process. (...) As such a person is then busy with self-correction. (...) I consider this to be the most meaningful activity that you (...) can provide.* (Expert 3)

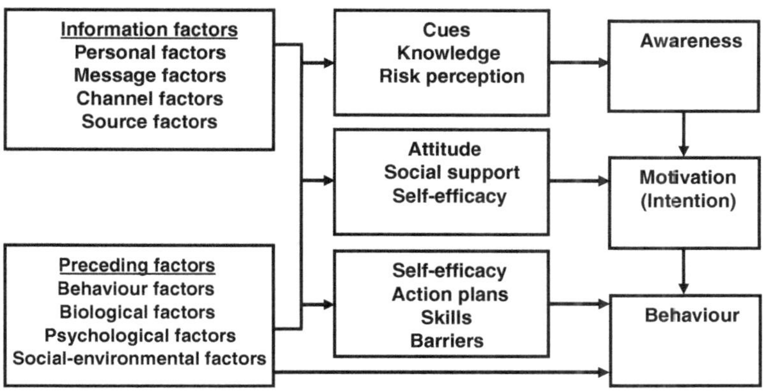

Figure 1 The I-Change model (2.0) [38].

This latter view was widely shared. It was stated that employees with CANS must put priority on their own health problem. Experts stated that it is important to be aware of the relationship between complaints and their causes and that individuals realize that they need to change their behaviour.

Knowledge about the complaints

Experts agreed that providing relevant knowledge can be a part of a self-management intervention. This can also create cues that prompt people to become aware. Awareness with regard to possible risk factors and how participants can influence these risk factors themselves, can be a cue to take action. In general, experts believed it is important that employees with CANS get information about their complaints, e.g. regarding symptoms such as pain, tingling, muscle spasms and loss of coordination. Moreover, most experts found it important that the intervention deals with possible risk factors related to the complaints. This also facilitates risk perception of the employees. The diversity of these topics is often not known and all these topics should be addressed. For employees with CANS, clarity of information is important. Experts agreed that the risk factors related to CANS are multifactorial and that causes can vary from person to person:

> *Quite often the causes simply arise from the relationship with the boss or employer... but the cause can also arise from a large number of other things. That your office material or equipment is not right, or your monitor is not good. Or just because you don't feel comfortable in the group, or you're having family problems.* (Expert 15)

Experts found it important to address the reasons why employees can be overloaded. They also found it important to address possible risk factors related to the persistence of the complaints, which employees are often unaware of. Employees must be aware that the body gives signals of overload. These signals should be a cue to take action. Experts stated that employees often carry on too long and often fail to take action until it is too late.

Experts believed it to be important to discuss the potential risk factors related to CANS, for instance, by giving some general examples and explaining the effects of several risk factors on the onset of complaints. The employee's behaviour was seen as an important factor related to the onset of symptoms. Some experts suggested possible risk factors that are important to discuss in the intervention: (work) stress, posture, workplace (materials and equipment), work tasks (repetitive tasks, extreme workload, extreme positions of joints), social factors (colleagues, relationship with supervisor), personal circumstances, and lack of physical activity.

In one focus group there was some discussion about the role that work plays as a cause of the onset of symptoms:

> *I agree that you have to do something about the pain, I don't agree that all of these non-specific complaints are caused by work. They are relevant to carrying out the work, they impede the work, and perhaps it's difficult to recover from these complaints if no accommodation is made in the work environment. But I don't know if it's always the cause ... but it is work-related.* (Expert 12)

This quote indicates that work is considered a factor in the onset and chronic character of symptoms and that complaints are believed to have at least a relationship with work. However, experts indicated that the actual work itself is not necessarily the cause of the complaints.

Some experts indicated that employees with CANS generally have high demands (on themselves) and are often perfectionists. One expert stated that particular highly educated employees develop CANS and that the content of the work may also play a role:

> *It's also a combination of stress and a high level of pressure at work. I also often see data typists, these people listen to music and are thus inputting things ... that's very repetitive work but these people often have less problems. And what I really have noticed is that these dedicated ITers, who also work on the computer at home for an extra 8 hours, have no complaints at all. It's often a combination of self-imposed stress and actual stress and repeated movements. Because of the deadlines and self-imposed stress they work through the pain.* (Expert 14)

Some experts also indicated that, in employees with CANS, the problem is less related to the workplace itself than to the behaviour (i.e. experiences and the intensity) of the employee at work. Generally, employees with complaints for ≥ 12 weeks have already tried many different options related to work adaptations. Regarding the causes, one expert stated:

> *It more closely resembles a burn-out than an irritation of a tendon or capsule. The intensity at which people work affects the development of complaints much more than the physical conditions of the work environment. After 12 weeks it really is more about the psychological aspects.* (Expert 14)

Taken together, experts stated that it is important to inform employees with CANS about all possible causes and potential risk factors, and to stimulate them to analyse their own situation. Moreover, experts stated that the intervention should focus on psychosocial aspects, especially during the self-management sessions. Moreover, it was stated that working conditions and environmental factors can be discussed in the eHealth module.

Motivation

Motivation for making changes

Experts agreed that self-management begins with the intention to take action; this is a prerequisite for a chance of success. Motivation is an important condition, participants must see the need for a change and the need to have control in their disease management.

> *Then it doesn't matter whether someone is working somewhere for a sheltered workplace or whether that person is a manager at the Shell Corporation. Both will go well, as long as the motivation is present to do something about it.* (Expert 11)

Experts agreed that self-management should start from a personal problem experienced by an employee. This ensures sufficient motivation. One has to recognize the possibilities to make changes. It is very important that people come up with their own solutions, are in control, and feel empowered. In the situation that healthcare professionals are involved, it is important that they support the client, but that the client stays in control and indicates his/her needs. One expert stated:

> *Self-management is by definition oriented towards decision-making. Therefore, you need a problem, which means that this person her/himself has to have a problem. Then you can come with (amongst others) some knowledge, or with advice and counselling, that can be instrumental - but self-management starts with a problem that you yourself have.* (Expert 1)

A barrier of self-management is that clients may be (too) passive. Therefore, healthcare professionals must be aware of this and facilitate the client to stay in control. According to most experts, it is important that healthcare professionals involved in self-management also undergo a change themselves.

Attitude towards the complaints

Experts stated that employees with CANS must be proactive rather than reactive. One must take action and make changes. People have to think about what they need to make a successful change; it is important that they think in terms of possibilities rather than problems. Concerning 'positive thinking' one expert remarked:

> *People often adopt the attitude that 'I can't do this anymore' - whereas you have to turn them around to adopt the attitude that 'I simply have this condition at this moment in time but I can still do other things'. Therefore, they have to actually see the opportunities rather than the limitations.* (Expert 7)

Experts believed that by providing information about CANS and by understanding the course of the disorder, the attitude of employees with CANS can be influenced. For example, in the chronic stage the pain can be present continuously, the course can also be erratic, and it can take a long time before the changes made have an effect. Therefore, to change the attitude towards pain, providing information about pain is considered important; for example, about what (chronic) pain is and what the function of pain is. Employees should be aware of this and understand it. Learning to deal with the pain is important. Attention should also be paid to the emotions that arise with pain, the cognitive aspects surrounding pain, and the use of pain medication. Regarding the experienced pain one expert said:

> *It's quite different when people suffer pain for 12 weeks than when you hit your thumb (with a hammer). I work with companies, which I visit every two weeks, where people can sign up, and then you might see only those who have had problems for two days. This is a completely different situation than when I see someone after about three months; in the latter situation, far more explanation is needed.* (Expert 14)

Social support and asking for help

According to the experts, people suffering from CANS for ≥ 12 weeks are in the chronic stage of CANS. Often, they do not know what they can do to reduce their symptoms. One expert indicated that there is a hidden need for reassurance in this group:

> *The first non-verbalized need - is that of reassurance. There are many people who say that it will never get better. When repetitive strain injury first appeared 15 years ago, the major newspapers went along with this: if you ever develop it, you will never get better. (...) What I did was to try to say that this is the situation right now, at this moment in time it's not going very well, but you don't have rheumatism or any other similar condition.* (Expert 14)

Experts said that in the group sessions people can recognize themselves and their problems and feel supported. Experts found that the exchange of experiences is a particularly important advantage of the group sessions:

> *... and then they learn a lot from each other, and see that 'yes' you also have this, I also experience it in the same way ... and then someone tells how he dealt with it and then the other person thinks – 'I'm going to try the same thing'. My experience is that discussing something like this takes an enormous amount of time.* (Expert 16)

The experts noted that it is sometimes difficult to properly formulate a request for support, and to discuss experiences and needs with the supervisor at the right moment. Therefore, employees should acquire the tools to communicate with their supervisor. One expert indicated that workers themselves must decide whether and how they want to talk with their supervisor, or perhaps choose another possible solution:

> *I believe that people have to think about that on their own - if you personally want to change something in your work environment then you have to consider that you will have to discuss this point. That's the approach which you have chosen for yourself, because you could choose different solutions which would not involve the need for this discussion.* (Expert 5)

According to some experts, relationships at work may play a role in the onset or persistence of complaints. It is important to reflect on the work environment and relationships:

> *... important is the work situation, the employer, how the work is organized and how the different spheres of influence work out. It's valuable to provide information in recognisable themes, perhaps also use role playing... but make it on a larger scale than only focusing on the employee with arm, neck and shoulder complaints.* (Expert 10)

Experts believed that employees with complaints can feel very unhappy if an employer does not cooperate. Social support was considered very important. Workers should be able to obtain social support from colleagues, managers, friends, family and/or healthcare professionals. One expert stated that support at the workplace, as well as in the private sphere, is one of the most important issues to be addressed. Knowing how to obtain these resources of social support, without feeling threatened, is an important skill. Employees are not always aware that this lack of workplace support may be an extra burden. In addition, there may be psychosocial factors at home, whether temporary or not, affecting the complaints or the personal capacity. Experts considered it important that employees are aware of these possible factors.

Experts mentioned communication as an important topic which can stimulate social support. Good communication starts with self-reflection: How do I communicate? In addition, suggestions for good communication were considered important, including training of communication skills. Employees with CANS are often highly engaged with their job and do not easily say 'no'. More assertiveness towards the employer may be required. It is also important that employees acquire the tools and skills to communicate with their supervisor, e.g. about their needs and experiences. Employees may also feel that their supervisor does not listen to them, so it is useful to examine how employees communicate their needs and experiences:

> *I occasionally meet people who say 'I want another computer mouse but I don't think my direct manager allows me to'. Then I ask whether he/she already made this request to his/her boss. That piece of competence - to approach your boss with your request for help - is important.* (Expert 7)

Behaviour

Self-efficacy and empowerment

Experts saw a role for a self-management program for employees with CANS and agreed with each other that the intervention should focus on increasing the employee's self-efficacy and empowerment. Employees must have the confidence to handle situations they are confronted with in the right way. Participants of a self-management program should also be challenged to take the lead in the management of their complaints. To achieve this, information may be provided, skills can be trained, and participants must identify possible solutions themselves. By offering a wide range of information and knowledge, and by practicing skills, each individual employee can select for themselves the relevant topics and then take action. Regarding the breadth of the information that should be provided, one expert said:

> *I would say that it must not only be about the arm, shoulder and neck, but primarily about work, about yourself, and how you manage to restore yourself to a good balance. And starting to work and continue working on a healthy way.* (Expert 10)

Taking action

No ready-made solutions should be offered. Participants should be facilitated to find a tailored solution. Participants themselves must take action and find solutions; in this way they will also be highly motivated. Participants must consider various solution options and make choices between them. One expert stated that three possible solutions must be available before one can make a 'real' choice. According to experts, an additional eHealth module could have added value because it may provide ideas for possible solutions. It is important that participants consider their own solutions; these will differ for each individual depending on the underlying problem (s) and personal situation. One expert explained:

> *I do believe that - which also is the challenge - to let it come from themselves. To use what they experience as support. Each person has his/her own manner.* (Expert 6)

It was assumed that the target group of the intervention, i.e. workers with longer-term CANS, are open to such an approach. Employees with CANS have often taken various steps with the aim to reduce their complaints.

Setting goals and making choices

Setting goals was indicated as important. Experts considered it important to split the main goal into sub-goals. Achieving some success in between can also work as a motivating factor. It is also important that participants feel strengthened. People gain confidence as they tackle a part of the problem and gain control over this problem. This increases the chance that, once the program has ended, the participants will continue working in this way.

> *I also think it's very rewarding if you really do have actual complaints and you have learned through reflecting on these complaints, discussing them with people, looking up information on the subject, and by trying out various things - and that you realize that the complaints become less severe over time. I can understand that this approach works well. Also, in different but similar situations, you can perhaps also use the same approach through which you can achieve success.* (Expert 5)

According to experts, another role of a self-management intervention is to ensure that employees are aware of the possible facilities and treatment options (with regard to their complaints) within and outside their organization or company. In this way, employees can more easily find the right facilities and care. Overall, experts believed that participants should be able to make their own choices. One expert stated:

> *For one person it mainly concerns the development of talent, identifying your own strengths and then using these optimally. For another person it involves the physiotherapist coming by and then, together with your employer, you determine where you can find the financial resources to obtain a better monitor.* (Expert 15)

Important skills and behaviour

Besides communication skills, according to some experts, other important skills can be related to physical activity, private life, load and capacity, setting limits, taking breaks, relaxation and ergonomics. Experts stated that participants must realize that what is good for one person may not be good (or not useful) for another.

Physical activity Some experts in the focus group who had employees with CANS tried to improve their complaints through sports/exercise and tried to upgrade their physical capacities. Experts agreed that the importance of physical activity should be emphasized and participants should be encouraged to undertake more physical activity. Exercises were also considered important. Experts said that physical activity and exercise must be gradually increased, because muscles may not be in optimal condition; in some cases activity should be supervised by a physical therapist. One expert stated:

> *One of the causative factors is also the lack of movement, and fear of movement.* (Expert 3)

Private life Experts stated that it is important that employees have sufficient relaxation in their spare time. A good balance between work and home activity was considered important. Concentrating on one's hobbies and interests can help with this. In addition, the home situation can also be a physically stressful factor, as indicated by one participant:

> *A lot of people work at home - many people work on the computer or are gaming online, have painted the ceiling, or have laid paving stones for a sidewalk.* (Expert 15)

Load and capacity Physical capacity can vary greatly from person to person. Employees can influence this by adjusting/lowering the load, or increasing their physical capacity. According to experts, employees should give priority and listen to signals from their own body. Employees should correctly estimate their capacity, set their limits, and ask for help from others when needed. One needs to find a good balance between one's load and one's capacity:

> *That is therefore the balance. which means that you know from experience that if you don't set this limit, then you will develop very serious complaints.* (Expert 5)

Setting limits As mentioned, employees must set their own limits; this was considered as an important skill. Experts also indicated that setting limits is not a convenient term in relation to self-management. In fact, in an intervention focused on self-management, participants should find their own solutions.

Experts stated that the experienced problems should therefore give rise to looking for solutions and alternatives. Employees with CANS should realize that if they carry on without changing anything their complaints will worsen, and then alternatives and solutions will also be more difficult to find. Setting their own limits could be a part of this solution. However, this is not always easy, for example in certain occupations:

> *I also see this during clean-ups or in the cantina where people have to repeatedly perform the same activities. Then you cannot easily say that you need to take your time. (...) I recognize this situation quite clearly in administrative work. In all work situations there is this constant pressure to keep working at all costs.* (Expert 2)

Taking breaks Taking regular breaks was considered important. Employees need to take a break at certain time intervals and not wait until they experience symptoms. One expert reported that, in some companies, taking a break is obligatory because of the increased risk of developing complaints when persisting with work. Employees are, for example, also encouraged to get up and move around during the breaks. About the role of taking breaks one expert stated:

> *There is a logic underlying the link between the development of complaints and the duration of the period when this actually occurs. There are intermediate stages, which precede the actual appearance of the complaints. If someone becomes aware of the fact that he has complaints after one and a-half hours, he could also have become aware of this within three-quarters of an hour when the first complaints became evident, if he'd known how the symptoms would manifest. I think that someone has to take breaks earlier.* (Expert 3)

Relaxation Experts believed it is important that participants receive information about stress and relaxation. Also, information on the negative effects of stress and information on stress in relation to the development of symptoms are considered important. Information on activities in relation to muscle tension is also helpful. Some experts stated that practical advice on how to relax (muscles) is essential.

Ergonomics Information on the ergonomics of the workplace is valuable: e.g. how to adjust the desk, chair and monitor, and the proper use of keyboards and/or mouse. One expert remarked:

> *On a completely different level, it's just about the competence to adjust your office chair.* (Expert 10)

Other aspects such as lighting, sound, climate, working posture, and work techniques were also important topics. Also, the ergonomics of the workplace at home was considered a matter of concern, because many people use a laptop at home where posture is often far from optimal. Within the framework of alternative workplace strategies this topic must also be addressed.

Combination of self-management sessions and eHealth

Experts indicated that the combination of group sessions and eHealth can work extremely well. The sessions and eHealth can strengthen and complement each other. Topics may be initiated in the sessions and participants can, if interested, sort these out in the eHealth module. Additional assignments or exercises can also be offered in the eHealth module. In general, experts endorsed the additional value of the eHealth: as one expert stated:

> *I really do view eHealth as a very definite support to this. (...) In fact, it can be considered as an additive you can offer to the palette ... and a great way in which you can provide a lot of information. Through this approach people can very selectively choose what they need.* (Expert 8)

The self-management intervention was seen as a roadmap, in which participants work on their personal goals, and have interaction with other participants. The eHealth module lends itself to provide more information. Participants could then use this information in the sessions in order to achieve their goals. Participants can use the eHealth to solve the formulated problems and fulfil their action plans. Because CANS has a multifactorial origin, experts expected that eHealth can offer the opportunity to sift through a considerable amount of information. The eHealth module is ideally suited to address all dimensions of the related topics. It is important to determine in advance which topics should be addressed in the self-management sessions, and which topics should be covered in the eHealth. Regarding what should be addressed in the meetings and the eHealth one expert stated:

> *For example, about office skills and adjustment to the office chair. Perhaps you actually don't do this in the sessions - but rather (a discussion of) a very distinct office chair and a description of the five most popular office chairs.* (Expert 10)

Generally the experts saw the self-management sessions as the main focus of the intervention, with the support of the eHealth module. The eHealth is thought to contain additional information, including scientific publications. In the eHealth it is also possible to look at topics from another perspective. Experts indicated that it is important to facilitate use of the eHealth module, e.g. by referring to this in the self-management sessions.

According to the experts, the eHealth should be self-explanatory with short and concise information. It should be attractive and could include a forum or an online community. An overview of the experts' opinions on the conditions and requirements concerning the layout and design of the eHealth module are presented in Table 2. The most important items regarding the intervention as reported by the experts are presented in Table 3.

Discussion

Experts seem to see a role for a self-management program for employees with CANS. However, as shown in Table 3, many items are indicated to be important by the experts. Experts emphasized that an intervention that aims at understanding or, moreover, decreasing CANS in employees, should focus on increasing employees' self-efficacy and empowerment. Employees with CANS have difficulty in managing their own health problem and their work. Informed awareness and behavioural change are considered important for this group of employees. Complaints will not always go away, but a self-management program can offer support to these employees.

Experts indicated that self-management begins with the intention to take action. Self-management starts from awareness of a personal problem of the employee. It is very important that people come up with their own solutions, are in control, and feel empowered. Providing knowledge can also be a part of a self-management intervention. It can consist partly of creating awareness with regard to possible risk factors, cues to prompt people to become aware, and about how participants can influence these risk factors themselves. According to the experts, self-management also involves self-efficacy; people must develop confidence that they can handle situations that they are confronted with in an appropriate way. The view of the experts on self-management finds support in literature [20,39,40].

Experts indicated that the combination of group sessions and eHealth can work extremely well. The sessions

Table 2 Conditions and requirements concerning the design, layout and interactivity of the eHealth module

Design	The eHealth should be designed in such a way that people can work with it themselves and can search for possible solutions. It should be self-explanatory.... *and with as little distraction as possible. The person has to immediately understand the correct button to be clicked on... and a short demonstration film, that sort of thing, is also often crucial. That its use does not represent a barrier to continue... and indeed, you must not want to fill in a website, no long texts. Visual support as much as possible, then you have to achieve something with a drawing/record or something interactive* (Expert 9)
	There must be a guiding line: for example, phases or themes. Some parts can be obligatory and other parts can be optional.
	The information should be short and concise. With the use of tabs: so that it is possible to distinguish between the main themes and to distinguish several levels.
	If possible, the eHealth should be designed as an independent program, so that in the implementation phase it can be used without the group meetings. In some sub-groups the eHealth itself may give sufficient support.
Layout	The layout should be attractive. *Irrespective whether or not people find the concept of eHealth appealing, the way you present it - the interface - its attractiveness is very important.* (Expert 13)
	Paying attention to apparently 'smaller' details is important: for example, the font that is used. What seems trivial may have considerable influence.
	Preferably use images, video and/or voice messages.
Interactivity	There is some discussion as to whether the website should be interactive. On the one hand this makes the website more attractive, but eHealth then becomes more complicated - which is not desirable for this purpose. These considerations should be evaluated. *If you say interactive then you first have to have a goal to reach - and only then can you say interactive or not.* (Expert 13)
	Implementing a diary feature is a possibility: *Regarding a diary - hopefully most participants won't have any objection to fill in a diary on the computer. If they already do that, then it's a good preparation for the next session. If people want to share the diary with each other – then they can.* (Expert 10)
	But another expert stated: *What is of course also interesting, is that there are people with complaints that arise from regular computer use* (Expert 10)
	Therefore, use of the computer for additional features needs to be considered, in order to prevent more hours spent behind the computer.
	Experts have different opinions about adding a forum/community with participants and experts. A community with healthcare providers is frequently used nowadays, and an online consultation is also an option. However, a forum/community has the disadvantage that participants might 'whine' about their complaints. Moreover, participants can contact each other in the group meetings and with small groups it is difficult to have an active community online.

Table 3 Most important item as reported by the experts

Group 1	
Expert 1	*On looking back, I think that you look back together with your colleagues. The colleague has done many things that she/he reflects on her/his own activities so that she/he feels stronger or learns from it. You only achieve the effect if you ask to reflect.*
Expert 2	*I think it's very important that you convey some degree of enthusiasm, so that they become convinced that you yourself to a large extent possess the key to the solution. And that you need some additional help with this - then they can go and do it on their own.*
Expert 3	*I think that knowledge on the symptoms and on the consequences of the symptoms for the activities that these people are carrying out is important information.*
Expert 4	*A little understanding, development of insight into the risk factors, and in this way to be able to work out what to do with it in more detail.*
Expert 5	*I have written down 'socially desirable behaviour, assertiveness and social skills'.*
Group 2	
Expert 6	*One thing that I find important is that people learn to feel what their body is telling them - and learn to listen to their body. And also to once again come into contact with themselves - a little bit of mindfulness.*
Expert 7	*For me it is important that people can establish a connection between what they are doing and the effect of what they are doing on their body. (...) And perhaps quite simple, but to celebrate successes. People sometimes find it quite normal that an action is successful. Subsequent processes are sometimes small steps but ones which are important to someone - for these you certainly require courage, perseverance, insight. Therefore, you may also celebrate the success that you have actually accomplish.*
Expert 8	*I say: the user interface of the eHealth. Therefore, that what people see is attractive.*
Expert 9	*I think what is important is the retention, the retention of the effect of the treatment. That there is a way to prevent relapse.*
Expert 10	*Perhaps the deeper question is what I consider to be more important, the pain in my arm or my work. (...) And about work load and capacity to work, the making of choices, most certainly with those people whom you know will always have minor complaints - they have to set priorities. Then the question which remains is what do I think is the most important.*
Expert 11	*I think I should say work ethics, norms and values. When do you find yourself (to be) a good employee. What are your criteria?*
Group 3	
Expert 12	*What I just said - the evaluation process, and what I said in the beginning - safety and support. That is very important.*
Expert 13	*I would in any case include physical activity, the stimulation of more physical activity in the program.*
Expert 14	*I think, whether you focus on the work environment or on the physical aspect, in both cases cognition is essential. How do people personally think about these things. There are many incorrect prejudices and opinions. Often there is too little knowledge about the human body.*
Expert 15	*What we just said - that people acquire insight into how behavioural changes work and how do I personally view such changes. In which phase are you - and how is that going - so that they also understand why their goals are not being reached. That you then - once again - can do something. Insight into behavioural change is very important.*
Expert 16	*The role of the supervisor in the development and solving of the problem.*
Expert 17	*I think that you also really do have to support the use of the website.*

and eHealth can strengthen and complement each other. To our knowledge, no group-based self-management intervention including eHealth currently exists. In a systematic review on the use of information technology for diabetes self-management, no single intervention combined group sessions with eHealth [41]. Topics may be initiated in the sessions and participants can, if interested, sort this out in the eHealth module. In general, experts endorse the additional value of an eHealth module. It is important to determine in advance which topics should be addressed in the self-management sessions and which can be covered in the eHealth module.

During data analyses, it appeared that the identified main categories emerging from the data, showed similarities with the I-Change model (2.0) Therefore, the main categories emerging from the data were clustered according to the three phases (Awareness, Motivation and Behaviour) of the I-Change model [38]. The I-Change model also assumes that behaviour is the result of intentions and abilities and explicitly makes a distinction between three phases of motivational change and their corresponding determinants [38]. In the pre-motivational phase (Awareness), people need to become aware of their risk behaviour. In the motivational phase (Motivation), people need to become motivated to change their behaviour; in this phase, an intention is formed. In the post-motivational phase (Behaviour) people need to translate intentions into actions, so several preparatory actions to facilitate the actual behaviours need to be planned and executed [38]. The I-Change model is built on the Attitude – Social influence – Efficacy (ASE) Model [42] (comparable to the theory of planned behaviour [43-45]), on which the original intervention of Detaille et al. [32,33] was based, and has incorporated ideas from several social cognitive models [38]. As can be seen in Figure 1, the I-Change model assumes that motivational factors are determined by various factors, such as awareness factors, preceding factors and information factors [38]. By using the I-Change model we were able to relate the outcomes of this study to the stages of behavioural change.

In general, experts found it important that the intervention deals with the possible (multifactorial) risk factors related to the complaints and the underlying problems; this is because employees with CANS are often unaware of the diversity of the possible risk factors. Moreover, earlier focus groups with employees revealed that not all employees are aware of the actual cause of their complaints [17]. The multifactorial risk factors of CANS are supported in the literature [4-7,46]. The earlier focus groups with employees with CANS also indicated that basic information about the complaints, including potential risk factors, is needed [17]. The importance of other topics identified in the focus groups with employees [17], such as information on symptoms (including chronic pain), as well as workload and physical capacity, are also endorsed. According to the experts, employees with CANS should be more proactive. Also, in the intervention, difficulties should be identified and participants should make their own choices and obtain reassurance.

Employees with CANS find it difficult to deal with their complaints and may have difficulty in managing prolonged work activities and paying sufficient attention to their physical posture [17]. Dealing with and acceptance of complaints are topics that also arise in relation to other chronic musculoskeletal disorders, such as low back pain [47]. Finding a balance between all the requirements related to activities at work is challenging; therefore, information about the work environment related to CANS, including workplace adjustments, is required [17]. Experts indicated several areas related to the work environment, including workplace ergonomics, that should be addressed in the intervention; therefore, the work environment seems to be an important topic, especially in the eHealth.

The importance of exercises is generally recognized by employees with CANS [17] and is also indicated by patients with low back pain as a way to manage complaints [47]. Some experts recommended that employees with CANS might improve their complaints through sports/exercise and should upgrade their physical capacities. On the other hand, in our focus groups with employees, some participants stopped stressful sports activities because they thought these activities would aggravate their complaints [17]. Experts recognized the value of physical activity and the importance of exercises. Both experts and employees with CANS also indicated the importance of having information on and exercises about (muscle) relaxation [17], which is supported by others [48].

Addressing the negative effects of stress, and information about stress in relation to CANS, is considered important by experts. Employees do not always find it easy to deal with the stress and pressure of work [17]. Experts stated that employees must set their own limits and that this is an important skill. Related to the setting of limits, employees with CANS have a relatively high threshold before asking for help, whereas others think they should tighten up their limits [17]. Focus groups with employees identified a relationship with stress in the development and worsening of their complaints [17]. In fact, work stress is associated with common health complaints, such as musculoskeletal pain [49]. Moreover, (work) stress is associated with musculoskeletal problems of the upper extremity [50]. Also, employees with CANS indicated that taking into account one's own limits is important [17].

Experts considered communication skills to be important. Employees with CANS did not always find it easy to talk about their complaints and/or to bother others about their problems [17]. Generally, there are no major problems encountered with communication, but employees with CANS considered providing communication tools for discussion with others about CANS to be important [17].

Social support is considered valuable by the experts. Patients with low back pain considered emotional support and encouragement as essential [47], and social support was also considered important by patients with rheumatoid arthritis [51], which emphasizes the importance of this topic. In general, employees with CANS experienced sufficient support from their colleagues and from those at home [17]. Most employees experienced sufficient support from their supervisor; however, some employees who participated in earlier focus groups experienced insufficient or no support from the supervisor [17]. This could indicate that knowing how to obtain social support is also an important skill.

Experts found it important to address the importance of finding a good balance between work and home. This is endorsed by some participants in the focus group with employees complaining that there is a lack of balance between their work and private life [17]; this can also occur in other chronic conditions, for example a neuromuscular disease [52].

Limitations of the study

This study has several limitations. First, a total of 17 experts in the field of CANS, self-management and/or eHealth participated; this is probably a rather arbitrary selection of all experts on these topics in the Netherlands. We decided to divide the different areas of expertise into the three focus groups, thereby ensuring that in all focus groups all topics could be discussed. The alternative, i.e. placing all experts of one area together in one group, might have produced more discussion about each of the topics - but separately. By having mixed focus groups all experts participated in the discussions on all topics, which made it possible to establish the relationships between the topics. Although we did not set a point of saturation in advance, it is highly likely that saturation was reached because the same issues were identified and discussed in all three focus groups. Data were coded by one researcher. Multiple coding involves the cross-checking of coding strategies and the interpretation of data by independent researchers [53]. However, as Barbour [53] stated, the degree of concordance between researchers is not very important; the main value of multiple coding is to supply alternative interpretations [53]. It is important that a transparent and systematic process is followed which can be carried out by one researcher, by a team, or by involving independent experts [53]. By discussing the emerging main categories and looking for alternative interpretations for our findings in a small research group, we investigated the potentially competing explanations.

As mentioned in the Introduction, for the specific group of participants with CANS, more prolonged computer use (due to following an eHealth program) could worsen their physical problems. However, this was not specifically mentioned by the experts.

Content of the intervention

Important topics of the intervention indicated by experts are the possible causes of complaints, addressing potential symptoms, identifying difficulties and problems, making choices, and reassurance and self-awareness. The intervention should also address behaviour such as setting limits, taking breaks and ensuring sufficient relaxation. Ergonomics, social relationships and social support, the importance of physical activity and exercises, and a good balance between work and home activity are also considered important. The topics identified in this focus group study generally meet the needs of employees with CANS [17] which are related to exercises, muscle relaxation, working with pain, work environment, social environment and personal factors (including work style), all of which are supported by earlier studies [6,7,18,19,54-63].

Conclusions

The present study provides valuable insight into experts' opinion on a self-management program for employees with CANS. Experts seem to see a role for a self-management program for employees with CANS and the intervention should focus on increasing the employee's self-efficacy and empowerment. Experts indicated that the combination of group sessions and an eHealth module can work extremely well. Moreover, experts from different fields provided valuable information regarding the development of a self-management program for employees with CANS, which can be used in the adaptation of a self-management program following the intervention mapping protocol [35]. This information can also be used to develop other interventions and for the treatment of employees with CANS.

Appendix: Interview guide for the focus group sessions

Introduction (5 min)

- Brief introduction about the research project and the aim of the focus group.

Introductory questions (20 min)

- Introduction of the participants (name, type of work, experience with CANS, self-management and eHealth).
- What is self-management for employees suffering from CANS?
- Does a self-management program for employees suffering from CANS for more than 12 weeks make sense?

Content of the intervention (55 min)

- Which topics should be addressed in a self-management intervention for employees with CANS?
- What kind of information about the onset and persistence of CANS needs to be discussed in the intervention?
- What kind of information about dealing with and reducing complaints should be included in the intervention?
- What kind of skills should employees with CANS have developed after the intervention?

Break (10 min)

Development of the intervention (30 min)

- Which requirements should a good eHealth module fulfill for the target group?
- What are potential pitfalls and/or important points in the development of an eHealth module?
- Which requirements should a good self-management program for the target group fulfill?
- What are effective methods to use in the self-management program?

Self-management program including eHealth (20 min)

- Which topics, or what kind of topics, should be covered in the self-management sessions and which

topics, or what kind of topics, should be addressed in the eHealth?
- How can the self-management program and eHealth module complement each other?

Closure (10 min)

- What would you say is the most important topic or item in the goal or the development of the intervention?
- Which topics did you miss during this meeting, but are important in the process of developing the intervention?

Abbreviations

CANS: Complaints of the arm, neck and/or shoulder; WMO: Dutch law on 'Medical Research involving Human Subjects'.

Competing interests

This study was fundec by ZonMw, the Netherlands Organisation for Health Research and Development (208030004).
The authors declare that they have no competing interests.

Authors' contributions

YH, JE, JBS and RN developed the initial study proposal and acquired funding for the study. All authors contributed to the development of the interview guide and analysis of the results. NH moderated the focus groups. All authors provided valuable input to the design of this paper, which was drafted by NH. All authors commented on the draft versions. All authors have read and approved the final manuscript.

Acknowledgements

The authors thank Luc Driessen (LD) for assisting with the focus groups and transcription, and Saran Detaille (SD) for reading the transcripts, checking the emergent themes, and discussing the supporting quotes.

References

1. Huisstede BM, Wijnhoven HA, Bierma-Zeinstra SM, Koes BW, Verhaar JA, Picavet S. Prevalence and characteristics of complaints of the arm, neck, and/or shoulder (CANS) in the open population. Clin J Pain. 2008;24(3):253–9. Epub 2008/02/22.
2. Huisstede BM, Bierma-Zeinstra SM, Koes BW, Verhaar JA. Incidence and prevalence of upper-extremity musculoskeletal disorders. A systematic appraisal of the literature. BMC Musculoskelet Disord. 2006;7:7. Epub 2006/02/02.
3. van Tulder M, Malmivaara A, Koes B. Repetitive strain injury. Lancet. 2007;369(9575):1815–22. Epub 2007/05/29.
4. van Eijsden-Besseling MD, Peeters FP, Reijnen JA, de Bie RA. Perfectionism and coping strategies as risk factors for the development of non-specific work-related upper limb disorders (WRULD). Occup Med. 2004;54(2):122–7. Epub 2004/03/17.
5. Feleus A, Bierma-Zeinstra SM, Miedema HS, Verhagen AP, Nauta AP, Burdorf A, et al. Prognostic indicators for non-recovery of non-traumatic complaints at arm, neck and shoulder in general practice-6 months follow-up. Rheumatology. 2007;46(1):169–76. Epub 2006/06/27.
6. Bongers PM, IJmker S, van den Heuvel S, Blatter BM. Epidemiology of work related neck and upper limb problems: psychosocial and personal risk factors (part I) and effective interventions from a bio behavioural perspective (part II). J Occup Rehabil. 2006;16(3):279–302. Epub 2006/07/20.
7. Staal JB, de Bie RA, Hendriks EJ. Aetiology and management of work-related upper extremity disorders. Best Pract Res Clin Rheumatol. 2007;21(1):123–33. Epub 2007/03/14.
8. Karels CH, Bierma-Zeinstra SM, Verhagen AP, Koes BW, Burdorf A. Sickness absence in patients with arm, neck and shoulder complaints presenting in physical therapy practice: 6 months follow-up. Man Ther. 2010;15(5):476–81. Epub 2010/06/24.
9. Macfarlane GJ, Hunt IM, Silman AJ. Role of mechanical and psychosocial factors in the onset of forearm pain: prospective population based study. BMJ. 2000;321(7262):676–9. Epub 2000/09/15.
10. Andersen JH, Kaergaard A, Mikkelsen S, Jensen JF, Frost P, Bonde JP, et al. Risk factors in the onset of neck/shoulder pain in a prospective study of workers in industrial and service companies. Occup Environ Med. 2003;60(9):649–54. Epub 2003/08/26.
11. Marcus M, Gerr F, Monteilh C, Ortiz DJ, Gentry E, Cohen S, et al. A prospective study of computer users: II. Postural risk factors for musculoskeletal symptoms and disorders. Am J Ind Med. 2002;41(4):236–49. Epub 2002/03/29.
12. Bernard B, Sauter S, Fine L, Petersen M, Hales T. Job task and psychosocial risk factors for work-related musculoskeletal disorders among newspaper employees. Scand J Work Environ Health. 1994;20(6):417–26. Epub 1994/12/01.
13. van den Heuvel SG, van der Beek AJ, Blatter EM, Hoogendoorn WE, Bongers PM. Psychosocial work characteristics in relation to neck and upper limb symptoms. Pain. 2005;114(1–2):47–53. Epub 2005/03/01.
14. Nicholas RA, Feuerstein M, Suchday S. Workstyle and upper-extremity symptoms: a biobehavioral perspective. J Occup Environ Med/Am Coll Occup Environ Med. 2005;47(4):352–61. Epub 2005/04/13.
15. Martimo KP, Shiri R, Miranda H, Ketola R, Varonen H, Viikari-Juntura E. Self-reported productivity loss among workers with upper extremity disorders. Scand J Work Environ Health. 2009;35(4):301–8. Epub 2009/05/28.
16. Harrington CB, Siddiqui A, Feuerstein M. Workstyle as a predictor of pain and restricted work associated with upper extremity disorders: a prospective study. J Hand Surg. 2009;34(4):724–31. Epub 2009/04/07.
17. Hutting N, Heerkens YF, Engels JA, Staal JB. Nijhuis-van der Sanden MWG. Experiences of employees with arm, neck or shoulder complaints: a focus group study. BMC Musculoskelet Disord. 2014;15:141.
18. Meijer EM, Sluiter JK, Frings-Dresen MH. Is workstyle a mediating factor for pain in the upper extremity over time? J Occup Rehabil. 2008;18(3):262–6. Epub 2008/08/09.
19. Keijsers E, Feleus A, Miedema HS, Koes BW, Bierma-Zeinstra SM. Psychosocial factors predicted nonrecovery in both specific and nonspecific diagnoses at arm, neck, and shoulder. J Clin Epidemiol 2010;63(12):1370–9. Epub 2010/05/01.
20. Lorig KR. Self-management of chronic illness: a model for the future. Generations. 1993;17(3):11–4.
21. Newman S, Steed L, Mulligan K. Self-management interventions for chronic illness. Lancet. 2004;364(9444):1523–37. Epub 2004/10/27.
22. McGowan P. Self-management: a background paper. New perspectives: international conference on patient self-management. 2005.
23. Carnes D, Homer KE, Miles CL, Pincus T, Underwood M, Rahman A, et al. Effective delivery styles and content for self-management interventions for chronic musculoskeletal pain: a systematic literature review. Clin J Pain. 2012;28(4):344–54. Epub 2011/10/18.
24. Nolte S, Osborne RH. A systematic review of outcomes of chronic disease self-management interventions. Qual Life Res Int J Qual Life Asp Treat Care Rehab. 2013;22(7):1805–16. Epub 2012/11/01.
25. Du S, Yuan C, Xiao X, Chu J, Qiu Y, Qian H. Self-management programs for chronic musculoskeletal pain conditions: a systematic review and meta-analysis. Patient Educ Couns. 2011;85(3):e299–310. Epub 2011/04/05.
26. Kuijpers W, Groen WG, Aaronson NK, van Harten WH. A systematic review of web-based interventions for patient empowerment and physical activity in chronic diseases: relevance for cancer survivors. J Med Internet Res. 2013;15(2):e37. Epub 2013/02/22.
27. Gaikwad R, Warren J. The role of home-based information and communications technology interventions in chronic disease management: a systematic literature review. Health Informatics J. 2009;15(2):122–46. Epub 2009/05/29.
28. Vonk Noordegraaf A, Huirne JA, Pittens CA, van Mechelen W, Broerse JE, Brolmann HA, et al. eHealth program to empower patients in returning to normal activities and work after gynecological surgery: intervention mapping as a useful method for development. J Med Internet Res. 2012;14(5):e124. Epub 2012/10/23.
29. Ahern DK. Challenges and opportunities of eHealth research. Am J Prev Med. 2007;32(5 Suppl):S75–82. Epub 2007/05/01.
30. Eysenbach G. The law of attrition. J Med Internet Res. 2005;7(1):e11. Epub 2005/04/15.
31. Health Council of the Netherlands. Beeldschermwerken (Computer use at work) [Dutch]. The Hague: Health Council of the Netherlands; 2012.
32. Detaille SI, van der Gulden JW, Engels JA, Heerkens YF, van Dijk FJ. Using intervention mapping (IM) to develop a self-management programme for

employees with a chronic disease in the Netherlands. BMC Public Health. 2010;10:353. Epub 2010/06/23.

33. Detaille SI. Building a self-management program for workers with a chronic somatic disease (PhD thesis). Nijmegen: Ipskamp Drukkers B.V; 2012.
34. Bartholomew LK, Parcel GS, Kok G. Intervention mapping: a process for developing theory- and evidence-based health education programs. Health Educ Behav. 1998;25(5):545–63. Epub 1998/10/13.
35. Bartholomew L, Parcel G, Kok G, Gottlieb N, Fernández M. Planning health promotion programs. An intervention mapping approach. 3rd ed. San Francisco: Jossey/BAss; 2011.
36. Krueger RAC, Casey MA. Focus groups. A practical guide for applied research. Thousand Oaks: Sage Publications Inc.; 2009.
37. Lacey ALD. Qualitative data analysis. Yorkshire and the Humber: The NIHR Research Design Service for the East Midlands; 2007.
38. de Vries H, Mesters I, Riet JV, Willems K, Reubsaet A. Motives of Belgian adolescents for using sunscreen: the role of action plans. Cancer Epidemiol Biomarkers Prev. 2006;15(7):1360–6. Epub 2006/07/13.
39. Lorig KR, Mazonson PD, Holman HR. Evidence suggesting that health education for self-management in patients with chronic arthritis has sustained health benefits while reducing health care costs. Arthritis Rheum. 1993;36(4):439–46. Epub 1993/04/01.
40. Johnston V, Jull G, Sheppard DM, Ellis N. Applying principles of self-management to facilitate workers to return to or remain at work with a chronic musculoskeletal condition. Man Ther. 2013;18(4):274–80. Epub 2013/05/07.
41. El-Gayar O, Timsina P, Nawar N, Eid W. A systematic review of IT for diabetes self-management: are we there yet? Int J Med Inform. 2013;82(8):637–52. Epub 2013/06/25.
42. De Vries H, Mudde A. Predicting stage transitions for smoking cessation applying the attitude – social influence – efficacy model. Psychol Health. 1998;13:369–85.
43. Ajzen I. The theory of planned behavior. Organ Behav Hum Decis Process. 1991;50:179–211.
44. Brug J, Assema P, Lechner L. Gezondheidsvoorlichting en gedragsverandering. Een planmatige aanpak. Van Gorcum: Assen; 2008.
45. Ajzen I. Attitudes, personality and behavior. Milton Keynes: Open University Press; 2005.
46. Beumer A, De Bie RA, Ten Cate A, Doornbos N. Multidisciplinaire richtlijn aspecifieke klachten arm, Nek en/of schouders [Multidisciplinary guideline non-specific complaints of arm, neck and/or shoulders] (Dutch). Amersfoort: Koninklijk Nederlands Genootschap voor Fysiotherapie (KNGF); 2012.
47. Kawi J. Chronic low back pain patients' perceptions on self-management, self-management support, and functional ability. pain management nursing. Official J Am Soc Pain Manage Nurses. 2014;15(1):258–64.
48. Toivanen H, Helin P, Hanninen O. Impact of regular relaxation training and psychosocial working factors on neck-shoulder tension and absenteeism in hospital cleaners. J Occup Med. 1993;35(11):1123–30. Epub 1993/11/01.
49. Toivanen S. Exploring the interplay between work stress and socioeconomic position in relation to common health complaints: the role of interaction. Am J Ind Med. 2011;54(10):780–90. Epub 2011/06/22.
50. Bongers PM, Kremer AM, ter Laak J. Are psychosocial factors, risk factors for symptoms and signs of the shoulder, elbow, or hand/wrist?: A review of the epidemiological literature. Am J Ind Med. 2002;41(5):315–42. Epub 2002/06/20.
51. Detaille SI, Haafkens JA, van Dijk FJ. What employees with rheumatoid arthritis, diabetes mellitus and hearing loss need to cope at work. Scand J Work Environ Health. 2003;29(2):134–42. Epub 2003/04/30.
52. Minis MA, Satink T, Kinebanian A, Engels JA, Heerkens YF, van Engelen BG, et al. How persons with a neuromuscular disease perceive employment participation: a qualitative study. J Occup Rehabil. 2014;24(1):52–67. Epub 2013/05/07.
53. Barbour RS. Checklists for improving rigour in qualitative research: a case of the tail wagging the dog? BMJ. 2001;322(7294):1115–7. Epub 2001/05/05.
54. Bernaards CM, Ariens GA, Knol DL, Hildebrandt VH. The effectiveness of a work style intervention and a lifestyle physical activity intervention on the recovery from neck and upper limb symptoms in computer workers. Pain. 2007;132(1–2):142–53. Epub 2007/09/05.
55. Esmaeilzadeh S, Ozcan E, Capan N. Effects of ergonomic intervention on work-related upper extremity musculoskeletal disorders among computer workers: a randomized controlled trial. Int Arch Occup Environ Health. 2014;87(1):73–83.
56. Andersen JH, Thomsen JF, Overgaard E, Lassen CF, Brandt LP, Vilstrup I, et al. Computer use and carpal tunnel syndrome: a 1-year follow-up study. JAMA. 2003;289(22):2963–9. Epub 2003/06/12.
57. Wahlstrom J. Ergonomics, musculoskeletal disorders and computer work. Occup Med. 2005;55(3):168–76. Epub 2005/04/29.
58. van Eijsden-Besseling MD, van den Bergh KA, Staal JB, de Bie RA, Smeets RJ, van den Heuvel WJ. The influence of work and treatment related factors on clinical status and disability in patients with non-specific work-related upper limb disorders. Work. 2010;37(4):425–32. Epub 2010/11/26.
59. van Eijsden-Besseling MD, van den Bergh KA, Staal JB, de Bie RA, van den Heuvel WJ. The course of nonspecific work-related upper limb disorders and the influence of demographic factors, psychologic factors, and physical fitness on clinical status and disability. Arch Phys Med Rehabil. 2010;91(6):862–7. Epub 2010/06/01.
60. van den Heuvel SG, van der Beek AJ, Blatter BM, Bongers PM. Do work-related physical factors predict neck and upper limb symptoms in office workers? Int Arch Occup Environ Health. 2006;79(7):585–92. Epub 2006/05/20.
61. Bernaards CM, Ariens GA, Simons M, Knol DL, Hildebrandt VH. Improving work style behavior in computer workers with neck and upper limb symptoms. J Occup Rehabil. 2008;18(1):87–101. Epub 2008/01/05.
62. Feuerstein M, Harrington CB. Secondary prevention of work-related upper extremity disorders: recommendations from the Annapolis conference. J Occup Rehabil. 2006;16(3):401–9. Epub 2006/06/28.
63. Martimo KP, Shiri R, Miranda H, Ketola R, Varonen H, Viikari-Juntura E. Effectiveness of an ergonomic intervention on the productivity of workers with upper-extremity disorders–a randomized controlled trial. Scand J Work Environ Health. 2010;36(1):25–33. Epub 2009/12/05.

13

Does the low-level occupational exposure to volatile organic compounds alter the seasonal variation of selected markers of oxidative stress?

Peter Grešner*, Radosław Świercz, Magdalena Beata Król, Ewa Twardowska, Jolanta Gromadzińska and Wojciech Wąsowicz

Abstract

Background: In this study we tested whether the seasonal variations in levels of selected biomarkers of oxidative stress in female nail technicians occupationally exposed to low levels of volatile organic compounds (VOCs) differ significantly from those observed among healthy unexposed controls. Airborne levels of selected VOCs in nail salons were also analyzed and tested for associations with seasonal variations of the levels of biomarkers among nail technicians.

Methods: The study enrolled 145 female nail technicians and 145 healthy unexposed female controls. The airborne VOCs and levels of biomarkers were assessed by GC-MS chromatography and absorption/fluorescence spectrophotometry, respectively.

Results: Plasma levels of thiobarbituric acid reactive species, ceruloplasmin, the activity of glutathione peroxidase (GPx1) and the SOD1/GPx1 activity ratio presented significant differences between the so-called "hot" and "cold" seasons in the case of nail technicians as well as in unexposed controls ($p < <0.0001$ for all four biomarkers). The pattern of these variations among nail technicians was found to be significantly different compared to that of the control subjects ($p < <0.0001$). Although such differences might intuitively be attributed to occupational exposure of nail technicians to VOCs, which was found to be higher during the "cold" season compared to the "hot" one, our study provided only limited evidence in favor of the hypothesis, that the different pattern of seasonal variations of biomarkers among nail technicians might have resulted from seasonal fluctuations in their occupational exposure to VOCs.

Conclusion: Further investigation is thus needed in order to elucidate the effect of low-level occupational exposure to VOCs on seasonal variations of biomarkers of oxidative stress.

Keywords: Oxidative stress, Seasonal variation, Occupational exposure, Volatile organic compound, Nail technicians

* Correspondence: pgresner@imp.lodz.pl
Department of Toxicology and Carcinogenesis, Nofer Institute of Occupational Medicine, 3, Sw. Teresy str., 91-348 Lodz, Poland

Background

An increasing amount of evidence is available suggesting that prolonged occupational exposure to volatile organic compounds (VOCs; including ethanol, acetone, toluene or xylene) may result in increased levels of biomarkers of oxidative stress, DNA damage and dysregulation of cellular antioxidant defense and trigger processes leading possibly to carcinogenesis [1–8]. It is, however, a bit astounding, that some studies report these adverse outcomes to be observable also if no biological and occupational exposure limits are being exceeded [9, 10].

Licensed nail technicians present an occupational group which has raised in number recently due to increased popularity of nail salon services throughout the western countries. Illustratively, the number of nail technicians registered in USA has increased by 345 % since 1991 reaching over 393.000 in 2005 [11]. Services provided by these technicians involve a number of chemical products comprising toxic substances including VOCs. The mixture of VOCs most frequently found in nail salons consist predominantly of ethanol, acetone, toluene, xylene and several acetates. The International Agency for Research on Cancer (IARC) has classified ethanol as a group I carcinogen and exposure to this compound has been recognized as a strong risk factor for several forms of cancer. The ethanol-induced carcinogenesis involves induction of oxidative stress, as one of possible mechanisms [12]. On the other hand, acetone, toluene and xylene have not been classified by IARC as neither carcinogenic nor genotoxic to humans, but evidence on increased levels of markers of oxidative stress, chromosomal aberrations or cancer incidence among workers occupationally exposed to these substances, even at exposures far below occupational limits, has been growing recently. Although precise mechanisms underlying these effects are currently unknown, the role of oxidative stress is anticipated, as well (see [13]).

Recent studies report various adverse health-related effects of occupational exposure to chemical products used in nail industry, including skin, eyes and upper airways mucosa irritation [11, 14–16], headaches [16, 17], musculoskeletal and reproductive system disorders [11, 15–19] and asthma [11, 14]. Nevertheless, despite the undoubted occurrence of VOCs in such occupational exposure, based on available studies it rather cannot be assumed that nail technicians are being overexposed to VOCs [20]. On the other hand, the use of chemical products in close vicinity to technician's breathing zone and eyes during working procedures may constitute a source of considerable health risks. Occupational exposure limits (OELs) for chemical substances in Poland are set by Central Institute for Labor Protection – National Research Institute in Warsaw. Values of the most frequently used forms of OEL, the time-weighted average (TWA)-OEL, defining an average exposure to a substance during a 8-h workday, can be retrieved from the Institute's online archive [21]. However, in our recent study we have shown that despite the low level of occupational exposure to VOCs, far below the respective TWA-OELs, nail technicians may be subject to dysregulation of the levels of selected biomarkers of oxidative stress and DNA damage (increased activities of glutathione peroxidase 1 and ceruloplasmin, increased ratio of glutathione peroxidase 1 and superoxide dismutase 1, decreased level of oxidatively-generated DNA damage) [13]. Intriguingly, studies on human subjects, as well as those performed upon animal models, seem to suggest, that the levels of biomarkers of oxidative stress present a distinct seasonal patterns of variations, with the summer season being associated with significantly higher levels compared to the winter one [22–30].

In this study we aimed to investigate whether the levels of selected markers of oxidative stress in nail technicians occupationally exposed to VOCs present any kind of seasonal variation and if so, whether these changes differ significantly from those found in general control population. To this end, we evaluated a panel of biomarkers of oxidative stress (the plasma levels of thiobarbituric acid-reactive species (TBARS) and ceruloplasmin (Cp), the blood plasma activity of glutathione peroxidase (GPx3), the red blood cells' activities of GPx1, zinc-copper superoxide dismutase (SOD1) and the SOD1/GPx1 ratio) in female nail technicians working in nail salons during the late spring/summer (the so-called "hot") and late autumn/winter (the so-called "cold") season and test their differences against healthy unexposed controls. Moreover, airborne concentrations of selected organic solvents in workrooms of respective nail salons were measured and analyzed in order to find out whether these concentrations change throughout the year and whether they might be associated with possible seasonal variations of the levels of biomarkers in nail technicians.

Methods

Recruitment of study and control subjects

The study group consisted of nail technicians occupationally exposed to low levels of VOCs, recruited from nail and/or beauty salons providing manicure and/or artificial nail sculpturing services selected randomly within downtown as well as suburb areas of the city of Lodz in central Poland. In total, three hundred and eighteen nail/beauty salons were contacted during the recruitment. Ultimately, the study group consisted of 145 female nail technicians of white descent aged 21 to 64 years (median age at the time of enrollment 34 years; interquartile range (IQR): 27–42 years.) from 109 different nail and/or beauty salons. All enrolled nail technicians were scheduled for blood withdrawal and workroom air sampling. If any health-related problems happened to occur to nail technicians on scheduled days, other days were scheduled to ensure all enrolled nail technicians were healthy at the time of measurements.

The control group consisted of 145 healthy female volunteers, aged 19 to 59 years (median age at the time of enrolment 33 years; IQR: 27–42 years), who agreed to undergo examinations. All control subjects were also of white descent, citizens of the Lodz district, without any history of occupational exposure to organic solvents or airborne acrylates, not involved in nail industry.

Both the nail technicians and controls were enrolled in two waves: the first one was between May and July (i.e., the late spring/summer period, hereinafter referred to as the so-called "hot" season") involving 66 nail technicians from 45 different nail salons (median age: 33 years; IQR: 28–41 years) and 101 control subjects (median age: 32 years; IQR: 26–42 years), and the other one between November and February (i.e., the late autumn/winter period, hereinafter referred to as the so-called "cold" season") involving 79 nail technicians from 64 different nail salons (median age: 34 years; IQR: 27–42) and 44 controls (median age: 34 years; IQR: 27–42 years). Supplementary information on lifetime tobacco-smoking history was collected from each individual enrolled in the study. All individuals were classified as never- or ever-smokers based on the criterion suggested by Pomerleau et al. [31], according to which the ever-smokers class consisted of current or former smokers with the lifetime history of smoking higher than 19 cigarettes. Additionally, precise lifetime tobacco consumption was expressed by means of the pack-years (i.e., the number of cigarette packs smoked per day times the number of years as a smoker; PY). The summary characteristics of both groups involved in the study is provided in Table 1.

Ethical issues

Prior to any further measurements, written and informed consent for participation in this study was obtained from each participant. All procedures performed in this study were in accordance with the ethical standards of the institutional and/or national research committee and with the 1964 Helsinki Declaration and its later amendments or comparable ethical standards. The study was approved by the Bioethics Committee of the Nofer Institute of Occupational Medicine (resolution no. 5/2011).

Blood withdrawal

To avoid the effect of daytime itself on the oxidative stress status, blood withdrawal was performed always in the morning before work, at around 8:00 – 9:00 am. A sample of peripheral blood was collected from each participant involved in the study by venipuncture into tubes containing either EDTA or heparin as anticoagulants. Heparinized blood was centrifuged (10 min, 1500 × g, 4 °C) in order to isolate blood plasma and red blood cells (RBCs). Further on, blood plasma was frozen at −80 °C and subsequently used in order to determine the level of TBARS, the activity of GPx3 and plasma level of Cp. In lysed RBCs the GPx1 and SOD1 activity assays were performed.

Assays of biomarkers of oxidative stress

The whole panel of biomarkers of oxidative stress was assayed in each subject enrolled in the study.

The blood plasma level of TBARS was determined using the method previously described by Wasowicz et al., based on the reaction of 2-thiobarbituric acid (TBA) with malondialdehyde, which is a naturally occurring side-product of lipid peroxidation [32]. The assay was conducted on a PerkinElmer LS50-B fluorescence spectrometer (PerkinElmer, Shelton, CT, USA) and the concentration of TBARS in blood plasma was expressed in μM.

The activity of RBCs' SOD1 was determined spectrophotometrically according to method described earlier by Beauchamp and Fridovich. The method consists in SOD1-mediated inhibition of the reduction of nitro blue tetrazolium (NBT) and the enzymatic activity of SOD1

Table 1 Characteristics of the groups of subjects involved in the study

	"Hot" season (May-July)		"Cold" season (November-February)	
Feature	Nail Technicians	Controls	Nail Technicians	Controls
Total number	66	101	79	44
Age [years]	33 [28–41]	32 [26–42]	34 [27–42]	34 [27–42]
Smoking status [never/ever]	26/40 [0.39/0.61]*	69/32 [0.68/0/32]	42/37 [0.53/0.47]	29/15 [0.66/0.34]
Pack-years	0.15 [0.0–22.5]**	0.0 [0.0–25.0]	0.0 [0.0–13.5]	0.0 [0.0–3.8]

Numerical data for age and pack-years presented as median [range]. Smoking status [never/ever-smokers] expressed as absolute [relative] counts. Age and pack-years were tested for significant differences among the groups using the Kruskal-Wallis H test with subsequent post-hoc comparisons performed using the z test. Smoking status was tested for significant differences among the groups using the log-linear analysis of contingency tables

*$p < 0.0005$ (nail technicians vs. control subjects during the "hot" season)

**$p < 0.01$ (nail technicians vs. control subjects during the "hot" season)

was expressed in units per mg haemoglobin (U/mg Hb) with 1 unit corresponding to amount of enzyme that reduces the rate of NBT reduction to 50 % per 1 min [33].

The GPx activities in peripheral blood plasma (GPx3) and RBC (GPx1) were determined according to method described by Paglia and Valentine based on spectrophotometric assessment of the oxidation of NADPH in the presence of exogenous glutathione reductase, NADPH, utilizing *tert*-butyl hydroperoxide as a substrate [34]. The enzymatic activity was expressed in units per milliliter (U/mL) and unit per gram of haemoglobin (U/g Hb) for plasma and RBC, respectively, with 1 unit equal to 1 μmol NADPH oxidized per 1 min.

Oxidase activity of ceruloplasmin in blood plasma was determined according to method described earlier by Sunderman and Nomoto [35]. The method consists in Cp-mediated oxidation of *p*-phenylenediamine hydrochloride yielding a color product measured spectrophotometrically at 535 nm. The rate of formation of the color product, corrected for nonenzymatic oxidation of *p*-phenylenediamine hydrochloride, is proportional to the blood plasma concentration of Cp, expressed in g/l.

All assays were optimized and performed using a Thermo Scientific Evolution 3000 UV/VIS spectrophotometer (Thermo Scientific, Wlatham, MA, USA).

Air sampling and chromatographic determination of airborne solvents

Air samples from nail salon workrooms were collected using the Sensidyne GilAir-3SC EX Atex air sampling pumps (Sensidyne, Clearwater, FL, USA) equipped with Anasorb 747 sorbent tubes (SKC, Dorset, UK). All measurements were performed as stationary but in the case of each nail technician the sampling pump was placed on a working table directly within the nail technician's working field, close to her breathing zone, in order to assure that the collected air sample mimicked the air the nail technician was breathing during the treatment. Each air sampling was performed on a weekday in busy hours during a period in which nail treatments were scheduled and lasted from 41 to 234 min (median 116 min; IQR 89–142 min). A single workroom air sample was collected per salon. If there were more nail technicians in one salon enrolled in the study, air sampling was scheduled on a day when all of them were at work and performing nail treatments. Prior to each sampling, sampling pumps were calibrated using a soap bubble flow meter and were operated during sampling at flow rate of 100 mL/min. After sampling, the tubes were stored at −20 °C prior to desorption and analysis which were performed according to method described previously by Gjolstad et al. [36] with minor modifications. Briefly, solvent tubes were desorbed in 1.5 mL of carbon disulfide and N,N-dimethylformamide (98:2, v/v) and sonicated for 30 min. Airborne solvents were quantified by means of external standard calibration with volumetrically prepared solution in carbon disulfide and dimethylformamide. Sorbent from an unexposed tube was added in order to correct for desorption efficiency. Chromatographic determination of solvents in workroom air samples was performed using Agilent's 6890 N gas chromatograph with 5973 Network mass selective detector and HP-5MS capillary column (Model 19091S-433; 30 m × 0.25 mm × 0.25 μm was used (Agilent Technologies, Palo Alto, CA, USA). In all analytical measurements, helium was used as carrier gas. The column temperature was initially held at 35 °C for 3 min, raised at 20 °C/min to 80 °C and then held at 80 °C for 7 min and finally raised at 5 °C/min up to 150 °C. The total runtime was 26.25 min. Mass spectrometer operated in SCAN mode with an associated m/z range set from 40 to 250. Peak integration was based on extracted ion and retention times for standard. All chemicals used in chromatographic assays except for ethanol (Witko, Poland), acetone, N,N-dimethylformamide (both from Polish Chemicals, Poland) and carbon disulfide (Analityk, Poland) were from Sigma-Aldrich (USA).

Statistical analysis

Normal distribution of numerical data was tested by means of the Shapiro-Wilk *W* test. Since the data on levels of biomarkers of oxidative stress met all relevant criteria for normal distribution but were found to be significantly right-skewed, they were logarithmically transformed prior to further analysis. Transformed data fulfilling all the criteria for normal distribution are presented as mean ± standard deviation (SD) and expressed in ln-units. Analysis of outliers was performed on the basis of estimated Cook's distances. Inter-seasonal and between-group differences in biomarkers of oxidative stress were tested for significance employing the multivariate analysis of covariance (MANCOVA) with the Wilk's Lambda statistics. Univariate ANCOVA was also performed for each individual biomarker of oxidative stress. All analyses of covariance were adjusted to age and smoking-habits as confounders, but employing two different approaches: the analyses either involved (1) each subject's age and lifetime pack-years as confounders in order to control for these additional two factors likely affecting the resultant oxidative stress, or (2) were performed following the stratification of all enrolled subjects according to their smoking status (i.e., never- or ever-smokers) involving only subject's age as confounder in each stratum analyzed separately. Post-hoc univariate comparisons were performed using the Scheffé test.

Measured airborne concentrations of organic solvents departed from normal distribution and are thus provided as medians [range]. Between-season differences in airborne levels of organic solvents were tested for significance using the Mann–Whitney U test. Assessment of the combined exposure to the mixture of organic solvents with similar toxicological effects was performed using the American Conference of Governmental Industrial Hygienists (ACGIH) formula for evaluating the additive effect by means of the formula $\Sigma(C_i/N_i)$, where C_i and N_i are the measured airborne concentration and time-weighted average occupational exposure limit (TWA-OEL) for i^{th} component. Polish TWA-OELs were used for the purposes of this study.

Simple inter-group comparisons of non-paired data were performed using the Mann–Whitney U, Student's t, or two-sided exact mid-P test, depending on type and distribution of data. Comparison of more than two groups were performed using log-linear analysis of contingency tables (discrete data) or the Kruskal-Wallis H-test (continuous data). The associations between airborne levels of organic solvents and biomarkers of oxidative stress were assessed by partial correlations analysis (forward stepwise regression) and expressed by means of semi-partial correlation coefficients r_{sp}.

All statistical calculations were performed using the Statistica 10 software package (StatSoft, Tulsa, USA).

Results

Seasonal variation in the levels of biomarkers of oxidative stress in nail technicians and controls

Seasonal variations in age-and-PY-adjusted levels of biomarkers of oxidative stress in nail technicians and control subjects are presented in Fig. 1. The multivariate analysis revealed the season, the group and their mutual interaction as factors significantly affecting the levels of investigated biomarkers of oxidative stress ($p << 0.0001$ for all three factors). Further univariate analyses revealed significant seasonal variations in four out of six investigated biomarkers of oxidative stress: blood plasma levels of TBARS and Cp, RBC's activity of GPx1, and the ln-ratio of SOD1/GPx1 ($p << 0.0001$ (the main effects) for all biomarkers). Furthermore, the season and the group

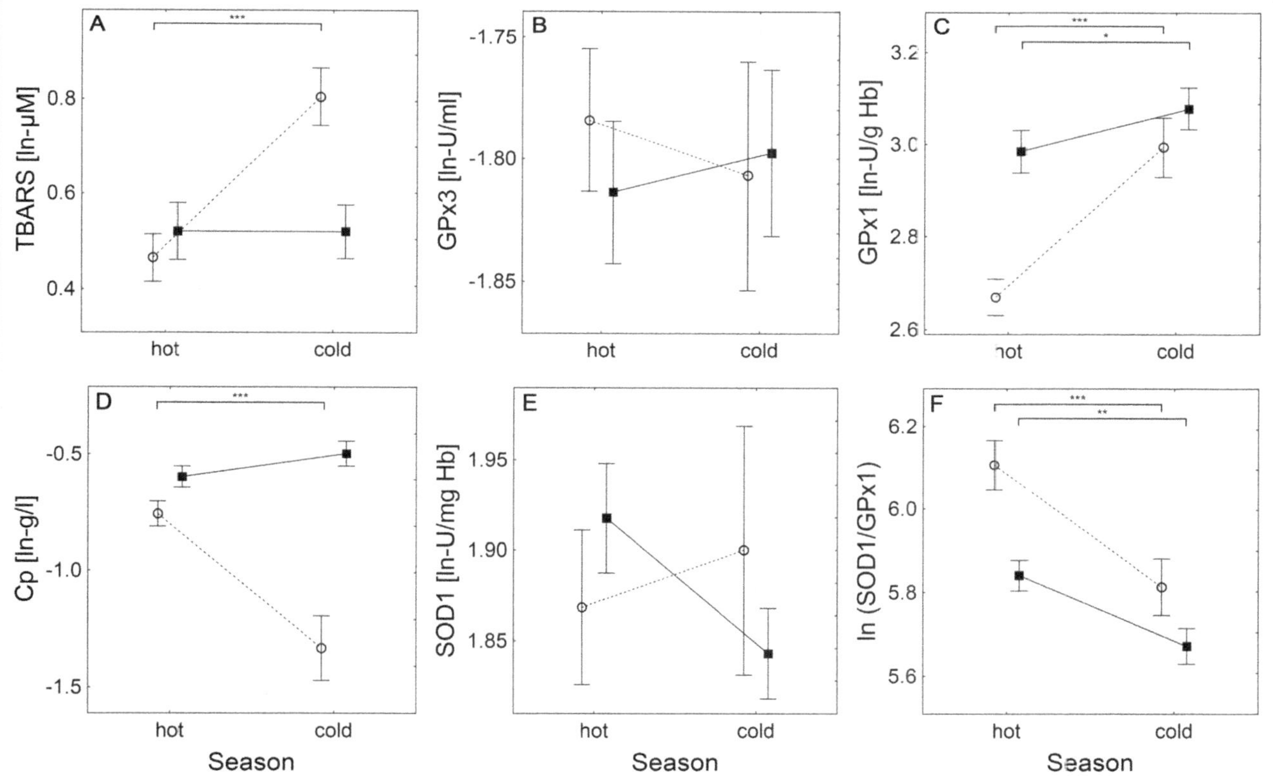

Fig. 1 Levels of biomarkers of oxidative stress in nail technicians (solid line, ■) and control subjects (dashed line, ○) during the "hot" and "cold" season. Individual panels show data for the plasma levels of TBARS (**a**), the activity of GPx3 (**b**), the activity of GPx1 (**c**), the plasma level of Cp (**d**), the activity of SOD1 (**e**) and the SOD1/GPx1 activity ratio (**f**). All data are presented as *ln*-transformed means (central points) ± SD (error bars). Natural-base logarithm transformation was employed in order to normalize the distribution of raw data for the purpose of MANCOVA analysis. Asterisks indicate the respective levels of significance of inter-season differences observed among nail technicians and/or control subjects. The activity of SOD1 (panel **e**) was found to be significantly affected by the interaction between the season and the group of given individual ($p < 0.05$) although no significant inter-seasonal differences were found * $p < 0.05$; ** $p < 0.0005$; *** $p << 0.0001$

were found to interact significantly with each other in the case of all these biomarkers (the levels of significance for the group/season interaction: $p < <0.0001$ in the case of TBARS, GPx1 and Cp; $p < 0.05$ in the case of the ln-ratio of SOD1/GPx1) indicating, that the seasonal variations in investigated biomarkers of oxidative stress differ significantly between the two groups involved.

In fact, the blood plasma levels of TBARS (Fig. 1a) were found to be significantly increased during the "cold" season compared to the "hot" one in controls ("hot" vs. "cold" season: 0.46 ± 0.25 vs. 0.80 ± 0.20 ln-μM, $p < <0.0001$) but not in nail technicians, in the case of which no significant differences between the two seasons were observed ("hot" vs. "cold" season: 0.52 ± 0.24 vs. 0.52 ± 0.25 ln-μM, *NS*). In contrast to the "hot" season, during the "cold" one, the levels of TBARS in controls differed significantly from that of nail technicians ($p < <0.0001$).

In the case of the RBC's GPx1 (Fig. 1c), the "cold" season was associated with significantly increased activities of this enzyme in both the controls ("hot" vs. "cold" season: 2.67 ± 0.20 vs. 2.99 ± 0.21 ln-U/g Hb, $p < <0.0001$) and nail technicians ("hot" vs. "cold" season: 2.98 ± 0.19 vs. 3.08 ± 0.20 ln-U/g Hb, $p < 0.05$). Although the levels of GPx1 differed significantly between controls and nail technicians during the "hot" season ($p < <0.0001$), the much more pronounced increase observed in controls resulted in the level of GPx1 activity reaching almost the one found in nail technicians, without any significant differences between these two groups during the "cold" season.

Concerning the blood plasma levels of ceruloplasmin (Fig. 1d), the seasonal changes between "hot" and "cold" season were observed only among controls with the "cold" season being associated with significantly lower values compared to the "hot" one ("hot" vs. "cold": -0.76 ± 0.27 vs. -1.33 ± 0.46 ln-g/L, $p < <0.0001$), but not among nail technicians in the case of which the ceruloplasmin levels were slightly but insignificantly increased during the "cold" season ("hot" vs. "cold": -0.60 ± 0.19 vs. -0.50 ± 0.24 ln-g/L, *NS*). Nail technicians presented increased blood plasma levels of ceruloplasmin compared to control subjects, irrespective of the season ("hot": $p < 0.01$; "cold": $p < <0.0001$).

In the case of the ln-ratio of SOD1/GPx1 (Fig. 1f), the seasonal variability was observed in both the controls ("hot" vs. "cold": 6.11 ± 0.30 vs. 5.81 ± 0.22, $p < <0.0001$) as well as nail technicians ("hot" vs. "cold": 5.84 ± 0.15 vs. 5.67 ± 0.19, $p < 0.0005$) with the "cold" season being associated with significantly lower values. Nevertheless, the difference was much more pronounced among controls. The value of the SOD1/GPx1 ln-ratio was significantly lower compared to control subjects, irrespectively of the season ("hot": $p < <0.0001$; "cold": $p < <0.05$).

In the case of the RBC's activity of SOD1, no significant main effect of either the season or the group to which the given subject belonged was observed, although the resultant level of this biomarker was found to be affected by significant interaction between these two main factors ($p < 0.05$). Based on data presented in Fig. 1e it is obvious that inter-seasonal changes in SOD1 activity, although insignificant, differ in their direction, with the "cold" season resulting in slight reduction of SOD1 activity among nail technicians ("hot" vs. "cold": 1.92 ± 0.12 vs. 1.84 ± 0.11 ln-U/mg Hb, *NS*), but slight increase among controls ("hot" vs. "cold": 1.87 ± 0.22 vs. 1.90 ± 0.23 ln-U/mg Hb, *NS*), instead. Nevertheless, none of these inter-seasonal, as well as none of the between-group changes, reached the level of statistical significance.

The blood plasma activity of GPx3 (Fig. 1b) was found to be independent of the season in both the controls and the nail technicians, with no significant differences between these two groups being observable, either.

Individual's smoking status was not found to interact significantly with the season and further modulate the above described seasonal changes in TBARS, GPx1, Cp, SOD1 and SOD1/GPx1, or the lack of changes in the case of GPx3: the pattern of seasonal changes observed among controls and nail technicians enrolled in this study was found to be the same in both the never-smokers and ever-smokers stratum, irrespective of whether univariate or multivariate analysis of covariance was employed (*data not shown*).

Airborne levels of organic solvents in nail salon workrooms during the "hot" and "cold" seasons

The measured airborne concentrations of organic solvents in air samples from nail salon workrooms are summarized in Table 2. During the "cold" season, total pool of organic solvents in nail salon workrooms as well as the combined exposure of nail technicians to mixture of organic solvents were significantly higher compared to the "hot" one (24.22 mg/m^3 vs. 7.60 mg/m^3, $p < <0.0001$ for total measured pool; 0.057 vs. 0.019, $p < 0.0005$ for combined exposure). During both seasons, ethanol, 2-propanol and ethyl acetate were the three most abundant organic solvents found in air samples from the nail salon workrooms and, moreover, were found to be also significantly increased during the "cold" season compared to the "hot" one ($p < <0.0001$, $p < 0.01$ and $p < 0.05$, respectively). Intriguingly, toluene and isopropyl acetate were found to be significantly lower during the "cold" season ($p < 0.05$ and $p < <0.0001$, respectively), yet these organic solvents were found to be two orders of magnitude less abundant in workroom air samples, and thus their inter-seasonal differences were far less pronounced. The inter-seasonal differences in airborne levels of acetone, 2-butanone and n-butyl acetate were insignificant. Nevertheless, median airborne levels of all organic solvents analyzed

Table 2 Airborne concentrations of organic solvents in nail salons, combined occupational exposure of nail technicians during the "hot" and "cold season

	TWA-OEL	"Hot" season	"Cold" season
Ethanol [mg/m^3]	1900	1.57 [0.06–16.12]	6.96 [0.35–54.77]****
Acetone [mg/m^3]	600	0.81 [0.03–43.23]	0.57 [0.05–61.69]
Toluene [mg/m^3]	100	0.02 [0.004–0.30]	0.01 [0.000–0.62]*
2-propanol (isopropyl alcohol) [mg/m^3]	900	1.31 [0.11–21.30]	3.44 [0.12–37.70]**
2-butanone (methyl ethyl ketone) [mg/m^3]	200	0.04 [0.007–0.92]	0.05 [0.002–1.63]
Ethyl acetate [mg/m^3]	200	1.36 [0.07–27.28]	3.96 [0.03–44.54]*
Isopropyl acetate [mg/m^3]	600	0.02 [0.010–0.10]	0.01 [0.000–0.22]****
n-butyl acetate [mg/m^3]	200	0.23 [0.021–4.87]	0.17 [0.00–18.53]
Total [mg/m^3]	-	7.60 [0.57–70.62]	24.22 [1.55–132.28]****
$\Sigma(C_i/N_i)$	1.0	0.019 [0.002–0.170]	0.057 [0.002–0.254]***

Airborne levels of organic solvents measured in air samples collected from nail salon workrooms during the "hot" ($N = 45$) and the "cold" ($N = 64$) season. Data presented as median [range] airborne concentrations were tested for significant inter-seasonal differences using the Mann–Whitney *U* test. TWA-OEL stands for the Polish time-weighted average occupational exposure limit of the respective organic solvent. $\Sigma(C_i/N_i)$ stands for the ACGIH measure of the additive effect of combined exposure of the mixture of organic solvents, with respective threshold value equal 1

$^{*}p < 0.05$; $^{**}p < 0.01$; $^{***}p < 0.0005$; $^{****}p < 0.0001$

in this study were found to be far below the respective Polish TWA-OELs.

Correlation analysis

Results of stepwise partial correlation analysis, in which associations between airborne levels of organic solvents and biomarkers of oxidative stress (adjusted for age distribution) were analyzed, are presented in Table 3. The activity of cytosolic GPx1 was positively correlated with airborne ethanol ($r_{SP} = 0.26$, $p < 0.05$), but negatively with airborne toluene ($r_{SP} = -0.25$, $p < 0.05$) levels. Moreover, the blood plasma concentration of Cp correlated positively with airborne ethyl acetate ($r_{SP} = 0.22$, $p < 0.05$), but negatively with isopropyl acetate ($r_{SP} = -0.25$, $p < 0.05$). The activity of RBC's SOD1 was negatively correlated with airborne acetone ($r_{SP} = -0.25$, $p < 0.05$).

Discussion

In this study, we investigated the seasonal variations in selected biomarkers of oxidative stress (the plasma levels of TBARS and Cp, activities of GPx3, GPx1 and SOD1, and the SOD1/GPx1 ratio) in the group of nail technicians occupationally exposed to VOCs and unexposed control subjects. Significant differences between the so-called "hot" and "cold" seasons were observed in the case of plasma levels of TBARS and Cp, the activity of GPx1 and the SOD1/GPx1 ratio suggesting that these biomarkers of oxidative stress may be subject to seasonal variations. More importantly, statistical analysis revealed a significant interaction between the effect of the season and the occupational exposure, as we found the pattern of these variations among nail technicians to be different compared to that of the control subjects. In the "cold" season, the plasma levels of TBARS were found to increase significantly compared to the "hot" season, but only among controls with no changes being observable among nail technicians. In both investigated groups, the "cold" season was associated with increased activity of GPx1 compared to the "hot" one nevertheless, the difference was more pronounced among controls. In the case of Cp, its plasma level in the "cold" season was found to drop significantly among controls, but was found to be significantly increased among nail technicians with the amplitude of inter-seasonal change being several times less the one observed among controls.

Table 3 Results of partial correlation analysis between airborne levels of organic solvents and biomarkers of oxidative stress in nail technicians

	TBARS [ln-μM]	GPx3 [ln-U/mL]	GPx1 [ln-U/g Hb]	Cp [ln-g/L]	SOD1 [ln-U/mg Hb]
Ethanol [ln-mg/m^3]	0.1813	0.0677	**0.2628***	−0.1064	0.1004
Acetone [ln-mg/m^3]	−0.0661	0.0915	−0.0567	0.2263	**−0.2537***
Toluene [ln-mg/m^3]	−0.0147	−0.1793	**−0.2519***	−0.1047	−0.0036
2-propanol [ln-mg/m^3]	−0.0583	−0.0456	0.0085	0.0543	0.1263
2-butanone [ln-mg/m^3]	0.0589	0.0219	−0.0473	0.0380	0.1546
Ethyl acetate [ln-mg/m^3]	−0.1057	0.1658	−0.0081	**0.2208***	0.0110
Isopropyl acetate [ln-mg/m^3]	0.0080	0.0431	−0.0513	**−0.2522***	0.2146
n-butyl acetate [ln-mg/m^3]	0.1906	0.0407	−0.1070	−0.0057	−0.1063

Presented are the semi-partial correlation coefficients (r_{sp}) for each given pair of airborne level of organic solvent and level of analyzed biomarker. Forward stepwise regression procedure upon *ln*-transformed data was employed. Significant associations are indicated in bold with respective level of significance indicated by the superscript. The portion of variability explained by the association: ethanol vs. GPx1: 6.9 %; acetone vs. SOD1: 6.4 %; toluene vs. GPx1: 6.3 %; ethyl acetate vs. Cp: 4.9 %; isopropyl acetate vs. Cp: 6.4 %

$^{*}p < 0.05$

Finally, the SOD1/GPx1 ratio was found to drop significantly in the "cold" season in both examined groups when compared to the "hot" one, nevertheless, the difference was more pronounced among controls. The activity of SOD1 seems to present opposite directions of changes due to seasonal variations in the two groups, although no significant changes for this biomarker were found.

In the literature, a couple of studies involving human subjects [22, 23, 25, 37] as well as animal models [22, 26–30] investigating the seasonal variability of the levels of biomarkers of oxidative stress can be found, suggesting that the summer (i.e., the "hot") season is likely associated with increased levels of biomarkers of oxidative stress (including the plasma level of TBARS, the activities of antioxidant enzymes, the level of DNA damage) compared to the winter (i.e., the "cold") one. Although the precise mechanism of such seasonal variability remains poorly understood, authors suggest that the balance may be shifted towards increased oxidative stress during the summer (i.e., the "hot") season due to an increased sunlight radiation and/or increased ambient temperature and humidity during this season [23, 28, 37]. Endothelial activation [22], altered melatonin levels [25], intensified temperature-dependent lipid peroxidation due to altered iron content in certain proteins [38], altered levels of glucocorticoids and altered ADP sensitivity and oxidative capacity of mitochondria associated with circannual changes in metabolism [30] are all among proposed molecular mechanisms leading plausibly to such shift towards increased oxidative stress. In the present study, we did not observe such consistently increased levels of biomarkers of oxidative stress during the "hot" season among the control subjects. During the "hot" season, increased activity levels were found only for plasma ceruloplasmin and plasma GPx3, with the latter one showing only slight and insignificant change compared to the "cold" season. On the other hand, plasma levels of TBARS and the activity of GPx1 were significantly decreased during the "hot" season. It is somehow puzzling why the seasonal variation in biomarkers of oxidative stress observed in our study presented a pattern which seems to be incompatible with the patterns of variation reported previously by the above cited studies. Thorough survey of the currently available literature, however, revealed, that in available studies there is also a certain degree of inconsistency, as reports on significantly lower levels of activities of antioxidant enzymes or lack of any changes in plasma TBARS during the summer season compared to the winter one can be found [22, 28, 29]. For example, the changes observed in the group of control subjects involved in studies by Rossner et al. [39, 40] also seems not to be in line with the hypothesis that the summer season is associated with increased levels of the biomarkers: comparing the levels of biomarkers of oxidative stress and oxidatively generated damage to lipids and DNA measured during the three consecutive seasons (winter, summer, winter), among control subjects, a trend of gradual increase of the values was observed, instead of the summer-season values being significantly higher compared to the values from previous and subsequent winter seasons. It might thus implicate that some other factors, not considered in the hereby cited studies, are involved in the modulation of the resultant levels of biomarkers. As suggested by Moller et al., such plausible factors may include average daily influx of sunlight during a certain period (around 50 days) prior to sample withdrawal, with the highest importance being attributed to the average sunlight influx during last 3–6 days prior to the measurement [23]. No such parameter was controlled or monitored in any of the above mentioned studies, neither was it in the hereby presented study, what may, at least to some degree, explain the observed discrepancies between the studies. Moreover, it has to be kept in mind, that TBARS, for example, is not a malondialdehyde-specific biomarker and that this assay may in principle detect any thiobarbituric acid-reactive compound, not necessarily derived from lipid peroxidation. Nevertheless, this aspect is surely worth thorough examination.

More importantly, examining the outcomes obtained in this study, it seems plausible that the seasonal variations in biomarkers of oxidative stress among nail technicians occupationally exposed to VOCs present markedly different patterns when compared to those observed among control subjects. At first glance, it seems apparent, that amplitude of inter-seasonal changes of the plasma levels of TBARS, the activity of GPx1, the plasma levels of Cp and the SOD1/GPx1 ratio in nail technicians observed in our study was attenuated to some degree, reaching only 0.1 %, 29.1 %, 17.7 % and 57.7 % of the respective amplitudes observed among unexposed controls. Moreover, the direction of inter-seasonal changes of plasma levels of Cp and the activity of SOD1 among nail technicians seems to be reversed compared to the one observed among controls. It seems reasonably to state, that the pattern of inter-seasonal changes of these biomarkers observed in nail technicians is not only significantly different compared to the one observed among control subjects enrolled in this study, but it seems to be different also compared to the pattern of seasonal variations reported in the previously published studies cited above.

At this point, one would probably consider as what might be the plausible causes of such different patterns of seasonal variability of investigated biomarkers among nail technicians when compared to unexposed controls. Undoubtedly, occupational exposure of nail technicians to VOCs would be among the major factors probably thought of as being responsible for this kind of differences. But first, it has to be stated, that based on the maximum combined exposure to the mixture of VOCs observed in our study, which was below 20 % and 25 % of TWA-OEL during the "hot" and "cold" season, respectively, we do not have any reasonable evidence to conclude that this occupational group is overexposed to VOCs, at least as long as the current occupational standards are considered. This conclusion seems to hold true also when occupational exposures to individual VOCs investigated in our study are considered separately: since the airborne levels of all VOCs investigated in our study were all far below the respective TWA-OELs, no overexposure to any VOC investigated in this study can be assumed. Similar outcomes were reported previously by several other studies [17, 20, 36, 41–43].

Even though the occupational exposure to VOCs among nail technicians was found to be very low, we found it to be significantly increased during the "cold" season compared to the "hot" one: the differences were apparent in the case of the combined exposure to the mixture of VOCs (3.0-times higher during the winer; $p < 0.0005$), as well as in the case of the airborne levels of the three most abundant VOC found in workroom air samples - ethanol (4.4-times higher; $p < 0.0001$), 2-propanol (2.6-times higher; $p < 0.01$) and ethyl acetate (2.9-times higher; $p < 0.05$). A question arises as what can be the cause of such increased airborne levels of organic solvents in nail salons during the "cold" season. Available studies indicate that in occupied houses, the ventilation behavior varies throughout the year and that it may significantly influence the rate of air exchange in rooms [44]. Moreover, studies by Goldin et al. [42] and Reolofs et al. [20] provide evidence of increased CO_2 content in some 75 % of nail salons indicating that the vast majority of nail salons do not meet the minimum ventilation requirements. Even though no records of window opening or any ventilation measurements in nail salons were performed in this study, based on this data, one can now speculate that the pattern of seasonal variation of the levels of biomarkers of oxidative stress found in nail technicians enrolled in our study may be attributable to their increased occupational exposure to VOCs due to limited workroom ventilation during the "cold" season and that this effect might have outmatched the effects supposedly imposed by increased temperature, humidity and sunlight during the "hot" season, observed among control subjects. This hypothesis, however, seems not to be supported by the outcomes of the correlation analysis performed in this study, as this analysis provided very limited evidence corroborating the possible correlation between the airborne levels of VOCs and the levels of biomarkers of oxidative stress among nail technicians. The airborne ethanol and ethyl acetate, the two of three most abundant VOCs, were the only exception, as they were found to be positively correlated with the activity of GPx1 and blood plasma levels of Cp, respectively. Nevertheless, these correlations, despite being statistically significant ($p < 0.05$), were relatively weak, explaining only some 7 % and 5 % of the seasonal variability of the respective biomarker in nail technicians. This may indicate, that the background underlying the seasonal changes observed in nail technicians might be more complex than just simple associations with airborne levels of VOCs during work-time and that possible differences in some other factors (including lifestyle-related factors, such as moderate physical activity, diet, coffee intake, alcohol consumption, etc.) not involved in this study may have contributed to observed outcomes. It might also be of importance, that airborne ethanol in nail salons was found to correlate significantly with the DNA strand breakage ($r_{SP} = 0.287$; $R^2 = 0.082$; $p < 0.001$) and oxidatively generated DNA damage ($r_{SP} = -0.259$; $R^2 = 0.067$; $p < 0.05$) in nail technicians ([13] and *unpublished data*), pointing to some plausible role of this organic solvent in predicting the level of investigated biomarkers among nail technicians. Although this compound has long been considered a potent inductor of reactive oxygen species both in vitro and in vivo [45], yet this aspect definitely requires more research.

Unfortunately, the number of studies investigating the effect of prolonged low-level occupational and/or the environmental exposure to VOCs on levels of biomarkers of oxidative stress is scarce so far, and they provide inconclusive outcomes. In studies involving occupationally exposed bus drivers, Rossner et al. failed to identify airborne VOCs as an independent factor predicting the levels of biomarkers of oxidative stress [39, 40]. On the other hand, low-level exposure to airborne toluene was found to be the only independent factor responsible for increased levels of biomarkers of oxidative stress and DNA damage among painters exposed to various xenobiotics in paints [9, 10]. In general population, the low-level environmental exposure to airborne VOCs was found to correlate significantly with biomarkers of oxidative stress (including DNA damage), although this correlation was limited to older subjects only [46]. It is therefore obvious, that this issue is not sufficiently understood and that further research is needed.

When interpreting our outcomes, one has to keep in mind, that only static and short-term breathing-zone area measurements were performed in order to assess the occupational exposure of nail technician, which might have led to slight underestimation of the real exposure. In addition to this, the measured exposures presented in our study need to be considered as approximations of the workday exposure to VOCs in nail salons, as they were averaged over 2 h on average only, not over a period of 6 h, which is required in Poland in order to make the reliable comparison with respective TWA-

OELs. It also needs to be emphasized, that the "hot" and "cold" season groups investigated in our study consisted of unpaired subjects, what may have introduced some additional between-group variation. Although this variation was dealt with by using statistical methods suited for analysis of unpaired data (instead of methods developed for testing the significance of differences in paired data), this aspect still has to be kept in mind. Last but not least, no sunlight radiation, ambient temperature and humidity monitoring during the "hot" and "cold" season was conducted within the framework of our study, due to which we were unable to precisely infer how the occupational exposure to VOCs interfered with the effect of temperature, humidity and sunlight radiation and/or their variations between the two seasons under discussion.

Conclusion

To sum up, in this study we provide evidence, that nail technicians present significantly different pattern of seasonal variation in selected biomarkers of oxidative stress compared to control subjects. Although such differences might intuitively be attributed to occupational exposure of nail technicians to VOCs which we found to be higher during the "cold" season compared to the "hot" one, our study did not provide convincing evidence in favor of such hypothesis and thus further studies must be conducted in order to elucidate possible factors underlying such differences between control subjects and nail technicians observed in our study.

Abbreviations

% DNA, relative amount of DNA in the comet tail; ACGIH, American Conference of Governmental Industrial Hygienists; ALSs, alkaline-labile sites; Cp, ceruloplasmin; FPGs, formamidopyrimidine glycosylase-sensitive sites; GPx, glutathione peroxidase; IARC, International Agency for Research on Cancer; IQR, Interquartile Range; MANCOVA, multivariate analysis of covariance; PY, pack-years; RBCs, red blood cells; SD, standard deviation; SOD1, zinc-copper superoxide dismutase; SSBs, single strand DNA breaks; TBARS, thiobarbituric acid-reactive species; TWA-OEL, time-weighted average occupational exposure limit; VOCs, volatile organic substances

Acknowledgements

Not applicable.

Funding

The study was supported by the National Science Centre grant No. PB/2011/01/B/NZ7/04681 and the Nofer Institute of Occupational Medicine fund no. IMP 1.18/2013.

Authors' contribution

PG, JG and WW designed and conceived the study. PG, RS, MBK, and ET performed the experiments. PG analyzed the data. PG, JG and WW wrote the paper. All authors read and approved the final manuscript.

Competing interests

The authors declare that they have no competing interests.

References

1. Manikantan P, Balachanadar V, Sasikala K, Mohanadevi S, Arun M, Kumar AK, Khan Mustaq Ahamed SA, Krishnan BB, Kumar SS. Cytogenetic methods for assessing human exposure to toluene in Coimbatore, South India. Asian Pac J Cancer Prev. 2010;11:1687–93.
2. Tunca BT, Egeli U. Cytogenetic findings on shoe workers exposed long-term to benzene. Environ Health Perspect. 1996;104(Suppl):1313–7.
3. Bogadi-Sare A, Brumen V, Turk R, Karacic V, Zavalic M. Genotoxic effects in workers exposed to benzene: with special reference to exposure biomarkers and confounding factors. Ind Health. 1997;35:367–73.
4. Gerin M, Siemiatycki J, Desy M, Krewski D. Associations between several sites of cancer and occupational exposure to benzene, toluene, xylene, and styrene: results of a case-control study in Montreal. Am J Ind Med. 1998;34:144–56.
5. Lundberg I, Milatou-Smith R. Mortality and cancer incidence among Swedish paint industry workers with long-term exposure to organic solvents. Scand J Work Environ Health. 1998;24:270–5.
6. Liu Y, Zhou Q, Xie X, Lin D, Dong L. Oxidative stress and DNA damage in the earthworm Eisenia fetida induced by toluene, ethylbenzene and xylene. Ecotoxicology. 2010;19(8):1551–9.
7. Singh MP, Mishra M, Sharma A, Shukla AK, Mudiam MKR, Patel DK, Ram KR, Chowdhuri DK. Genotoxicity and apoptosis in Drosophila melanogaster exposed to benzene, toluene and xylene: attenuation by quercetin and curcumin. Toxicol Appl Pharmacol. 2011;253:14–30.
8. Coskun O, Oter S, Korkmaz A, Armutcu F, Kanter M. The oxidative and morphological effects of high concentration chronic toluene exposure on rat sciatic nerves. Neurochem Res. 2005;30:33–8.
9. Moro AM, Charão M, Brucker N, Bulcão R, Freitas F, Guerreiro G, Baierle M, Nascimento S, Waechter F, Hirakata V, Linden R, Thiesen FV, Garcia SC. Effects of low-level exposure to xenobiotics present in paints on oxidative stress in workers. Sci Total Environ. 2010;408:4461–7.
10. Moro AM, Brucker N, Charão M, Bulcão R, Freitas F, Baierle M, Nascimento S, Valentini J, Cassini C, Salvador M, Linden R, Thiesen F, Buffon A, Moresco R, Garcia SC. Evaluation of genotoxicity and oxidative damage in painters exposed to low levels of toluene. Mutat Res. 2012;746:42–8.
11. Roelofs C, Azaroff LS, Holcroft C, Nguyen H, Doan T. Results from a community-based occupational health survey of Vietnamese-American nail salon workers. J Immigr Minor Health. 2008;10:353–61.
12. Yu HS, Oyama T, Isse T, Kitagawa K, Pham TT, Tanaka M, Kawamoto T. Formation of acetaldehyde-derived DNA adducts due to alcohol exposure. Chem Biol Interact. 2010;188:367–75.
13. Grešner P, Stepnik M, Król MB, Swiercz R, Smok-Pieniazek A, Twardowska E, et al. Dysregulation of markers of oxidative stress and DNA damage among nail technicians despite low exposure to volatile organic compounds. Scand J Work Environ Health. 2015;41:579–93.
14. Lazarov A. Sensitization to acrylates is a common adverse reaction to artificial fingernails. J Eur Acad Dermatol Venereol. 2007;21:169–74.
15. Quach T, Nguyen K-D, Doan-Billings P-A, Okahara L, Fan C, Reynolds P. A preliminary survey of Vietnamese nail salon workers in Alameda County, California. J Community Health. 2008;33:336–43.
16. Park S-A, Gwak S, Choi S. Assessment of occupational symptoms and chemical exposures for nail salon technicians in daegu city, Korea. J Prev Med Public Health. 2014;47:169–76.
17. Quach T, Gunier R, Tran A, Von Behren J, Doan-Billings P-A, Nguyen K-D, Okahara L, Lui BY-B, Nguyen M, Huynh J, Reynolds P. Characterizing workplace exposures in Vietnamese women working in California nail salons. Am J Public Health. 2011;101(Suppl):S271–6.
18. Reutman SR, Rohs AM, Clark JC, Johnson BC, Sammons DL, Toennis CA, Robertson SA, Mackenzie BA, Lockey JE. A pilot respiratory health assessment of nail technicians: symptoms, lung function, and airway inflammation. Am J Ind Med. 2009;875:868–75.
19. Harris-Roberts J, Bowen J, Sumner J, Stocks-Greaves M, Bradshaw L, Fishwick D, Barber CM. Work-related symptoms in nail salon technicians. Occup Med (Lond). 2011;61:335–40.
20. Roelofs C, Do T. Exposure assessment in nail salons: an indoor air approach. ISRN Public Health. 2012;2012:1–7.

21. Central Institute for Labor Protection - National Research Institute. www.ciop.pl.
22. Konior A, Klemenska E, Brudek M, Podolecka E, Czarnowska E, Beręsewicz A. Seasonal superoxide overproduction and endothelial activation in guinea-pig heart; seasonal oxidative stress in rats and humans. J Mol Cell Cardiol. 2011;50:686–69.
23. Moller P, Wallin H, Holst E, Knudsen LE. Sunlight-induced DNA damage in human mononuclear cells. FASEB J. 2002;16:45–53.
24. Møller P, Folkmann JK, Forchhammer L, Bräuner EV, Danielsen PH, Risom L, Loft S. Air pollution, oxidative damage to DNA, and carcinogenesis. Cancer Lett. 2008;266:84–97.
25. Morera AL, Intxausti A, Abreu-Gonzalez P. Winter/summer seasonal changes in malondialdehyde formation as a source of variance in oxidative stress schizophrenia research. World J Biol Psychiatry. 2009;10:576–80.
26. Belló-Klein A, Morgan-Martins MI, Barp J, Llesuy S, Belló AA, Singal PK. Circaannual changes in antioxidants and oxidative stress in the heart and liver in rats. Comp Biochem Physiol C Toxicol Pharmacol. 2000;126:203–8.
27. Bernabucci U, Ronchi B, Lacetera N, Nardone A. Markers of oxidative status in plasma and erythrocytes of transition dairy cows during hot season. J Dairy Sci. 2002;85:2173–9.
28. Bhat S, Rao G, Murthy KD, Bhat PG. Seasonal variations in markers of stress and oxidative stress in rats. Indian J Clin Biochem. 2008;23:191–4.
29. Chigerwe M, Beck AD, Kim SS, Coons DM. Comparison of plasma oxidative status biomarkers in neonatal dairy calves during summer and fall seasons. J Vet Sci Technol. 2013;S11:006.
30. Mujkosová J, Ferko M, Humeník P, Waczulíková I, Ziegelhoffer A. Seasonal variations in properties of healthy and diabetic rat heart mitochondria: Mg2+–ATPase activity, content of conjugated dienes and membrane fluidity. Physiol Res. 2008;57 Suppl 2:S75–82.
31. Pomerleau CS, Pomerleau OF, Snedecor SM, Mehringer AM. Defining a never-smoker: results from the nonsmokers survey. Addict Behav. 2004;29:1149–54.
32. Wasowicz W, Neve J, Peretz A, Nève J. Optimized steps in fluorometric determination of thiobarbituric acid-reactive substances in serum: importance of extraction pH and influence of sample preservation and storage. Clin Chem. 1993;39:2522–6.
33. Beauchamp C, Fridovich I. Superoxide dismutase: improved assays and an assay applicable to acrylamide gels. Anal Biochem. 1971;44:276–87.
34. Paglia DE, Valentine WN. Studies on the quantitative and qualitative characterization of erythrocyte glutathione peroxidase. J Lab Clin Med. 1967;70(0022–2143 (Print)):158–69.
35. Sunderman Jr FW Nomoto S. Measurement of human serum ceruloplasmin by its p-phenylenediamine oxidase activity. Clin Chem. 1970;16:903–10.
36. Gjolstad M, Thorud S, Molander P. Occupational exposure to airborne solvents during nail sculpturing. J Environ Monit. 2006;8:537–42.
37. Møller P, Knudsen LE, Loft S. The Comet assay as a rapid test in biomonitoring occupational exposure to DNA-damaging agents and effect of confounding factors 1. Cancer Epidemiol Biomarker Prev. 2000;9:1005–15.
38. Miura T, Muraoka S, Fujimoto Y. Temperature-dependent lipid peroxidation of rat brain homogenate. Res Commun Mol Pathol Pharmacol. 1998;100:117–28.
39. Rossner P, Svecova V, Milcova A, Lnenickova Z, Solansky I, Sram RJ. Seasonal variability of oxidative stress markers in city bus drivers. Part I. Oxidative damage to DNA. Mutat Res. 2008;642:14–20.
40. Rossner P, Svecova V, Milcova A, Lnenickova Z, Solansky I, Sram RJ. Seasonal variability of oxidative stress markers in city bus drivers. Part II. Oxidative damage to lipids and proteins. Mutat Res. 2008;642:21–7.
41. Yang JH, Han D-H. Occupational exposure of nail technicians to airborne chemicals and biological monitoring. J Korean Soc Occup Environ Hyg. 2010;20:53–62.
42. Goldin LJ, Ansher L, Berlin A, Cheng J, Kanopkin D, Khazan A, Kisivuli M, Lortie M, Bunker Feterson E, Pohl L, Porter S, Zeng V, Skogstrom T, Fragala MA, Myatt TA, Stewart JH, Allen JG. Indoor air quality survey of nail salons in Boston. J Immigr Minor Health. 2013;8:508–14.
43. Alaves VM, Sleeth DK, Thiese MS, Larson RR. Characterization of indoor air contaminants in a randomly selected set of commercial nail salons in Salt Lake County, Utah, USA. Int J Environ Health Res. 2013;23:419–33.
44. Wallace L, Emmerich S, Howard-Reed C. Continuous measurements of air change rates in an occupied house for 1 year: effect of temperature, winds, fans and windows. J Expo Anal Environ Epidemiol. 2002;12:296–306.
45. Comporti M, Signorini C, Leoncini S, Gardi C, Ciccoli L, Giardini A, Vecchio D, Arezzini B. Ethanol-induced oxidative stress: basic knowledge. Genes Nutr. 2010;5:101–9.
46. Hong E, Lee E, Kim Y, Oh E, Kim YW, Moon KW, Choi JW, Lee J, Roh J. The correlations between oxidative stress markers and indoor volatile organic compounds among the general population in Ansan and Incheon cities, Korea. Toxicol Environ Health Sci. 2009;1:37–48.

Tuberculin skin test and Quantiferon test agreement and influencing factors in tuberculosis screening of healthcare workers

Monica Lamberti[1], Rossella Uccello[1*†], Maria Grazia Lourdes Monaco[1†], Mariarosaria Muoio[1†], Daniela Feola[1], Nicola Sannolo[1], Albert Nienhaus[2,3] and Paolo Chiodini[4]

Abstract

Objective: A systematic review and meta-analysis was conducted to evaluate the agreement between Tuberculin Skin Test (TST) and Quantiferon (QFT) in screening for tuberculosis (TB) infection among healthcare workers (HCWs) and to estimate associations between TST and QFT agreement and variables of interest, such as *Bacillus Calmette-Guérin* (BCG) vaccination and incidence of TB.

Methods: Cross-sectional and longitudinal studies on HCWs, published in English until October 2013, comparing TST and QFT results, were selected. For each study *Cohen's κ* value and a 95% confidence interval were calculated. Summary measures and indexes of heterogeneity between studies were calculated.

Results: 29 studies were selected comprising a total of 11,434 HCWs. *Cohen's κ* for agreement between TST and QFT for 24 of them was 0.28 (95% CI 0.22 to 0.35), with the best value in high TB incidence countries and the lowest rate of BCG vaccination.

Conclusion: Currently, there is no gold standard for TB screening and the most-used diagnostic tools show low agreement. For evidence-based health surveillance in HCWs, occupational physicians need to consider a number of factors influencing screening results, such as TB incidence, vaccination status, age and working seniority.

Keywords: Tuberculosis, Tuberculin skin test, Quantiferon TB Gold, Healthcare workers, Health surveillance, Meta-analysis, Cohen's k

Introduction

Occupational exposure to biological agents is a major risk for healthcare workers (HCWs) thus in health surveillance much has to be dedicated to infectious disease screening. Tuberculosis (TB) is an ongoing risk in low-income countries due to abandonment of vaccination campaigns, immigrations flows, wide diffusion of primary or secondary immunosuppression, poor efficacy of vaccine currently in use [1,2] so that tuberculosis remains a major public health problem.

According to the World Health Organization (WHO), in 2012 there were an estimated 8.6 million cases of TB (range 8.3–9.0 million) globally, equivalent to 122 cases per 100,000 population. Most of the estimated case numbers in 2012 occurred in Asia (58%) and Africa (27%); smaller proportions occurred in the Eastern Mediterranean region (8%), the European region (4%) and the Americas (3%). One third of the world's population is estimated to be latently infected with *Mycobacterium tuberculosis*: people with latent TB infection (LTBI) do not show symptoms of TB and are not infectious, but they are at risk of developing active disease and becoming infectious. Several factors increase the risk of progressing from infection to active TB, for example, HIV infection or immunosuppressive treatment, malnutrition, diabetes and alcohol

* Correspondence: rossella.uccello@unina2.it
†Equal contributors
[1]Department of Experimental Medicine, Section of Hygiene, Occupational Medicine and Forensic, Medicine, Second University of Naples, Naples, Italy
Full list of author information is available at the end of the article

abuse. Preventing active TB by addressing these risk factors as well as proper diagnosis and treatment of LTBI in selected risk groups is thus important for the individual and for public health [3].

It is clear that LTBI diagnosis is mostly based on screening programs that address the general population or occupational categories such as healthcare workers. Actually, there is a lack of gold-standard for LTBI diagnosis: traditionally, TB infection screening is conducted by tuberculin skin testing (TST). Some years ago interferon-gamma release assays (IGRAs) became commercial available. IGRAs are used as a confirmatory test for TST in a two steps procedure or as a replacement of the TST particularly in situations in which the TST is not recommended [4]. TST remains the major tool used around the world for diagnosis of TB infection because of well-established algorithms for test interpretation. In addition TST is easy to use and it has a good cost-effectiveness. Although widely used, TST has limitations; its sensitivity may be reduced by malnutrition, severe TB diseases and immunodeficiency. Decreased TST specificity might occur in settings where *non-tuberculous mycobacteria* (NTM) are prevalent and in populations who have received *Bacillus Calmette-Guérin* (BCG) vaccine post-infancy or via multiple vaccinations [5], although its effect on TST reactions could be modest after 10 years. Additionally, completing the TST requires two healthcare visits, resulting in loss of reading in approximately 10% of cases [6]. This method is affected by inter-observer variability and the positive result does not distinguish recent from remote infection [6].

Most recent national guidelines present IGRAs (especially Quantiferon, QFT) as a new valid tool for diagnosis of latent tuberculosis, also because they are ex-vivo blood-based tests that, in contrast to the TST, can be repeated any number of times without sensitization or boosting, they require only one visit and do not need a baseline two-step protocol [5]. However, reviews have suggested that IGRA performance differs in high versus low TB incidence settings as well as in presence of some risk factors [6]. Moreover, IGRA reproducibility is influenced by several technical factors and immunomodulation [5]; subsequently, appropriate cut-offs and borderline zones need jet to be derived especially for interpreting of IGRA result in serial testing of HCWs in light of an individual's tuberculosis risk factors [7]. Although a single IGRA is more expensive than the intradermal investigation, the cost-effectiveness analysis depends on epidemiological and individual elements, as explained in several studies that also sought to elaborate specific models [8].

Several recent systematic reviews showed that HCWs are at an increased risk of exposure to *Mycobacterium tuberculosis* [1,2,9,10]. For this reason, periodic screening of HCWs is an important component of TB programs, according to the background TB incidence in the population, resulting in TB as an occupational disease.

In specific working population such as HCWs, serial testing for TB seems to be more appropriate in order to identify recent infections and to target infected individuals for preventive therapy [8]. Some guidelines from high-income low-incidence countries have not recommended IGRAs for serial testing of HCWs while others state that IGRAs may be used for serial testing of HCWs in place of the TST [11]: according to WHO guidelines [12] IGRAs should not be used in HCW screening programs for low- and middle-income countries (strong recommendation). This indication derives from reversion or conversion rates that reduce IGRA reproducibility.

Until now, there have been various systematic reviews of literature, evaluating prevalence or incidence of latent TB disease among HCWs [9] or IGRA performance [11] for tuberculosis screening in HCWs; agreement between TST and IGRA has been generally evaluated as secondary outcome. A systematic review and meta-analysis had compared the accuracy of Quantiferon TB Gold in Tube and the T-SPOT assays with the TST, but has not considered HCWs and not quantified the agreement between skin testing and IGRA [13].

The present study aims to conduct a systematic review with a meta-analysis of the impact of some factors on the agreement between the two tests (TST and QFT) for TB screening programs in HCWs, measured with *Cohen's* κ in order to be more rigorous and informative than narrative and systematic reviews [14,15]. The impact of some risk factors on the outcome of those tests has also been examined in order to derive an "evidence-based" protocol for healthcare workers at risk of tuberculosis.

Methods

Data sources and searches

A systematic review with meta-analysis, according to the PRISMA (Preferred Reporting Items for Systematic Reviews and Meta-Analyses) statement, was conducted [16].

Original articles were searched through PubMed, Embase, Web of Science and Scopus from 1 January 2004 to17 October 2013, using various combinations, in line with the specific database language, of the terms "workers" AND "tuberculosis" OR "TB infection" or "TB disease" OR "TB" AND "tuberculin skin test" OR "tuberculin skin testing" AND "Quantiferon". Additional studies were taken by means of reference lists from previous review articles, and citations of relevant original articles were screened.

Study outcomes and selection

Original articles were evaluated, including cross-sectional and longitudinal studies, meeting all the following criteria: screening of LTBI in HCWs with contemporary TST and

QFT, comparison between TST and QFT results, sample vaccination rates, English language. The following studies were excluded: duplicates, case reports or studies on close contacts, editorials, immunological or laboratory studies, NTM studies. Articles about HCWs affected by HIV, chronic rheumatological diseases or inflammatory bowel diseases were also eliminated in order to avoid other influence factors and to obtain a more homogeneous sample.

Epidemiological studies often did not apply to specific medical occupational groups, but instead calculated the risk of infection or disease for the *overall group of healthcare workers* with a highly heterogeneous definition of 'healthcare worker' that included both occupational groups with a potentially increased risk and groups without any contact with tuberculosis patients [10]. In studies physicians, nurses, midwives, laboratory personnel, radiographers, medical or nursing students were considered as HCWs; if the authors also included a few contacts or administrative workers, only data on HCWs was extrapolated wherever possible.

Three reviewers (RU, MM, MGLM) independently screened the citations (title and abstract) identified from all sources. Subsequently, full-text articles selected by titles and abstracts were reviewed to identify the final set of eligible studies. Disagreements were resolved by discussion.

Data extraction

The following characteristics of each study were listed: country, publication and screening years, sample size, type of study, incidence of TB disease in the general population, gender, mean HCW age, working age, type of tuberculin used for testing, BCG vaccination rates (Table 1).

According to several national guidelines, different types of purified tuberculin proteins (PPD) were used, PPD RT23 and PPD-S; 5 TU dose of PPD-S (0.1 ml) are accepted as bio-equivalent to 2 TU of PPD RT23 (0.1 ml) [17].

Different types of QFT have been considered, such as in the technological development of IFN-γ release assays over the years: from the first assay, known as Quantiferon-TB, to the last and more specific Quantiferon-TB-Gold in Tube (QFT-GIT), that replaced all other types, which are no longer marketed [18]. In order to provide clear information about IGRA/TST agreement, we considered all of them as "QFT".

In order to calculate overall agreement between the two main screening tools, data on TST induration (cutoff positivity $\geq$ 10 mm) and QFT positivity (cutoff positivity 0.35 IU/ml) in HCWs was considered among with the impact of variables of interest on that agreement (vaccination rates and TB incidence). In particular, studies were divided in two groups on the basis of the BCG vaccination rate using different cutoff values because no reference value was available. The incidence of all forms of TB disease in the general population were obtained from the WHO global TB database for each study year, or publication year, if unavailable. Studies were classified in three groups based on TB incidence in each country: low $\leq$20 cases/100,000, intermediate 21–99 cases/100,000, and high $\geq$100 cases/100,000. In order to best characterize TB incidence, the screening year(s) was/were identified in each study; studies lasting for two or more years had an incidence rate calculated by mean.

Any discrepancies were resolved by consensus with the help of the team coordinator, thus obtaining an inter-reviewer agreement of 100%.

Data synthesis and analysis

Study characteristics and results are presented in tables and plots. The primary outcome of the meta-analysis was the *Cohen's κ*. For each study the κ value and 95% confidence interval (CI) were calculated. Weighted mean effect size was used as a summary measure. Heterogeneity of studies was assessed by using Q statistics and I^2 [19]. The P value of Q statistics of less than 0.10 was considered significant [20]. I^2 values of 25%, 50%, and 75% correspond to cutoff points for low, moderate, and high degrees of heterogeneity. If overall heterogeneity was significant, a random-effect model was used, otherwise a fixed-effect model was used. Meta-regression was applied to test difference of study-level covariates. Meta-regression is a regression model that relates the effect to study-level covariates, while assuming additivity of within-study and between-studies components of variance. Restricted maximum likelihood estimators were used to estimate model parameters [21]. A permutation test (using 1,000 re-allocations) was used to assess the true statistical significance of an observed meta-regression finding [22]. Data was analyzed using Stata, version 11.0 (Stata Corp., College Station, TX). All statistical tests were two-sided and p-values <0.05 were regarded as significant.

Results

Description of included studies

Figure 1 shows the flow chart of the studies selection. From the initial 1,430 abstracts, 29 studies [23-51] met our inclusion criteria; 871 studies were discarded as not concerning HCWs, as expected, because a more sensitive than specific search string was preferred in order to obtain as many studies of the health sector as possible. Two hundred and eighty studies were rejected owing to the lack of all results about agreement between TST and QFT or about vaccination status; 13 were rejected for enrolling the same sample of HCWs. Characteristics of the selected studies in this review are shown in Table 1, data are presented by TB incidence. Most studies were

Table 1 Characteristics of studies

First author	Country	n	Gender (F/M)	Sample age[a]	Working seniority[a]	Type of study	TB incidence 2012[b]	Screening year	TB real incidence[c]	PPD dose	Type of PPD[d]	BCG vaccination (%)
Zwerling et al., 2012 [45]	Canada	388	288/100	34,4 (26,9-44,7) y M(range)	5 (2–12) y M(range)	Cross-sectional	4,5	2007-2011	4,8	5 U	PPD-S	36
Khoury et al., 2011 [40]	Minnesota, USA	611	Missing data	/	Start of work 100%	Cross-sectional	3,9	2005-2006	5,3	5 U	PPD-S (as in national guidelines)	82
Fox et al., 2009 [30]	Israel	100	69/31	31 ± 10 y m + SD	TST-: 3,7 ± 6,1 y TST+: 8,7 ± 10,1 y QFT-: 4,6 ± 7,3 y QFT+: 4,2 ± 5,8 y m + SD	Prospective	5,8	2007	6,1	5 U	PPD-S	37
Vinton et al., 2009 [29]	Australia	481	431/50	42 (20–66) y M(range)	/	Cross-sectional	6	2008	6,1	10 U	PPD-S	78
Larcher et al., 2012 [46]	Italy	549	397/152	38,3 (19–64) y m(range)	/	Cross-sectional	2,8	2006-2007	6,7	5 U	PPD-S (as in national guidelines)	38
Nienhaus et al., 2008[e] [25]	Germany	261	212/49	40 ± 10,4 y m ± SD	/	Cross-sectional	4,5	2006	6,8	2 U	PPD-RT23	38
Soborg et al., 2007[e] [23]	Denmark	139	115/24	<30 y 17% 30–39 y 30% 40–49 y 33% ≥ 50 y 20%	/	Cross-sectional	6,5	2007	6,9	2 U	PPD-RT23	76
Girardi et al., 2009 [31]	Italy	115	67/48	≤41 y 51% >41 y 49%	/	Cross-sectional	2,8	2004-2005	7,5	5 U	PPD-S	37
Freeman et al., 2012[e] [47]	New Zealand	325	270/55	18-30 y 49,2% 31–50 y 41,8% 51–60 y 8,9%	/	Cross-sectional	7,6	2007-2008	8,5	5 U	PPD-S (as in national guidelines)	67
Tripodi et al., 2009 [32]	France	148	109/39	20-29 y 28,4% 30–39 y 19.6% 40–49 y 27,7% 50 60 y 24,3%	≤10 y 52,7% > 10 y 47,3%	Cross-sectional	4,3	2006-2007	9,2	2U	PPD-S (Tubertest)	100
Alvarez-Leon et al., 2009 [33]	Spain	134	101/33	33,4 ± 9,4 y m ± SD	10,8 ± 8,2 y m ± SD	Cross-sectional	15	2007	18	2 U	PPD-RT23	35
Casas et al., 2009 [34]	Spain	147	113/34	43,3 (22–63) y M(range)	18,4 (1–43) y m(range)	Cross-sectional	15	2004-2005	19	2 U	PPD-RT23	16
Talebi-Taher et al., 2011 [41]	Iran	200	127/73	34,36 ± 8,26 y m + SD	1-10 y 69,5% 11–20 y 23% 21–30 y 7,5%	Cross-sectional	21	2009-2010	19,5	5 U	PPD SACHIN (Surat) India	100

Table 1 Characteristics of studies *(Continued)*

Hotta et al., 2007[e] [24]	Japan	207	132/75	20 (18–42) y M(range)	/	Cross-sectional	19	2006	24	3 U	PPD (equivalent to PPD-S)	93
Topic et al., 2009 [35]	Croatia	54	51/3	44 (21–63) y m(range)	/	Cross-sectional	17	2007	25	2 U	PPD-RT23	100
Ozdemir et al., 2010[e] [38]	Turkey	76	33/43	30,4 ± 5,4 y m + SD	3,9 ± 4,7 y m ± SD	Cross-sectional	24	2005	31	5 U	PPD-S	91
Torres Costa et al., 2011 [42]	Portugal	2884	2068/816	<25 y 10,4% 25–29 y 28,5% 30–39 y 27,4% 40–49 y 18,5% ≥50 y 15,2%	start of work 13,9% <1 y 4,9% 1–5 y 27,3% >5-10 y 16,1% 10–20 y 19,9% ≥20 y 18%	Cohort	24	2007	33	2 U	PPD-RT23	100
Rafiza et al., 2011 [43]	Malaysia	953	839/114	<24 y 30,7% 25–29 y 35,2% 30–34 y 15,6% > 35 y 18,5%	<1 y 14% 1–5 y 47% 6–10 y 17,5% ≥ 11 y 21,5%	Cross-sectional	81	2008-2009	83	2 U	PPD-RT23	100
Choi et al., 2008 [26]	South Korea	80	75/5	28 (23–45) y M(range)	26 (12–240) m M(range)	Cross-sectional	100	2006	90	2 U	PPD-RT23	100
Lee et al., 2009 [36]	South Korea	196	196/0	23,4 ± 1,4 y m + SD	/	Prospective	100	2007	92	2 U	PPD-RT23	93
Lee et al., 2010 [39]	South Korea	82	82/0	28 (22–53) y M(range)	51,5 (0,25-276) m M(range)	Cross-sectional	100	2009-2010	97	2 U	PPD-RT23	100
Moon et al., 2011 [44]	South Korea	173	102/71	32 (22–67) y M(range)	7 (0,2-42) y M(range)	Cross-sectional	100	2010	98	2 U	PPD-RT23	100
Jung et al., 2012 [48]	South Korea	153	48/105	21.9 ± 0.9 y m + SD	/	Cross-sectional	108	2010-2012	102	2 U	PPD-RT23	86
Jo et al., 2013 [50]	South Korea	493	383/110	30,6 ± 6,0 y m + SD	<1 y 8,3% 1–5 y 49,7% 6–10 y 23,1% 11–15 y 13,8% ≥ 15 y 5,1%	Cross-sectional	100	2012	108	2 U	PPD-RT23	81
Whitaker et al., 2013 [51]	Georgia	319	259/60	18-29 y 20% 30–39 y 26% 40–49 y 31% ≥ 50 y 23%	0-4 y 22% 5–14 y 26% 15–24 y 23% ≥ 25 y 29%	Prospective	125	2009-2011	128	5 U	PPD-S	90
Mirtskhulava et al., 2008 [27]	Georgia	265	229/36	42 (18–74) y m(range)	8 (1–42) y M (range)	Cross-sectional	125	2006	160	5 U	PPD-S	78
Lien et al., 2009 [37]	Vietnam	265	197/68	40 (20–58) y M(range)	<2 y 11% ≥2 < 5 y 17,7% ≥5 < 10 y 16,6% ≥10 y 54,7%	Cross-sectional	151	2007	202	5 U	PPD (Pasteur Institute, Vietnam)	33

Table 1 Characteristics of studies *(Continued)*

Pai et al., 2008 [28]	India	719	446/273	22 y M	/	Cohort	249	2004	212	1 U	PPD-RT23	71
He et al., 2012 [49]	Mongolia	917	659/258	18-29 y 22% 30–39 y 23% 40–49 y 35% ≥ 50 y 20%	10 (<1-50) y M(range)	Cross-sectional	223	2010	224	5 U	missing data	34

[a]Data shown through mean (m) + standard deviation (SD) or through mean (m) and range or through Median (M) and range or through percentage (%); / = missing data. Data are shown in months (m) or years (y).
[b]According to WHO data 2012, rates for 100.000 population.
[c]According to WHO data for each screening year, rates for 100.000 population.
[d]According to data reported in each study or cited national guidelines.
[e]Studies not included for the meta-analysis.

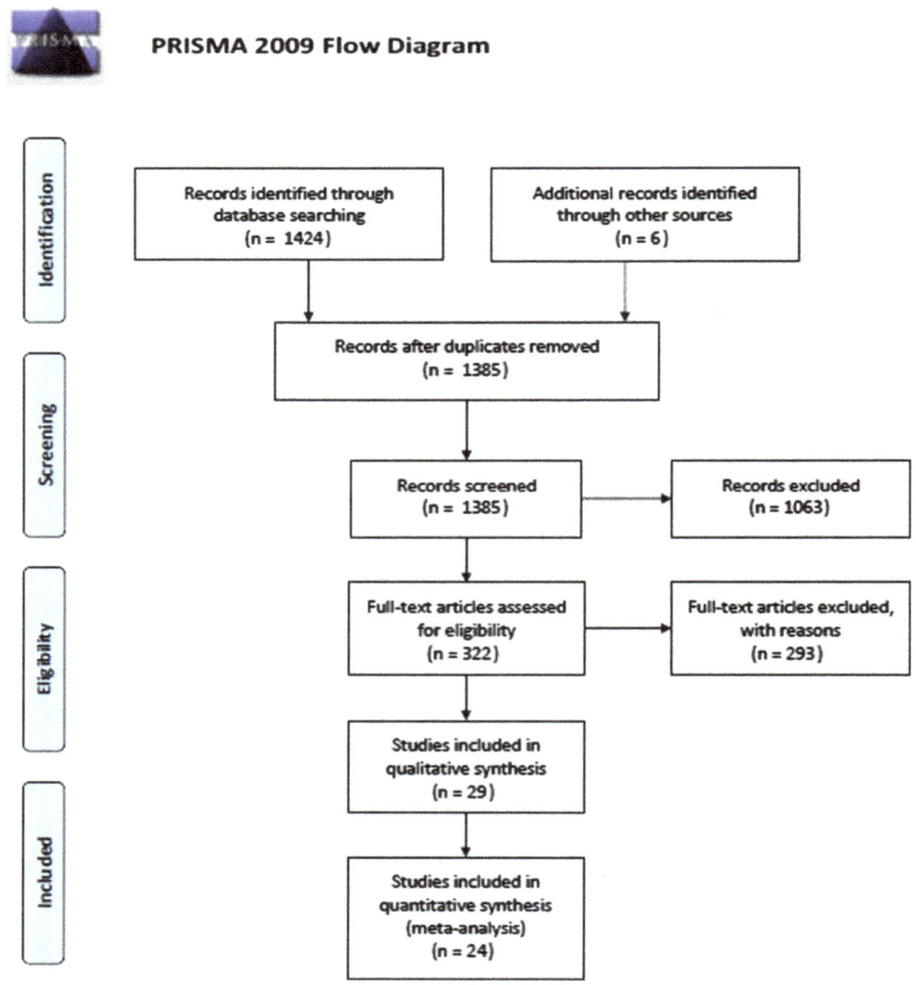

Figure 1 Flow-chart of studies selection. From the initial 1430 abstracts, 29 studies met our inclusion criteria. Study sizes ranged from 54 to 2884 HCWs, for a total of 10.314 HCWs across the 29 studies.

cross-sectional (25/29); in prospective studies, baseline information was taken. Study sizes ranged from 54 to 2,884 HCWs, for a total of 11,434 HCWs across the 29 studies. In total, there were 8,098 female and 2,725 male workers; for 611, gender was not indicated [40].

The age mostly represented in the sample was between 30 and 50 or between 18 and 30 when students were included. The overall mean or median age could not be calculated because the sample age was differently reported in the studies as mean, median or percentage.

Working seniority was defined by the number of years or months spent in contact with patients: it played an important role in TB screening results, but in 11 studies data was not shown; in the other 18, this information was heterogeneous (reported through mean, median or percentage). Therefore as with age a mean or median for working seniority could not be calculated; one study carried out a pre-employment evaluation in a healthcare occupational surveillance program [40].

Skin testing was conducted using different types and doses of tuberculin: the dose varied from 1 to 10U according to the national guideline. TST was performed using 2U of RT23 in most studies (14/29) while in 12/29 5U of PPD-S were used.

Among the 29 selected studies, 24 used 10 mm as cut-off for positivity [26-37,39-46,48-51], 2 of them reported 15 mm [24,38], other 2 studies considered 5 mm [25,47] and in only one was the cutoff 12 mm [23]. In order to calculate overall agreement, we considered only studies with 10 mm as cutoff positivity. BCG vaccination rates run from 16 to 100%, with a median of 81%.

On the basis of TB incidence identified by WHO information for each year of screening, studies were divided into three groups of incidence: the low TB incidence group was the most represented, being included in 10 studies, followed by the intermediate group with 7 studies and the high group with 7 studies (Figure 2). In a few cases, there was a relevant difference between the two incidence rates [31,32,46,35] owing to a delay in publication.

Agreement between TST and QFT

Table 2 shows data by TB incidence on subjects with both TST and QFT results, excluding indeterminate QFT results; for this reason the effective sample size was 10,314, or lower than in Table 1.

Screening results were reported as positive TST alone, positive QFT alone and crossed of TST and QFT. Out of the 10,314 tests performed, TST and QFT agreed for 6,893 of them and failed to do so for 3,421. TST positive QFT negative discordance occurred about four times more often than TST negative QFT positive discordance [2,711 (26.3%) versus 710 (6.9%)].

In order to evaluate TST and QFT agreement, a statistical analysis was conducted using *Cohen's* κ in each study. However, only for 24/29 studies, which used a TST positivity cutoff at 10 mm, overall agreement was

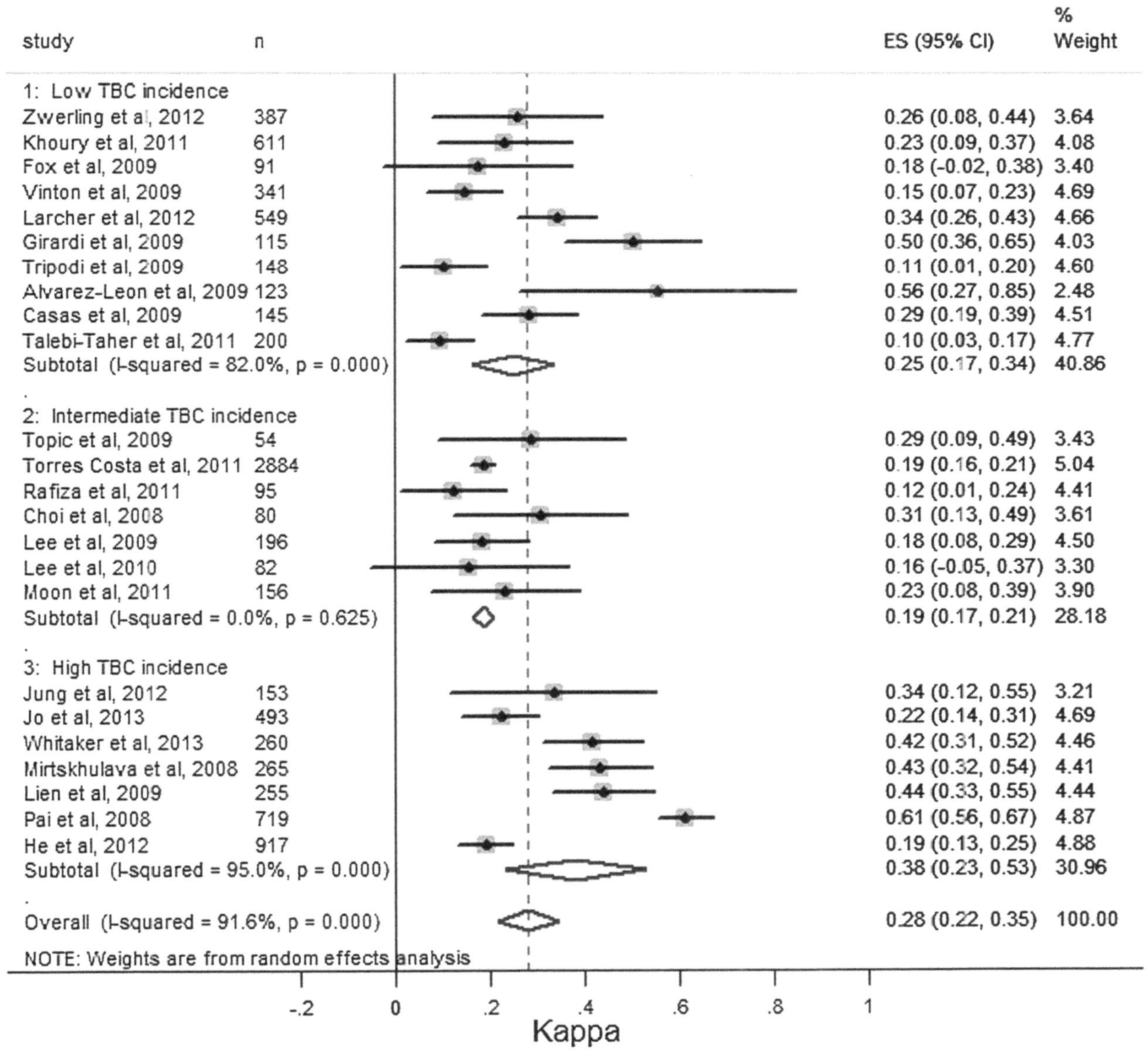

Figure 2 Meta-analysis of Cohen's k values for agreement between Tuberculin Skin Test (TST) and Quantiferon TB Gold-In-Tube (QFT) by Tuberculosis (TB) infection incidence classes. In order to calculate overall agreement, we considered only studies with 10 mm as cutoff positivity. ES: k value.

Table 2 Comparison of TST and QFT results in healthcare workers from different studies

First author	Sample size (n)	TST+ (n)	QFT+ (n)	TST+/QFT+ (n)	TST+/QFT- (n)	TST-/QFT+ (n)	TST-/QFT- (n)
Zwerling et al., 2012 [45]	387[a]	22	24	7	15	17	348
Khoury et al., 2011 [40]	611	50	12	8	42	4	557
Fox et al., 2009 [30]	91[a]	31	17	9	22	8	52
Vinton et al., 2009 [29]	341[a]	114	21	16	98	5	222
Larcher et al., 2012 [46]	549	160	81	57	103	24	365
Nienhaus et al., 2008[b] [25]	261	63	25	15	48	10	188
Soborg et al., 2007[b] [23]	139	47	2	2	45	0	92
Girardi et al., 2009 [31]	115	61	40	36	25	4	50
Freeman et al., 2012[b] [47]	317[a]	67	28	19	48	9	241
Tripodi et al., 2009 [32]	148	97	51	23	74	5	46
Alvarez-Leon et al., 2009 [33]	123[a]	9	8	5	4	3	111
Casas et al., 2009 [34]	145[a]	101	43	42	59	1	43
Talebi-Taher et al., 2011 [41]	200	105	17	14	91	3	92
Hotta et al., 2007[b] [24]	202[a]	120	3	3	117	0	82
Topic et al., 2009 [35]	54	34	17	15	19	2	18
Ozdemir et al., 2010[b] [38]	76	41	65	39	2	26	9
Torres Costa et al., 2011 [42]	2,884	2,102	953	850	1252	103	679
Rafiza et al., 2011 [43]	95a	56	13	11	45	2	37
Choi et al., 2008 [26]	80	36	16	13	23	3	41
Lee et al., 2009 [36]	196	93	28	22	71	6	97
Lee et al., 2010 [39]	82	31	19	10	21	9	42
Moon et al., 2011 [44]	156[a]	52	32	18	34	14	90
Jung et al., 2012 [48]	153	23	8	6	17	2	128
Jo et al., 2013 [50]	493	181	85	54	127	31	281
Whitaker et al., 2013 [51]	260[a]	145	112	90	55	22	93
Mirtskhulava et al., 2008 [27]	265	177	159	133	44	26	62
Lien et al., 2009 [37]	255[a]	163	135	114	49	21	71
Pai et al., 2008 [28]	719	298	288	226	72	62	359
He et al., 2012 [49]	917	439	638	350	89	288	190
Total	*10,314*	*4,918*	*2,940*	*2,207*	*2,711*	*710*	*4,686*

[a]we consider only subjects with both TST and QFT results, excluding undeterminate quantiferon results.
[b]Studies not included in the meta-analysis.

calculated. *K* values appeared in a wide range from 0.10 to 0.61, with a significant heterogeneity ($p < 0.0001$, $I^2 = 91.6\%$). Overall κ value, estimated using the random effect model, was 0.28 (95% CI 0.22 to 0.35), which is quite low reflecting that almost one third of TST and QFT results were discordant (Table 2).

Association between κ value and variables of interest

Studies were classified according to type and dose of PPD. No significant difference ($p = 0.717$) was found between studies with <5 TU ($\kappa = 0.27$, 95% CI 0.17 to 0.37) versus ≥5 TU ($\kappa = 0.29$, 95% CI 0.21 to 0.38).

According to TB incidence classification, TST and QFT agreement was calculated with *Cohen's* κ resulting in 0.25 (95% CI 0.17 to 0.34) in the low incidence group, 0.19 (95% CI 0.17 to 0.21) in the intermediate, and 0.38 (95% CI 0.23 to 0.53) in the high group. The best agreement was observed in the high incidence group, while the worst was seen in the intermediate one, with the highest rate of vaccination; comparing the three κ figures there was a significant difference between the intermediate and the high incidence group ($p = 0.041$).

Furthermore, studies were divided in two groups (lower and higher vaccination rate) to best elucidate BCG vaccination impact on agreement; considering a 90% cutoff value as a statistically significant difference ($p = 0.013$) was found, with an agreement of 0.34 (95% CI 0.25 to 0.43) in the lower rate group (15 studies), and 0.17

(95% CI 0.13 to 0.21) in the higher group (9 studies) (Figure 3).

Discussion

This meta-analysis had the aim of analyzing screening tools for diagnosis of TB infection among HCWs and examining the impact of some risk factors on the outcome of those tests in order to derive an "evidence-based" protocol for screening of healthcare workers at risk of tuberculosis. As already highlighted [11], overall agreement between TST and QFT was quite low. This result can be related to the different immunological targets of the two tests, so that any immunological dysfunction can variously influence their respective results. Moreover, QFT is often characterized by fluctuating results so that its reproducibility is unclear [52]; on the other hand, TST has an inter-observer variability.

TST and QFT also differ in specificity and sensitivity. A lower rate of positivity in the QFT can be explained by a higher specificity of QFT than TST that could come from the intrinsic difference in the methods used by the two tests. QFT uses antigens showing higher specificity to *Mycobacterium tuberculosis* and to only a limited number of NTM, in contrast with the tuberculin used in TST, which represents a mixture of more than 200 nonspecific antigens shared with NTM and with the strains developed from *Mycobacterium bovis* used for BCG vaccination [53].

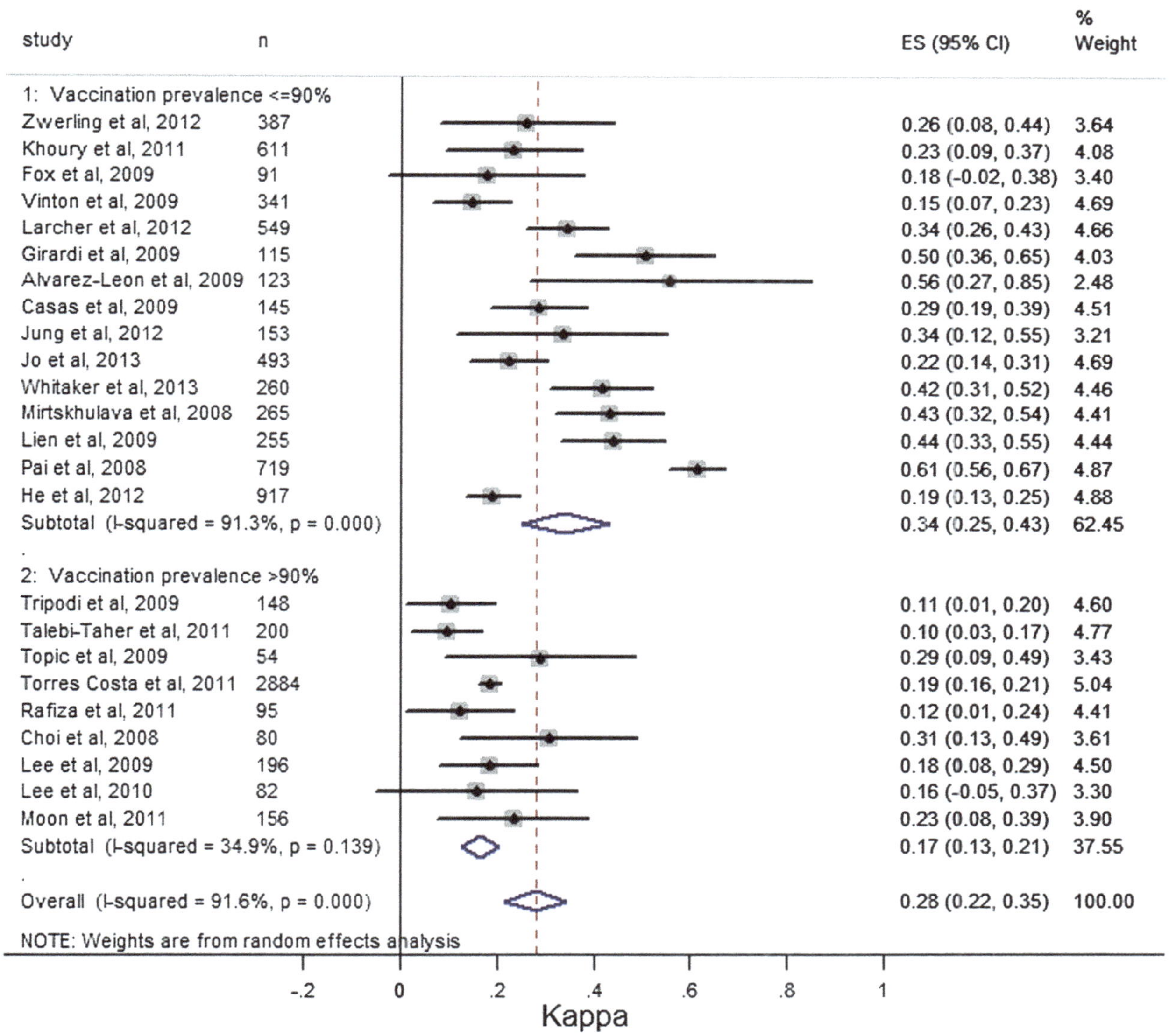

Figure 3 Meta-analysis of Cohen's k values for agreement between Tuberculin Skin Test (TST) and Quantiferon TB Gold-In-Tube (QFT) by Bacillus Calmette-Guérin (BCG) vaccination groups. ES: k value.

An important feature of the present systematic review was the high heterogeneity of the studies chosen owing to different impact of each variable (vaccination rates, incidence of TB in each country, age, working seniority, induration diameter cutoff and type of PPD) on the TST/QFT agreement. Again, this variability could be considered as a strength of the study because it offered an opportunity to best elucidate the agreement, taking these factors into account.

BGC vaccination status and incidence of TB, influencing TST and QFT agreement at the same time, could not be valued separately. BCG vaccination reduced the agreement, influencing the TST positivity (rather than QFT positivity) and increasing the risk of a false positive result, especially in recently vaccinated subjects. Although some studies [29,45,47,34] showed a QFT positivity amount lower than the TST positivity one, in the BCG vaccinated group, this result could not be explained with a cross-reaction between vaccination and QFT antigens, but with a TB infection among vaccinated subjects. In the high TB incidence group, a vaccination status lower than 90% was found and, at the same time, the higher observed agreement, although two studies in particular contributed to the decrease of the agreement [49,50]; in detail, some authors found high rates of TST-/QFT+ [49] and others found high rates of TST+/QFT- [50]. In the first case, the result could be explained by a high TB risk ward and a history of TB infection for some subjects; in the other study, false positive results can be explained by re-vaccination. Some authors also affirmed that repeated vaccination influenced quantitative TST positivity but decreased a probability of positive QFT in the case of three or more repeated doses [42]. Moreover, in the low TB incidence group, studies with higher agreement were characterized by the lower rate of vaccination.

Increasing age of HCWs is correlated with concordant TST and QFT positive results [33,34]; Discordant QFT positive TST negative results were associated with an age of over 40 [46,50] or over 50 [49,42] and anyhow this association increased each year [39], although data was not statistically elaborated due to heterogeneity of presentation.

In consideration of working seniority and TST/QFT results, most studies [27,44,42,49] found an association between increasing working years and positivity of both tests; this information cannot be accounted for alone but it has to be contextualized in the risk evaluation at each worksite (high or low TB risk ward). However, in this review there was no statistical analysis of overall age or working seniority possible because of heterogeneity of data presentation or missing information.

Among the studies considering 10 mm and 15 mm as cutoff diameters, three showed better agreement when shifting TST cutoff from 10 mm to 15 mm [29,35,43]; instead, in five studies there was no meaningful difference [33,24,26,44,27].

Some authors affirmed that the type of tuberculin could play a significant effect on skin response: both vaccinated and unvaccinated subjects receiving RT23 2 TU or 1TU were more likely to have a positive result than those receiving 5 TU PPD [54]. Others [55] considered that TST induration size was larger with PPD-S than with PPD RT23 at 48, 72 and 96 hours, resulting in a statistically lower number of false negatives with PPD-S than with PPD RT23. Despite this evidence, no significant difference was found between various types and doses of tuberculin in the chosen studies, confirming bio-equivalence of RT23 and PPD-S [17].

Study limitations and strength

This systematic review has several strengths. A more sensible than specific search string was elaborated, using multiple databases. Three reviewers (RU, MM, MGLM) independently assessed eligible articles for inclusion. Selection criteria were quite restrictive, so that information obtained was as comparable as possible in order to realize a meta-analysis of overall agreement between the two main screening tools and the influence of some factors (BCG vaccination, TB incidence). However, this was not possible for other variables of interest (age and working seniority) owing to heterogeneity in study design, outcomes and data presentation, despite the limited selection. Still, different national guidelines contribute different study characteristics, particularly on TST procedures and vaccine indications. Lastly, there was a lack of evidence at the highest level of hierarchy on reference standards: a majority of the studies included were cross-sectional. Our study would have appeared more relevant if we had considered longitudinal studies and TST/QFT agreement in serial testing, analyzing all factors that could impact on reversion and conversion. Nevertheless, longitudinal studies did not allow us to analyze both tests in each measurement because it is not always appropriate to repeat both TST and QFT in every HCW.

Conclusion

Screening for TB infection is a major objective of health surveillance programs. Nowadays, even if there is no gold standard, the most-used diagnostic tools are TST and IGRAs (such as QFT) that show a low agreement and are also influenced by few variables that partially justify their variability alone.

Choosing the proper protocol is a prerogative of the occupational physician, who needs to know about TB and BCG vaccination incidence in the general population and the immunological status and risk factors for each individual worker. TST remains the first-step exam, especially when a higher agreement can be expected, i.e.

when there is a low prevalence of vaccination or a high incidence of TB infection. Indeed, QFT is helpful in cases of a higher prevalence of vaccination. Further studies with a unique protocol of health surveillance carried out in variously burdened countries will best clarify the role of TST and QFT for HCW screening.

Competing interests
The authors declare that they have no competing interests.

Authors' contributions
LM had the idea for the study. LM and PC designed the study, developed the search strategy and established inclusion criteria. RU, MGLM and MM searched studies, reviewed abstracts and full-texts and extracted the study data. LM, RU, MGLM and MM wrote the manuscript. PC supervised extraction data and provided expertise in meta-analytic methods. AN, DF and NS contributed to interpretation of the results, drafting of the article and revisions of the manuscript. All authors contributed to and approved the final draft for publication.

Author details
[1]Department of Experimental Medicine, Section of Hygiene, Occupational Medicine and Forensic, Medicine, Second University of Naples, Naples, Italy. [2]Center of Excellence for Epidemiology and Health Services Research for Healthcare Professionals (CVcare), Institute for Health Service Research in Dermatology and Nursing, University Medical Center Hamburg-Eppendorf, Hamburg, Germany. [3]Principles of Prevention and Rehabilitation Department (GPR), Institute for Statutory Accident Insurance and Prevention in the Health and Welfare Services (BGW), Hamburg, Germany. [4]Medical Statistics Unit, Second University of Naples, Naples, Italy.

References
1. Baussano I, Nunn P, Williams B, Pivetta E, Bugiani M, Scano F. Tuberculosis among health care workers. Emerg Infect Dis. 2011;17(3):488–94. doi:10.3201/eid1703.100947.
2. Menzies D, Joshi R, Pai M. Risk of tuberculosis infection and disease associated with work in health care settings. Int J Tuberc Lung Dis. 2007;11 (6):593–605.
3. World Health Organization (WHO): Global tuberculosis Report 2013 [http://apps.who.int/iris/bitstream/10665/91355/1/9789241564656_eng.pdf]
4. Centers for Disease Control and Prevention (CDC). Guidelines for Preventing the Transmission of Mycobacterium tuberculosis in Health-Care Settings. MMWR. 2005;54(RR-17):1–141 [http://www.cdc.gov/mmwr/preview/mmwrhtml/rr5417a1.htm]
5. Pollock NR, McAdam AJ, Pai M, Nardell EA, Bernardo J, Banaei N, et al. Interferon γ-release assays for diagnosis of latent tuberculosis in healthcare workers in low-incidence settings:pros and cons. Clin Chem. 2014;60(5):714–8. doi:10.1373/clinchem.2012.201178. Epub 2013 Oct 7.
6. Trajman A, Steffen RE, Menzies D. Interferon-Gamma Release Assays versus Tuberculin Skin Testing for the Diagnosis of Latent Tuberculosis Infection: An Overview of the Evidence. Pulm Med. 2013;2013:601737. doi:10.1155/2013/601737.
7. Pai M, Kik SV, Banaei N. Occupational screening for tuberculosis. A testing time for interferon-γ release assays. Ann Am Thorac Soc. 2014;11(3):399–401. doi:10.1513/AnnalsATS.201401-019ED.
8. Pai M, Denkinger CM, Kik SV, Rangaka MX, Zwerling A, Oxlade O, et al. Gamma interferon release assays for detection of Mycobacterium tuberculosis infection. Clin Microbiol Rev. 2014;27(1):3–20. doi:10.1128/CMR.00034-13.
9. Joshi R, Reingold AL, Menzies D, Pai M. Tuberculosis among health-care workers in low- and middle-income countries: a systematic review. PLoS Med. 2006;3(12):e494. doi:10.1371/journal.pmed.0030494.
10. Seidler A, Nienhaus A, Diel R. Review of epidemiological studies on the occupational risk of tuberculosis in low-incidence areas. Respiration. 2005;72:431–46. doi:10.1159/000086261.
11. Zwerling A, van den Hof S, Scholten J, Cobelens F, Menzies D, Pai M. Interferon-gamma release assays for tuberculosis screening of healthcare workers: a systematic review. Thorax. 2012;67(1):62–70. doi:10.1136/thx.2010.143180.
12. World Health Organization (WHO): Use of tuberculosis interferon-gamma release assays (IGRAs) in low- and middle-income countries: Policy Statement. 2011, WHO/HTM/TB/2011.18. http://www.who.int/tb/laboratory/policy_statements/en.
13. Diel R, Goletti D, Ferrara G, Bothamley G, Cirillo D, Kampmann B, et al. Interferon-γ release assays for the diagnosis of latent Mycobacterium tuberculosis infection: a systematic review and meta-analysis. Eur Respir J. 2011;37(1):88–99. doi:10.1183/09031936.00115110.
14. Sun S. Meta-analysis of Cohen's kappa. Health Serv Outcomes Res Method. 2011;11:145–63. doi:10.1007/s10742-011-0077-3.
15. Trikalinos TA, Balion CM. Chapter 9: Options for Summarizing Medical Test Performance in the Absence of a "Gold Standard". J Gen Intern Med. 2012;27 Suppl 1:67–75. doi:10.1007/s11606-012-2031-7.
16. Moher D, Liberati A, Tetzlaff J, Altman DG, PRISMA Group. Preferred reporting items for systematic reviews and meta-analyses: the PRISMA statement. J Clin Epidemiol. 2009;62(10):1006–12. doi:10.1016/j.jclinepi.2009.06.005.
17. Comstock GW, Edwards LB, Philip RN, Winn WA. A comparison in the United States of America of two tuberculins, PPD-S and RT23. Bull WHO. 1964;31:161–70.
18. Centers for Disease Control and Prevention (CDC). Guidelines for Using the QuantiFERON®-TB Gold Test for Detecting Mycobacterium tuberculosis Infection, United States. MMWR. 2005;54(RR15):49–55 [http://www.cdc.gov/mmwr/preview/mmwrhtml/rr5415a4.htm]
19. Deeks JJAD, Bradburn MJ. Statistical methods for examining heterogeneity and combining results from several studies in meta-analysis. In: Egger MD-SG, Altman DG, editors. Systematic Reviews in Health Care. London: BMJ Publishing; 2001. p. 285–312.
20. Van Houwelingen HC, Arends LR, Stijnen T. Advanced methods in meta-analysis: multivariate approach and meta-regression. Stat Med. 2002;21:589–624. doi:10.1002/sim.1040.
21. Thompson SG, Sharp SJ. Explaining heterogeneity in meta-analysis: a comparison of methods. Stat Med. 1999;18:2693–708. doi:10.1002/(SICI)1097-0258(19991030).
22. Higgins JPT, Thompson SG. Controlling the risk of spurious findings from meta-regression. Stat Med. 2004;23:1663–82. doi:10.1002/sim.1752.
23. Soborg B, Andersen AB, Larsen HK, Weldingh K, Andersen P, Kofoed K, et al. Detecting a low prevalence of latent tuberculosis among health care workers in Denmark detected by M. tuberculosis specific IFN-gamma whole-blood test. Scand J Infect Dis. 2007;39(6–7):554–9. doi:10.1080/00365540601148483.
24. Hotta K, Ogura T, Nishii K, Kodani T, Onishi M, Shimizu Y, et al. Whole blood interferon-gamma assay for baseline tuberculosis screening among Japanese healthcare students. PLoS One. 2007;2(8):e803. doi:10.1371/journal.pone.0000803.
25. Nienhaus A, Schablon A, Bâcle CL, Siano B, Diel R. Evaluation of the interferon-gamma release assay in healthcare workers. Int Arch Occup Environ Health. 2008;81(3):295–300. doi:10.1007/s00420-007-0212-1.
26. Choi JC, Shin JW, Kim JY, Park IW, Choi EW, Lee MK. The effect of previous tuberculin skin test on the follow-up examination of whole-blood interferon-gamma assay in the screening for latent tuberculosis infection. Chest. 2008;133(6):1415–20. doi:10.1378/chest.07-2193.
27. Mirtskhulava V, Kempker R, Shields KL, Leonard MK, Tsertsvadze T, del Rio C, et al. Prevalence and risk factors for latent tuberculosis infection among health care workers in Georgia. Int J Tuberc Lung Dis. 2008;12(5):513–9.
28. Pai M, Dendukuri N, Wang L, Joshi R, Kalantri S, Rieder HL. Improving the estimation of tuberculosis infection prevalence using T-cell-based assay and mixture models. Int J Tuberc Lung Dis. 2008;12(8):895–902.
29. Vinton P, Mihrshahi S, Johnson P, Jenkin GA, Jolley D, Biggs BA. Comparison of QuantiFERON-TB Gold In-Tube Test and tuberculin skin test for identification of latent Mycobacterium tuberculosis infection in healthcare staff and association between positive test results and known risk factors for infection. Infect Control Hosp Epidemiol. 2009;30(3):215–21. doi:10.1086/595695.
30. Fox BD, Kramer MR, Mor Z, Preiss R, Rusanov V, Fuks L, et al. The QuantiFERON-TB-GOLD assay for tuberculosis screening in healthcare workers: a cost-comparison analysis. Lung. 2009;187(6):413–9. doi:10.1007/s00408-009-9182-2.
31. Girardi E, Angeletti C, Puro V, Sorrentino R, Magnavita N, Vincenti D, et al. Estimating diagnostic accuracy of tests for latent tuberculosis infection

without a gold standard among healthcare workers. Euro Surveill. 2009;14(43):29–37.
32. Tripodi D, Brunet-Courtois B, Nael V, Audrain M, Chailleux E, Germaud P, et al. Evaluation of the tuberculin skin test and the interferon-γ release assay for TB screening in French healthcare workers. J Occup Med Toxicol. 2009;4:30. doi:10.1186/1745-6673-4-30.
33. Alvarez-León EE, Espinosa-Vega E, Santana-Rodríguez E, Molina-Cabrillana JM, Pérez-Arellano JL, Caminero JA, et al. Screening for tuberculosis infection in spanish healthcare workers: Comparison of the QuantiFERON-TB gold in-tube test with the tuberculin skin test. Infect Control Hosp Epidemiol. 2009;30(9):876–83. doi:10.1086/598519.
34. Casas I, Latorre I, Esteve M, Ruiz-Manzano J, Rodriguez D, Prat C, et al. Evaluation of interferon-gamma release assays in the diagnosis of recent tuberculosis infection in health care workers. PLoS One. 2009;4(8):e6686. doi:10.1371/journal.pone.0006686.
35. Topić RZ, Dodig S, Zoricić-Letoja I. Interferon-gamma and immunoglobulins in latent tuberculosis infection. Arch Med Res. 2009;40(2):103–8. doi:10.1016/j.arcmed.2008.11.001. Epub 2009 Jan 20.
36. Lee K, Han MK, Choi HR, Choi CM, Oh YM, Lee SD, et al. Annual incidence of latent tuberculosis infection among newly employed nurses at a tertiary care university hospital. Infect Control Hosp Epidemiol. 2009;30(12):1218–22. doi:10.1086/648082.
37. Lien LT, Hang NT, Kobayashi N, Yanai H, Toyota E, Sakurada S, et al. Prevalence and risk factors for tuberculosis infection among hospital workers in Hanoi. Viet Nam PLoS One. 2009;4(8):e6798. doi:10.1371/journal.pone.0006798.
38. Ozdemir D, Annakkaya AN, Tarhan G, Sencan I, Cesur S, Balbay O, et al. Comparison of the tuberculin skin test and the quantiferon test for latent Mycobacterium tuberculosis infections in health care workers in Turkey. Jpn J Infect Dis. 2007;60(2–3):102–5.
39. Jong Lee K, Ae Kang Y, Mi Kim Y, Cho SN, Wook Moon J, Suk Park M, et al. Screening for latent tuberculosis infection in South Korean healthcare workers using a tuberculin skin test and whole blood interferon-gamma assay. Scand J Infect Dis. 2010;42(9):672–8. doi:10.3109/00365548.2010.485575.
40. Khoury NZ, Binnicker MJ, Wengenack NL, Aksamit TR, Buchta WG, Molella RG. Preemployment screening for tuberculosis in a large health care setting: comparison of the tuberculin skin test and a whole-blood interferon-γ release assay. J Occup Environ Med. 2011;53(3):290–3. doi:10.1097/JOM.0b013e31820c91c5.
41. Talebi-Taher M, Javad-Moosavi SA, Entezari AH, Shekarabi M, Parhizkar B. Comparing the performance of QuantiFERON TB Gold and Mantoux test in detecting latent tuberculosis infection among Iranian heath care workers. Int J Occup Med Environ Health. 2011;24(4):359–66. doi:10.2478/s13382-011-0046-7.
42. Torres Costa J, Silva R, Ringshausen FC, Nienhaus A. Screening for tuberculosis and prediction of disease in Portuguese healthcare workers. J Occup Med Toxicol. 2011;6:19. doi:10.1186/1745-6673-6-19.
43. Rafiza S, Rampal KG, Tahir A. Prevalence and risk factors of latent tuberculosis infection among health care workers in Malaysia. BMC Infect Dis. 2011;11:19. doi:10.1186/1471-2334-11-19.
44. Moon HW, Kim H, Hur M, Yun YM, Lee A. Latent tuberculosis infection screening for laboratory personnel using interferon-γ release assay and tuberculin skin test in Korea: an intermediate incidence setting. J Clin Lab Anal. 2011;25(6):382–8. doi:10.1002/jcla.20479.
45. Zwerling A, Cojocariu M, McIntosh F, Pietrangelo F, Behr MA, Schwartzman K, et al. TB screening in Canadian health care workers using interferon-gamma release assays. PLoS One. 2012;7(8):e43014. doi:10.1371/journal.pone.0043014.
46. Larcher C, Frizzera E, Pretto P, Lang M, Sonnleitner N, Huemer HP. Immunosurveillance for Mycobacterium tuberculosis of health care personnel in a third level care hospital. Med Lav. 2012;103(1):26–36.
47. Freeman JT, Marshall RJ, Newton S, Austin P, Taylor S, Chew TC, et al. Screening for Mycobacterium tuberculosis infection among healthcare workers in New Zealand: prospective comparison between the tuberculin skin test and the QuantiFERON-TB Gold In-Tube assay. N Z Med J. 2012;125(1349):21–9.
48. da Jung H, Jo KW, Shim TS. Prevalence of Latent Tuberculosis Infection among Medical Students in South Korea. Tuberc Respir Dis (Seoul). 2012;73(4):219–23. doi:10.4046/trd.2012.73.4.219.
49. He GX, Wang LX, Chai SJ, Klena JD, Cheng SM, Ren YL, et al. Risk factors associated with tuberculosis infection among health care workers in Inner Mongolia, China. Int J Tuberc Lung Dis. 2012;16(11):1485–91. doi:10.5588/ijtld.12.0193.
50. Jo KW, Hong Y, Park JS, Bae IG, Eom JS, Lee SR, et al. Prevalence of Latent Tuberculosis Infection among Health Care Workers in South Korea: A Multicenter Study. Tuberc Respir Dis (Seoul). 2013;75(1):18–24. doi:10.4046/trd.2013.75.1.18.
51. Whitaker J, Mirtskhulava V, Kipiani M, Harris DA, Tabagari N, Kempker RR, et al. Prevalence and incidence of latent tuberculosis infection in georgian healthcare workers. PLoS One. 2013;8(3):e58202. doi:10.1371/journal.pone.0058202.
52. Zhao X, Mazlagic D, Flynn EA, Hernandez H, Abbott CL. Is the QuantiFERON-TB blood assay a good replacement for the tuberculin skin test in tuberculosis screening? a pilot study at Berkshire Medical Center. Am J Clin Pathol. 2009;32(5):678–86. doi:10.1309/ajcpuhc34nbdgkkl.
53. Nahid P, Pai M, Hopewell PC. Advances in the diagnosis and treatment of tuberculosis. Proc Am Thorac Soc. 2006;3(1):103–10. doi:10.1513/pats.200511-119JH.
54. Wang L, Turner MO, Elwood RK, Schulzer M, FitzGerald JM. A meta-analysis of the effect of Bacille Calmette-Guérin vaccination on tuberculin skin test measurements. Thorax. 2002;57:804–9. doi:10.1136/thorax.57.9.804.
55. Morán-Mendoza O, Tello-Zavala MC, Rivera-Camarillo M, Ríos-Meza Y. Comparison of different methods and times for reading the tuberculin skin test. Int J Tuberc Lung Dis. 2013;17(10):1273–8. doi:10.5588/ijtld.13.0147.

15

Occupational exposure to blood borne pathogens among healthcare workers

Carlos Pérez-Diaz[1,2,3], Omar-Javier Calixto[3*], Álvaro A. Faccini-Martínez[3,4], Juan S. Bravo-Ojeda[3], Carlos A. Botero-García[5], Erika Uribe-Pardo[3], Yesid F. Mantilla-Florez[3], Fabian Benitez[3], Ada Duran[3] and Johana Osorio[6]

Abstract

Background: Occupational exposure to blood borne pathogens caused by percutaneous injuries or mucosal contamination is frequent among Healthcare Workers (HCW).

Methods: A cross-sectional analysis of HCW with an occupational exposure to blood reported to professional risk insurance agencies between 2009 and 2014 was performed. Comparisons between groups according to exposure level (mild, moderate, and severe) were evaluated.

Results: Two thousand, four hundred three reports were classified according exposure as mild 2.7 %, moderate 74.8 %, severe 21.9 %. Factors related: health sciences student with mild exposure events [adjusted odds ratio (AOR) 11.91, 95 % CI 5.13–27.61, $p < 0.00001$], and physician with moderate exposure events (AOR 1.90, 95 % CI 1.17–3.07, $p = 0.009$). Factors inversely related: physician with severe exposure events (AOR 0.54, 95 % CI 0.32–0.91, $p = 0.02$) and health sciences student with moderate exposure events (AOR 0.08, 95 % CI 0.04–0.15, $p < 0.00001$). It was found an important relationship between severe events with infectious diseases specialist assessment, and follow-up adherence. Additionally, a case of Human Immunodeficiency Virus seroconversion was presented (0.0004 %), no other seroconversions were observed.

Conclusions: Occupational exposure events must be managed according to established protocols, but adherence failure was evident with the exception of severe exposure cases. Thus, interventions to enhance occupational safety are required. Occupation must be considered as a risk factor during initial assessment of events.

Keywords: Health care worker, Blood borne pathogen, Occupational exposure

Background

Health Care Workers (HCW) refers to any person that performs a paid or non-paid labor activity in health care [1, 2]. This population is potentially exposed to infectious materials as corporal fluids and contaminated medical devices and surfaces. HCW include physicians, paramedics, nurses, dentists, technicians, students, and assistants whose role is related directly with health care. Additionally the personnel that is indirectly related with patients attention can also be exposed to blood or other fluids, as it is the case of cleaning, security, maintenance and volunteer personnel [1, 2].

Biohazard event is defined as the exposure to blood, tissues or any other potentially infectious fluid [1], one of the most obvious occupational risks in HCW daily practice and produces anxiety among them [3]. Exposure to blood borne pathogens caused by percutaneous injuries or mucous membranes contamination is a frequent event. It is considered, seroconversion risk for blood borne viruses are; 1–6 % to 22–31 % for Hepatitis B

* Correspondence: calixto.oj@hotmail.com
[3]Servicios y asesorías en infectología (SAI), Calle 50 # 13-62, 110231420, Bogotá, Colombia
Full list of author information is available at the end of the article

Virus (HBV) depending on serological status of the source, 1.8 % for Hepatitis C Virus (HCV), and 0.3 % for the Human Immunodeficiency Virus (HIV) [4]. Worldwide, the cases of infection associated to occupational activity in HCW represents 39 % of the cases of infection by HCV, 37 % of the cases of infection by HBV, and 4.4 % of the cases of infection by HIV [5]. For the region of the Americas it is considered that 57,000, 61,000 and 23,000 events occur with a positive source to HCV, HBV and HIV, respectively [5].

Universal precaution recommendations have been created for prevention, especially needles and sharp objects injuries, as well as preventing contact of fluids with mucous membranes [6].

In Colombia once the exposure event occurs the HCW must contact their insurance agency in order to be advice of initial treatment and risk assessment in the emergency room or presenting to a specialized consultation service. But there is not an integrated national record of these events, for that reason the objective of this study is to analyze the reports of exposure to blood and corporal fluids of five professional risk insurance companies in Colombia between years 2009 and 2014, as well as determining the factors associated to mild, moderate, and severe exposure classification.

Methods

Study design

The study was an epidemiological, retrospective, record-based review. This study included registries of Colombian HCWs who presented an episode of exposure to blood borne pathogens caused by percutaneous injuries or mucous membranes contamination reported to five professional risks insurance companies and evaluated in Servicios y Asesorías en Infectología (SAI), which performed the occupational exposure initial management and follow-up, between years 2009 and 2014. The present study protocol was approved by the Institutional Review Board, SAI.

The sample size was calculated taking into account the formula for this type of study based on expected prevalence of occupational exposure events in a local teaching hospital from Colombia (31.6 %) [31]. Based on an alpha risk of 5 % with a confidence level of 99 % and a two-sided configuration. As a result, the estimated sample size was 2294 subjects.

Needle puncture or sharp object injuries and cutaneous or mucosal splashes were surveyed by reports of exposures assessed in a specialized infectious diseases agency. The follow up consisted in guaranteeing and guiding the medical advice, and treatment of cases according to their classification in mild, moderate or severe exposure events. Sociodemographic, clinical and laboratory data were obtained from the event registries and double-check with medical registries by two investigators in order to control bias. These data was registered in an electronic database.

Statistical analysis

In the first place, a univariate descriptive analysis was performed. Categorical variables were analyzed through frequencies. The Kolmogorov-Smirnov test was performed to evaluate the normality. Parametric data is expressed with the mean and standard deviation (SD), and non-parametric data is described with median and interquartile range (IQR).

Subsequently, a bivariate analysis was performed to establish association between demographic and clinical characteristics of the patients. Parametric values were analyzed by chi-square test or Fisher exact test. A value of $p \leq 0.05$ was considered as significant.

A multiple logistic regression was considered by taking the exposure level classification as independent variables. As dependent factors: statistically significant associations in the bivariate analysis were used, as additional variables described in the literature.

The adequacy of the logistic models was evaluated through Hosmer-Lemeshow goodness-of-fit test. The Nagelkerke R2 was used to estimate the percentage of variance explained by the model. The adjusted odds ratio (AOR) was calculated with confidence intervals of 95 % (CI). Wald statistic test was used to evaluate the significance of different logistic regression coefficients for each independent variable. A step by step progressive elimination approach was used. Statistical analyses were made in the statistical program IBM SPSS Statistics 22.

Results

Characteristics of the 2403 participants, 82.4 % were females, with a mean age between 29.5 ± 9.2 years. Regarding their origin, 69.8 % came from urban areas, the remaining percentage of cases occurred in rural areas. Biohazard events were classified as mild in 2.7 %, moderate in 74.8 % and severe in 21.9 %. The main mechanisms were: needle puncture (hollow needle, blunt needle, or unspecified needle) 86.5 %, mucocutaneous splash 7.9 %, and injuries with contaminated sharp object 5.6 %. For further description of demographical data and injury mechanisms, see Table 1.

During follow up, it was found that 21.5 % received any type of prophylaxis for the HIV infection. However, prophylaxis in severe exposures was received in 94.6 % cases. The most used drug was zidovudine/lamivudine (AZT/3TC) in 87.1 %, followed by AZT/3TC plus lopinavir/ritonavir in 8.8 % and emtricitabine/tenofovir in

Table 1 Characteristics of the health care workers with occupational exposure

Sociodemographic characteristics	Mean ± SD	Median, IQR
Age (y)	29.5 ± 9.2	27, 28.8–48.3
	%(n/N)	
Female	82.4 (1980/2403)	
Urban area	69.8 (1677/2402)	
Occupation	%(n/N)	
Nursing	47.5 (1141/2403)	
Physician	13.9 (334/2403)	
Student	13.1 (315/2403)	
Cleaning personnel	9.6 (230/2403)	
Odontology	7.3 (175/2403)	
Bacteriology	4.9 (118/2403)	
Surgical instrumentation	2.6 (62/2403)	
Respiratory therapy	1.1 (27/2403)	
Contact Mechanism	%(n/N)	
Hollow needle	53.0 (1272/2403)	
Unspecified needle	22.8 (548/2403)	
Blunt needle	10.7 (256/2403)	
Mucocutaneous splash	7.9 (190/2403)	
Lancet puncture	4.1 (99/2403)	
Scalpel injury	1.3 (31/2403)	
Contaminated glass injury	0.2 (5/2403)	
Exposure Classification	%(n/N)	
Mild	2.7 (67/2403)	
Moderate	74.8 (1798/2403)	
Severe	21.9 (527/2403)	
Follow up	%(n/N)	
Medical follow-up	33.1 (796/2403)	
Infectious diseases specialist assessment	30.3 (728/2403)	
Prophylactic medication	21.5 (517/2403)	

IQR interquartile range, *SD* standard deviation, *y* years

2 %. Other included medication regimens used were abacavir/lamivudine, atazanavir, efavirenz, and raltegravir. And 7 (0.3 %) patients received human immunoglobulin due to exposition to HBV.

Additionally, 30.3 % of the cases reported assessment by infectious diseases specialist, and 33.1 % had a medical follow-up 6 months after the event. However, in patients classified as severe exposure, 99.2 and 68.9 % were assessed by infectious diseases specialist and received medical follow-up, respectively. A case of seroconversion to HIV was presented during the study time period, representing 0.0004 % of all the followed cases. Furthermore, there was no other disease transmission diagnosed during the follow up time.

Factors associated to the type of exposure

In bivariate analysis, mild exposure was significantly related to health sciences students ($p = <0.00001$). In contrast, being a nurse ($p = 0.015$), assessment by an infectious diseases specialist ($p = 0.025$), and presenting a medical follow-up during follow up ($p = <0.00001$) were associated inversely with mild exposure (Table 2).

Factors significantly related to moderate exposure events were physicians ($p = <0.00001$), and respiratory therapists ($p = 0.041$); however, the confidence interval of the group of respiratory therapy included the unit (CI95% 0.98–17.58). Meanwhile health sciences student ($p = 0.048$), and cleaning personnel ($p = <0.00001$), infectious diseases specialist assessment ($p = <0.00001$), and medical follow-up ($p = <0.00001$) were inversely related (Table 2).

Factors related severe exposure events were cleaning personnel ($p = <0.00001$), as well as infectious diseases specialist assessment ($p = <0.00001$), receiving post-exposure prophylaxis ($p = <0.00001$), and medical follow-up ($p = <0.00001$). Contrary, there was an inverse relationship between being a physician ($p = 0.001$) (Table 2).

As a result of a multivariate analysis it was found in mild exposure events, being a health sciences student was related to presenting a mild exposure event (AOR 11.91, 95 % CI 5.13–27.61, $p = <0.00001$). In contravention, having a medical follow-up was inversely related (AOR 0.19, 95 % CI 0.05–0.64, $p = 0.008$) (Table 3).

Moderate exposure, in multivariate analysis was associated with being a physician (AOR 1.90, 95 % CI 1.17–3.07, $p = 0.009$). While, health sciences students was inversely related to moderate exposure events (AOR 0.08, 95 % CI 0.04–0.15, $p = <0.00001$). Also, infectious diseases specialist assessment (AOR 0.01, 95 % CI 0.01–0.15, $p = <0.00001$), and medical follow-up (AOR 0.67, 95 % CI 0.47–0.94, $p = 0.020$), (Table 3).

Severe exposure in multivariate analysis showed relationship with infectious diseases specialist assessment (AOR 1160.89, 95 % CI 285.56–4719.37, $p = <0.00001$), and the medical follow-up (AOR 1.83, 95 % CI 1.28–2.63, $p = 0.001$). Although, physicians were inversely related to this classification (AOR 0.54, 95 % CI 0.32–0.91, $p = 0.021$) (Table 3).

Discussion

One of the most related factors to biohazard events in HCW is occupation; previously, different studies have reported that exposure to blood borne pathogens is more frequent in personnel that must manipulate vascular accesses or blood samples such as nursing personnel (nurses and nursing assistants), physicians, and laboratory personnel [7–20].

According to these findings in our registry it was clear that the most frequently related occupations were:

Table 2 Bivariate analysis of event according to exposure classification

Mild exposure	Yes %	No %	OR (CI 95 %)	p value
Female	76.6	82.6	0.69 (0.35–1.37)	0.287
Urban area	80.6	69.5	1.82 (0.99–3.36)	0.051
Physician	6.0	14.1	0.39 (0.14–1.07)	0.071
Student	34.3	12.5	3.66 (2.18–6.15)	<0.00001
Nursing	32.8	47.9	0.53 (0.32–0.89)	0.015
Bacteriology	4.5	4.9	0.91 (0.28–2.92)	1.000
Odontology	7.5	7.3	1.03 (0.41–2.56)	0.814
Surgical Instrumentation	6.0	2.5	2.49 (0.88–7.08)	0.092
Cleaning personnel	9.0	9.6	0.93 (0.40–2.17)	0.861
Respiratory therapy	0.0	1.2	1.03 (1.02–1.04)	1.000
Infectious diseases specialist assessment	17.9	30.7	0.49 (0.26–0.93)	0.025
Prophylactic medication	0.0	22.1	1.04 (1.03–1.05)	<0.00001
Medical follow-up	11.9	33.9	0.26 (013–0.56)	<0.00001
Moderate exposure	Yes %	No %	OR (CI 95 %)	p value
Female	82.7	81.4	1.90 (0.83–1.43)	0.525
Urban area	70.1	69.0	1.05 (0.86–1.29)	0.627
Physician	15.5	8.9	1.88 (1.38–2.56)	<0.00001
Student	12.3	15.5	0.77 (0.59–0.99)	0.048
Nursing	48.6	44.1	1.20 (0.99–1.45)	0.056
Bacteriology	4.9	4.9	1.01 (0.66–1.55)	0.968
Odontology	7.0	8.2	0.83 (0.59–1.18)	0.298
Surgical Instrumentation	2.8	2.0	1.38 (0.73–2.61)	0.320
Cleaning personnel	7.5	16.0	0.42 (0.32–0.56)	<0.00001
Respiratory therapy	1.4	0.3	4.15 (0.98–17.58)	0.041
Infectious diseases specialist assessment	10.7	90.1	0.13 (0.01–0.02)	<0.00001
Prophylactic medication	0.0	87.0	24.48 (19.67–30.47)	<0.00001
Medical follow-up	23.7	62.5	0.19 (0.15–0.23)	<0.00001
Severe exposure	Yes %	No %	OR (CI 95 %)	p value
Female	82.0	82.5	0.96 (0.73–1.28)	0.068
Urban area	67.6	70.5	0.87 (0.71–1.08)	0.200
Physician	9.3	15.2	0.57 (0.42–0.79)	0.001
Student	13.1	13.1	0.99 (0.75–1.33)	0.987
Nursing	45.5	48.1	0.90 (0.75–1.10)	0.308
Bacteriology	4.9	4.9	1.01 (0.64–1.57)	0.980
Odontology	8.3	7.0	1.21 (0.85–1.73)	0.288
Surgical Instrumentation	1.5	2.9	0.52 (2.46–1.10)	0.082
Cleaning personnel	16.9	7.5	2.50 (1.88–3.32)	<0.00001
Respiratory therapy	0.4	1.3	0.28 (0.07–1.19)	0.097
Infectious diseases specialist assessment	99.2	10.9	1065.13 (394.06–2879.05)	<0.00001
Prophylactic medication	98.1	0.0	188.50 (101.59–349.76)	<0.00001
Medical follow-up	68.9	23.3	7.28 (5.89–9.02)	<0.00001

CI confidence interval, *OR* Odds ratio

Table 3 Multiple logistic regression of event according to exposure classification

Mild classification logistic regression model				
Variable	β	AOR	CI 95 %	p value
Constant	−3.397	0.020	-	<0.0000001
Gender (female)	−0.234	0.792	0.381–1.647	0.532
Student	2.477	11.901	5.129–27.613	<0.0000001
Nursing	0.388	1.475	0.624–3.487	0.376
Infectious diseases specialist assessment	−0.065	0.937	0.411–2.134	0.877
Medical control	−1.684	0.186	0.054–0.642	0.008
Moderate classification logistic regression model				
Variable	β	AOR	CI 95 %	p value
Constant	3.845	46.750	-	<0.0000001
Gender (female)	0.347	1.414	0.924–2.164	0.110
Physician	0.641	1.898	1.174–3.068	0.009
Student	−2.532	0.080	0.042–0.149	<0.0000001
Respiratory therapy	0.251	1.286	0.184–8.984	0.800
Infectious diseases specialist assessment	−4.708	0.009	0.006–0.15	<0.0000001
Medical follow-up	−0.406	0.667	0.473–0.939	0.020
Severe classification logistic regression model				
Variable	β	AOR	CI 95 %	p value
Constant	−6.328	0.002	-	<0.0000001
Gender (female)	−0.362	0.697	0.416–1.166	0.169
Physician	−0.613	0.542	0.322–0.911	0.021
Cleaning personnel	0.173	1.189	0.662–2.135	0.563
Infectious diseases specialist assessment	7.057	1160.887	285 559–4719.372	<0.0000001
Medical follow-up	0.604	1.830	1.275–2.626	0.001

AOR Adjusted Odds Ratio, *CI* confidence interval

nursing, physician and health sciences student. Nursing with 47.5 % (1141 registries), although this value is not as high as reported in Spain (61.6–78 %) [17], Poland (68 %) [12], and Egypt (66.7 %) [11]. However, a similar percentage is found in other countries as Turkey (44 %) [7], and Georgia (39 %) [9]. This variation may be due to the current record includes professions not considered by these studies as students, cleaning personnel, laboratory personnel, and not only physicians and/or nurses.

To our knowledge there are few studies that have attempted to perform an analysis according to the severity classification proposed by the CDC, in our study statistically significant associations were found with each category; it was found and association to mild exposure event and being a student, that could be related to the population that presented more events with blunt needle (46.3 %) and mucosal splash (22.4 %) that is generally associated to mild exposure.

Physicians were associated to moderate severity exposure events, possibly explained by main exposure mechanisms as blunt needle puncture (32.1 %) and hollow needle puncture (30.2 %) in this occupational group.

Contrariwise being a physician was inversely associated to severe exposure events since physicians only represented 9.2 % of the cases. An interesting finding was that despite it was not evident an association in the logistic regression model, being part of the cleaning personnel was associated to severe exposure events, were 96.6 % of the reported events were associated to hollow needle puncture or unspecified needle puncture with unknown source.

A study including different occupational groups by Montufar-Andrade F, et al. [20]. conducted in Colombia, informed the occupational exposure in nursing (22.9 %), cleaning personnel (21.7 %), students in formation in 14.3 %, and physicians in 4.2 %, similarly to those found in our study. Additionally, In Turkey there was reported a 34 % of cleaning personnel in the exposure registries [7]. Regarding severe classification group, in Tunisia it was found that being part of the nursing personnel was a risk factor [14], and Colombian medical students in practice during surgical areas was associated to severe events [21].

Among factors reported previously associated to exposure to biological material in HCW are: working in the emergency room, working in the operating room, working in the ICU or in resuscitation area, inadequate illumination system, age under 25 years, lack of experience, workload >40 hours/week, lack of training in infection risk, and inconsistency in the use of gloves [16, 22–25]. Even, in some cases the use of gloves was only present in 47 % of the events [26]. Additionally, there was an association in HCW as students in formation, especially during surgical practices [21, 27–31], gynecology and obstetrics [21, 27–32], anesthesiology [31], internal medicine [27], or in the emergency room [29]. Those who were in surgical areas had the presence of severe exposure events [21], and nearly 20 % did not register the use of protective materials [28]. In the United Kingdom it was found that most physicians experienced events with suture (blunt) needles, while younger physicians presented exposure during laboratory sample recollection [33].

During the protocol period a case of HIV seroconversion occurred (0.0004 %); this case was recently described as the first case HIV seroconversion in a HCW from Colombia; the event occurred in 2005 and the patient did not receive post expositional prophylaxis [34], making clear the importance of a protocol for the proper and prompt attention of these events. On the other hand, no other additional infections were recorded in HCW.

Adherence is a major concern in HCW occupational exposure protocols with a large percentage of professionals that do not complete the prophylactic recommendations or fail to attend to follow-up and evaluation by an infectious diseases specialist [35, 36]; in an analysis of all the reports it was noticed that only 21.5 % received any type of post expositional prophylaxis with antiretroviral medication, 33.1 % assisted to medical follow-up, and 30.3 % assisted to an appointment with infectious diseases specialist. However it is noteworthy that those patients classified as severe exposure 94.6 % received post expositional prophylaxis, 99.2 % assisted to medical control and 68.9 % were evaluated by an infectious diseases specialist.

Factors associated with poor adherence to protocol in HCW are described as poor risk awareness or lack of time, and these arguments could lead to an important sub-registry [4, 19]. In Colombia a study conducted by Tapias-Vargas LE et al. [29] in a group of residents, it was found that 31 % of this HCW did not report the event, and therefore did not received any guidance or comprehensive assessment.

There are several limitations of the current study consists in the retrospective character of the data and absence of sampling methodology. Similarly, other factors previously reported abroad could not be analyzed based on registries used. Although reports from several regions of the country where analyzed, including urban and rural areas, we cannot ensure representativeness of all the HCW population nationwide and underreport could be also considered since HCW must contact initially agencies in order to access to the program. Additionally, the transversal nature of the study does not allow making an inference of causality of the associated factors presented.

Conclusion

Occupational exposure events must be managed according to established protocols, but adherence failure was evident with the exception of severe exposure cases in this study and generally on published literature, so these results can promote the study of determinants in lack of adherence in Colombian HCWs. This study added evidence of relevance in the initial management of occupation, thus allowed a more specific assessment in HCWs with severe exposure classification.

Abbreviations

AOR: adjusted odds ratio; CI: confidence intervals; HCW: healthcare workers; HBV: Hepatitis B Virus; HCV: Hepatitis C Virus; HIV: Human Immunodeficiency Virus; IQR: interquartile range; 3TC: lamivudine; SD: standard deviation; AZT: zidovudine.

Competing interests

All authors report no conflicts of interest relevant to this article.

Authors' contributions

OJC, AFM, JSBO, and CABG participated in the design of the study and drafting of the manuscript. AE, YFMF, FB, and AD carried out the review of participant's registries and database development. OJC and AFM review the database information. OJC carried out the statistical analysis. CMP and CPD drafted the design of study, and supervised the study implementation. All authors read and approved the final manuscript.

Acknowledgments

We thank Servicios y asesorías en infectología (SAI) for data provided.

Author details

[1]Infectious Diseases Department, Clinica Marly, Bogotá, Colombia. [2]Infectious Diseases Department, Hospital de la Samaritana, Bogotá, Colombia. [3]Servicios y asesorías en infectología (SAI), Calle 50 # 13-62, 110231420, Bogotá, Colombia. [4]School of Medicine, Universidad de la Sabana, Chia, Colombia. [5]School of Medicine, Universidad Militar Nueva Granada, Bogotá, Colombia. [6]School of Medicine, Fundación Universitaria Navarra, Neiva, Colombia.

References

1. Kuhar DT, Henderson DK, Struble KA, Heneine W, Thomas V, Cheever LW, et al. Updated US Public Health Service guidelines for the management of occupational exposures to human immunodeficiency virus and recommendations for postexposure prophylaxis. Infect Control Hosp Epidemiol. 2013;34:875–92.

2. Panlilio A, Cardo D, Grohskopf L, Heneine W, Ross C. Guidelines for the management of occupational exposures to HIV and recommendations for postexposure prophylaxis. MMWR. 2005;54:1–17.
3. Wald J. The psychological consequences of occupational blood and body fluid exposure injuries. Disabil Rehabil. 2009;31:1963–9.
4. CDC. Updated US public health service guidelines for the management of occupational exposure to HBV, HCV, and HIV and recommendations for PEP. MMWR Recomm Rep. 2001;50(RR-11):1–52.
5. Prüss-Üstün A, Rapiti E, Hutin Y. Estimation of the global burden of disease attributable to contaminated sharps injuries among health-care workers. Am J Ind Med. 2005;48:482–90.
6. Hamlyn E, Easterbrook P. Occupational exposure to HIV and the use of post-exposure prophylaxis. Occup Med (Chic Ill). 2007;57:329–36.
7. Gönen I. Percutaneous injuries among healthcare workers at a general hospital. J Microbiol Infect Dis. 2011;1:26–30.
8. Gumodoka B, Favot I, Berege ZA, Dolmans WM. Occupational exposure to the risk of HIV infection among health care workers in Mwanza Region, United Republic of Tanzania. Bull. Bull World Health Organization. 1997;75:133–40.
9. Butsashvili M, Kamkamidze G, Kajaia M, Morse DL, Triner W, Dehovitz J, et al. Occupational exposure to body fluids among health care workers in Georgia. Occup Med (Lond). 2012;62:620–6.
10. Kosgeroglu N, Ayranci U, Vardareli E, Dincer S. Occupational exposure to hepatitis infection among Turkish nurses: frequency of needle exposure, sharps injuries and vaccination. Epidemiol Infect. 2004;132:27–33.
11. Omar AA, Abdo M, Salama F, Al-mousa HH. Occupational Injuries Prone to Infectious Risks amongst Healthcare Personnel in Kuwait: A Retrospective Study. Med Princ Pract 2014; :1–6.
12. Różańska A, Szczypta A, Baran M, Synowiec E, Bulanda M, Wałaszek M. Healthcare workers' occupational exposure to bloodborne pathogens: a 5-year observation in selected hospitals of the Małopolska province. Int J Occup Med enviromental Heal. 2014;27:747–56.
13. Liu XN, Sun XY, van Genugten L, Shi YH, Wang YL, Niu WY, et al. Occupational exposure to blood and compliance with standard precautions among health care workers in Beijing, China. Am J Infect Control. 2014;42: e37–8.
14. Hajjaji Darouiche M, Chaabouni T, Jmal Hammami K, Messadi Akrout F, Abdennadher M, Hammami A, et al. Occupational blood exposure among health care personnel and hospital trainees. Int J Occup Environ Med. 2014; 5:57–61.
15. Helena Palucci Marziale M, Ludmilla Rossi Rocha F, Lúcia do Carmo Cruz Robazzi M, Maria Cenzi C, Ehmke Cardoso dos Santos H, Elisa Mendes Trovó M. Organizational influence on the occurrence of work accidents involving exposure to biological material. Rev Lat Am Enfermagem. 2013;21:199–206.
16. Leiss JK. Work experience, work environment, and blood exposure among home care and hospice nurses. Ind Health. 2012;50(6):521–8.
17. Blázquez RM, Moreno S, Menasalvas A, Guerrero C, Novoa A, Segovia M. Exposición a patógenos hemáticos en el personal sanitario. Enferm Infecc Microbiol Clin. 2001;19:156–60.
18. Hernández Navarrete MJ, Montes Villameriel FJ, Solano Bernad VM, Sánchez Matienzo D, del Val García JL, Gil Montalbán E, et al. Accidentes con material biológico en trabajadores sanitarios de 2 áreas de atención primaria (1990–1999). Aten Primaria. 2001;28:255–8.
19. Panunzio A, Nuñez-Barboza M, Molero-Zambrano T, Sirit Y, Zambrano M, Fuentes B, et al. Accidentalidad por fluidos biológicos en profesionales de laboratorios clínicos de Maracaibo, Venezuela. Rev Salud Pública. 2010;12: 93–102.
20. Montufar Andrade FE, Madrid Muñoz CA, Villa Franco JP, Diaz Correa LM, Vega Miranda J, Vélez Rivera JD, Accidentes ocupacionales de riesgo biológico en Antioquia, Colombia. Enero de 2010 a diciembre de 2011. Infectio 2014; 18(3):79–85.
21. Martínez Díaz LA, Cadena Afanador LP. Los accidentes biológicos entre estudiantes de medicina: el caso de la UNAB. Med UNAB. 2001;4:161–6.
22. Moon CS, Hwang JH, Lee CS, Park KH, Kim ES. Exposure to blood and body fluid among medical students in Korea. Am J Infect Control. 2010;38:582–3.
23. Yenesew MA, Fekadu GA. Occupational exposure to blood and body fluids among health care professionals in Bahir Dar town, Northwest Ethiopia. Saf Health Work. 2014;5:17–22.
24. Campins M, Torres M, Varela P, López Clemente V, Gascó A, de la Prada M, et al. Accidentes biológicos percutáneos en el personal sanitario: análisis de factores de riesgo no prevenibles mediante precauciones estándares. Med Clin (Barc). 2009;132:251–8.
25. Tesfay FA, Habtewold TD. Assessment of prevalence and determinants of occupational exposure to HIV infection among healthcare workers in selected health institutions in debre Berhan town, North shoa zone, Amhara region, Ethiopia, 2014. AIDS Res Treat. 2014;2014:731848.
26. Zhang M, Wang H, Miao J, Du X, Li T, Wu Z. Occupational exposure to blood and body fluids among health care workers in a general hospital, China. Am J Ind Med. 2009;52:89–98.
27. Osborn EH, Papadakis MA, Gerberding JL. Occupational exposures to body fluids among medical students. A seven-year longitudinal study. Ann Intern Med. 1999;130:45–51.
28. Alberth Cristian HG, Ossa RG. Accidentes por riesgos biológicos en los estudiantes de medicina y médicos internos de la Universidad Tecnológica de Pereira. Rev Médica Risaralda. 2003;9:1–10.
29. Tapias-vargas LF, Torres SA, Tapias Vargas L, Santamaria CM, Valencia Angel LI, Orozco Vargas LI. Accidentes biológicos en médicos residentes de Bucaramanga, Colombia. Rev Colomb Cir. 2010;25:290–99.
30. Eduardo Lozano C, Gissella González A, Del Pilar Cadena L. Caracterización de los accidentes por exposición a agente biológico en una población de estudiantes de medicina de Bucaramanga. Infectio. 2012;16:204–10.
31. Davanzo E, Frasson C, Morandin M, Trevisan A. Occupational blood and body fluid exposure of university health care workers. Am J Infect Control. 2008;36:753–6.
32. Fica CA, Jemenao PMI, Ruiz RG, Larrondo M, Hurtado C, Muñoz G, et al. Accidentes de riesgo biológico entre estudiantes de carreras de la salud: Cinco años de experiencia. Rev Chil infectología. 2010;27:34–9.
33. Naghavi SHR, Sanati KA. Accidental blood and body fluid exposure among doctors. Occup Med (Chic Il). 2009;59:101–6.
34. Montufar FE, Villa JP, Vélez JD, Zuleta JJ. Investigación de infección por VIH posterior a exposición ocupacional de riesgo biológico en trabajadores de la salud. Infectio. 2014;19:31–4.
35. Shokuhi S, Gachkar L, Alavi-Darazam I, Yuhanaee P, Sajadi M. Occupational exposure to blood and body fluids among health care workers in teaching hospitals in Tehran, Iran. Iran Red Crescent Med J. 2012;14:402–7.
36. Martins AMEDBL, Pereira RD Ferreira RC. Compliance with occupational post-exposure protocol for injuries among dental surgeons. Rev Saude Publica. 2010;44:528–40.

16

Health status and health-related quality of life of municipal waste collection workers

Marcial Velasco Garrido*, Cordula Bittner, Volker Harth and Alexandra Marita Preisser

Abstract

Background: Waste collection workers are exposed to several occupational stressors which may affect their quality of life. Our aim was to assess the health status and health-related quality of life (HRQoL) of municipal waste collection workers of a big German city.

Methods: Cross-sectional study with a non-random sample of 65 (62 male, 3 female) workers of the Hamburg sanitation department, volunteering to participate in the study. We assessed the prevalence of reported health complaints and health problems. HRQoL was assessed with the self-administered EQ-5D-5L questionnaire and its visual analogue scale (VAS).

Results: The most common health problems were musculoskeletal complaints (back pain reported by 67.2 %, other musculoskeletal complaints 15.4 %). Asthma or chronic obstructive pulmonary disease (COPD) was reported by 15.4 % of the workers. All participants reporting having a diagnosis of asthma or COPD had been or were active smokers. Our findings indicate an impaired HRQoL among the investigated occupational group. Regarding EQ-5D 68.3 % reported at least "slight" problems in one or more dimensions, and almost one third (31.7 %) reported "no problems" in any dimension. Problems were most frequently reported in the dimension "pain/ discomfort" (64.1 % of the workers). The mean VAS value was 80.9 (13.2). The presence of back pain was associated with limitations in HRQoL (RR 3.1; 95 %-CI 1.5-6.1). The EQ5D VAS score was statistically significantly lower among waste collectors with back pain (77.9 SD 14.1) compared to those with no back complaints (88.0 SD 7.6, $p < 0.01$).

Conclusions: Back complaints are common among municipal waste collectors and are associated with considerable impairments in their HRQoL. Interventions to enhance ergonomic work are needed in order to reduce back complaints and enhance HRQoL in this occupational group.

Keywords: Refuse collection, Waste collection, Back complaints, HRQoL, EQ-5D-5L, Cross-sectional study

Introduction

Municipal solid waste generation varies across countries in relation to income level and rate of urbanization, with the OECD countries accounting for 44 % of the 1.3 billion tonnes of waste generated yearly worldwide [1]. The duties of waste collectors usually include picking-up waste from its point of production, emptying refuse containers onto trucks, and delivering the waste to disposal and processing facilities. Despite the variety of collection methods, the job has, in general, been described as 'characterized by frequent lifting, carrying, pushing, and pulling of heavy objects' [2]. Besides the recurrent heavy physical activity, waste collectors are also exposed to bacteria, endotoxins, mould, allergens, particulate matter, irritant inhalants, vehicle exhaust, atmospheric conditions, noise, and psychomental stress. These multiple work demands and hazards result in a higher incidence of health problems and injuries compared to other occupations [2–4]. As one would expect, there is growing evidence that the incidence of respiratory problems and musculoskeletal complaints is higher among waste collectors than in other occupations [5, 6].

* Correspondence: m.velasco-garrido@uke.de
Institute for Occupational Medicine and Maritime Medicine (ZfAM), University Medical Center Hamburg-Eppendorf, Seewartenstrasse 10, 20459 Hamburg, Germany

Health-related quality of life (HRQoL) is a well-established aspect of health and general well-being, which can be measured with a variety of validated instruments [7]. In recent years, the issue of quality of life is increasingly being considered in occupational health research, with assessments of the relationship between occupational diseases and quality of life [8, 9]; and in relation to specific occupations [10–12].

The aim of our study was to assess (i) the prevalence of health problems and (ii) the HRQoL of waste collectors, and (iii) to investigate their associations.

Methods

Study design and participants

We conducted a descriptive cross-sectional study among workers of the Hamburg sanitation department. The study was part of a broader occupational and ergonomic field study which assessed the working conditions and job strain of municipal waste collectors with qualitative interviews, real-life observation and objective strain measurements (e.g. mobile spiroergometry) [13]. For the study, waste collectors were recruited by the human resources department of the municipal waste collection services of the City of Hamburg with the involvement of the safety engineer and collection tour planners. Participation in the field study was voluntary and rewarded with two days off. The sampling method was predefined by the ergonomic study and aimed at representing the broad spectrum of working conditions in the collection tours (i.e. areas with low and high population density, areas with frequent architectonic barriers, predominant type and size of container, etc.) and the two main work groups (street waste collectors and household waste collectors). The sample size was also determined by the ergonomic field study. The final study group consisted of 65 persons (62 male and 3 female) who were all active (i.e. not on sick leave) at the time of data collection (between January and August 2013). The majority of participants (71 %) were working in the household waste collection service.

Measurements

Participants were invited to our Outpatient Clinic for Occupational and Environmental Health for a health check including a general clinical examination, 12-channel resting-ECG, lung function testing (spirometry and body plethysmography), as well as spiroergometry as described elsewhere [14]. All participants signed a written informed consent document after the examining physician had explained the health check-up and the study. Before undergoing the clinical interview and clinical examinations, the participants were asked to answer a questionnaire regarding current and past health problems and to self-assess their HRQoL. The health problems questionnaire listed organ systems and asked (yes/no questions) whether the participant 'suffered or had suffered from any disease of that system, providing examples of the most common conditions for each system. It also included questions on smoking habits and medical treatments. The questionnaire was used to support the subsequent clinical interview.

HRQoL was self-assessed with the EQ-5D-5L instrument [15, 16] in its German version. The instrument consists of a descriptive system with five dimensions ('mobility', 'self-care', 'usual activities', 'pain/discomfort', 'anxiety/depression') and a visual analogue scale (VAS). In the descriptive system, the participant is asked to report his/her health state for each dimension on the present day (i.e. the day of answering the questionnaire) by ticking the most appropriate answer among five levels ('no problems', 'slight problems', 'moderate problems', 'severe problems', and 'extreme problems'; the word 'problems' is replaced by "pain or discomfort' in the fourth dimension and by 'anxious or depressed' in the fifth dimension). For each dimension, the answers are coded with a 1-digit number from '1' ('no problems') to '5' ('extreme problems'). The digits of the 5 dimensions are combined into a 5-digit number which describes the overall health state of the respondent [17]. For example '11111' indicates no problems in any of the dimensions; '21131' would indicate slight problems in mobility, moderate pain and discomfort and no problems in the other dimensions. In the EQ VAS, the self-rated health is visualized on a 20 cm vertical, visual analogue scale with endpoints labelled 'the best health you can imagine' ('100') and 'the worst health you can imagine' ('0') and to write the number marked in the scale on a box [17]. The time horizon for the VAS is also the present day.

The clinical interview was structured around the above-mentioned health problems questionnaire and aimed at ensuring the collection of relevant data on health problems.

Statistical analysis

Descriptive statistics are presented as median (interquartile range, IQR) or mean (standard deviation, SD) for continuous variables, and as frequency and percentage for categorical variables. The associations between health problems commonly reported and HRQoL were analysed calculating relative risk (RR) with 2x2 contingency tables and Fisher's exact test. Mean differences across groups were tested with unpaired Student's t. For multivariate analysis, logistic regression was performed adjusting for age, BMI and current smoking status, since these have been associated before with impairments in quality of life among adults [18, 19]. Two-tailed P values were calculated. Statistical analyses were carried out using PASW Statistics Software 18.0 (SPSS Inc., Chicago, IL, USA, IQR and Epi Info™ 7.1.3.3 (Centers for Disease Control and Prevention, Atlanta, GA, USA).

The study was approved by the Ethics Committee of the Hamburg Medical Association (register no. PV4524).

Results

Table 1 reports the characteristics of the study participants in comparison with the source population. Despite slight differences, the self-selected non-random sample was similar to the source population regarding age, gender distribution and years on the job. Vocational training prior to employment in the municipal waste collection services had been done more frequently by study participants. In general, waste collectors represent an aged collective, with the median age at 47.5 (IQR 10.6) years and 66.1 % of participants being above 45 years old.

Mean body mass index (BMI) was 28.3 kg/m^2 (SD 3.8). Overweight (BMI ≥25 kg/m^2) was highly prevalent among participants (83.1 %); obesity (BMI ≥30 kg/m^2) was present in 29.2 % of the waste collectors. The prevalence of smoking among the participants was 35.4 %; only 22.4 % reported to have never smoked.

Table 2 summarizes the results regarding health problems. A total of 89.2 % of the participants reported having at least one health problem. Considering vision limitations as a health problem raised the prevalence of health problems to 93.8 %. About one third reported currently being under medical treatment (29.2 %) or on long-term drug treatment (33.8 %). Most of the drug therapies (60 %) targeted cardiovascular diseases and cardiovascular risk factors. 11 % of the participants reported that they took antidepressant drugs.

The most common health problem was back pain, reported by 67.2 % of the participants. In the clinical examination, spinal percussion and/or palpation were painful in 11.5 % of the waste collectors and the finger-floor distance was over 10 cm in 19.3 % of the study group. Other musculoskeletal complaints were reported by 15.4 %.

According to the answers to the questionnaire, asthma and COPD had a prevalence of 7.7 % each. All participants reporting a diagnosis of asthma or COPD had been or were active smokers. Lung function tests yielded an obstructive pattern (FEV_1/FVC <70 %) in 21.5 % of the participants. Among those reporting a diagnosis of respiratory disease, 38.4 % showed an obstructive pattern (3 of them had reported a diagnosis of asthma and 2 of COPD).

All but one participant answered the EQ-5D questionnaire; one participant did not rate the "anxiety/depression" dimension. Almost one third (31.7 %) of the participant waste collectors rated their health status as 'without problems' in any 5 dimensions (i.e. 11111) (Table 3). The rest reported at least 'slight' problems in at least one dimension. The dimension for which problems were most frequently reported was 'pain/discomfort' with 46.9 %, and 17.2 % reported 'slight' or 'moderate' problems respectively. Almost one third (28.1 %) reported 'slight' or

Table 2 Reported diseases and health problems. [N = 65, multiple answers possible]

	Number	Percent
Back complaints	43	67.2
Vision problems or eye diseases	38	58.5
Long-term drug treatment	22	33.8
Allergies	21	32.3
Currently under medical treatment	19	29.2
Cardiovascular diseases	15	23.1
Respiratory diseases	13	20.0
Hearing problems or ear diseases	12	18.5
Gastrointestinal diseases	11	16.9
Other musculoskeletal complaints	10	15.4
Psychiatric problems	10	15.4
Dermatological problems	10	15.4
Vertigo, Syncope	8	12.3
Neurological diseases	5	7.7
Diabetes	3	4.6

Table 1 Participant characteristics compared to source collective

	Study participants (N = 65)				Source collective (N = 1,544)			
	Mean	SD	Number	Percent	Mean	SD	Number	Percent
Age (years)	45.5	8.3			46.5	9.4		
Gender								
Female			3	4.6			31	2.1
Male			62	95.4			1513	97.9
Previous vocational training								
Yes			52	80			1109	71.8
No			13	20			435	28.2
Years working for the municipal waste collection service	20.4	9.1			18.6	9.9		

Table 3 Frequency of health status (i.e. response patterns to the five-dimension descriptive part of EQ5D). [N = 63, frequency shown for patterns reported by more than one participant]

EQ5D Health Status	Number	Percent
11111	20	31.7
11121	14	22.2
21121	6	9.5
11122	4	6.3
11112	3	4.8
31231	3	4.8
11222	2	3.2
21122	2	3.2
21131	2	3.2

'moderate' problems in the dimension 'mobility'. The only dimension for which 'severe' problems were reported was 'anxiety/depression'. None of the participants reported any problems in the dimension 'self-care'.

The distribution of the VAS scores is shown in Fig. 1. All but 3 participants rated their HRQoL in the VAS. The mean EQ5D VAS score was 80.9 (SD 13.2); the lowest score was 50, the highest 100.

We explored the association between reported health problems and HRQoL in contingency tables for the conditions reported by at least one fifth of the participants (Table 4). Reported back complaints were associated with lower quality of life in the five-dimensional part of the EQ5D. The majority (87.8 %) of waste collectors with back pain had an HRQoL other than 11111. All participants reporting problems in the dimension 'mobility' had also reported back pain. The majority (88.4 %) of participants reporting back pain had also reported at least 'slight' problems in the dimension 'pain/discomfort'. Back complaints were also associated with lower VAS score. The VAS score among waste collectors without back pain was statistically significantly higher than the VAS score of participants with back pain (88.0 SD 7.6 vs. 77.9 SD 14.1, p = 0.0051). VAS score was also

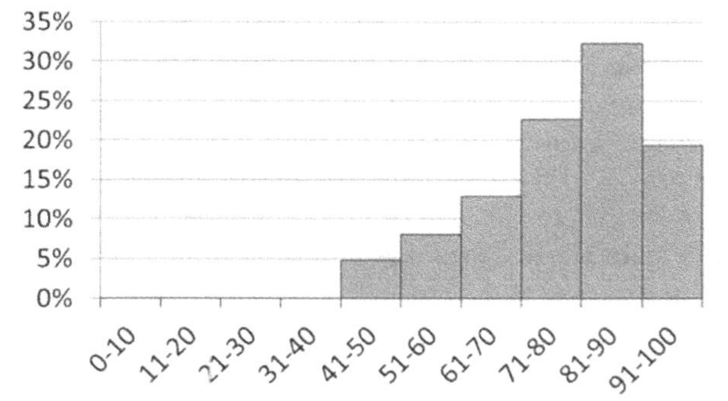

Fig. 1 Distribution of VAS-scores. [N = 62; 3 missing values]

statistically significantly lower among waste collectors under current medical treatment compared to those not in treatment (75.8 SD 14.8 vs. 85.0 SD 10.1, p = 0.0001) and among waste collectors reporting allergies compared to those with no allergy (75.9 SD 15.1 vs. 83.3 SD 11.7, p = 0.0408). For all other conditions listed in Table 4, there were no statistically significant differences in mean VAS score, although mean VAS score was always lower among waste collectors reporting the health problem or disease.

The association between back complaints and any limitation in quality of life (i.e. health status other than '11111') was still statistically significant after adjusting for age, BMI and current smoking status with logistic regression (OR 14.1; 95 %-CI 3.4-59.0).

Discussion

This is the first study to examine health status and quality of life using a validated instrument, the EQ-5D, of waste collection workers, although sample size was small. Interestingly, we observed a high prevalence of back complaints which was strongly associated with limitations in health related quality of life in this occupational group.

Previous studies have reported a higher prevalence of respiratory problems, including workplace-related respiratory complaints, among waste collectors than in the general population [3, 5, 6, 20]. This might be explained through the exposure against allergens and toxins contained in waste, seasonal allergens, and infectious agents [2]. Despite a higher prevalence of smokers and ex-smokers as in the German general population [21], we unexpectedly found a similar prevalence of asthma and COPD among our sample of waste collection workers as reported by the German general population [22]. However, on the basis of lung function testing, we identified 9 subjects with obstructive ventilatory abnormalities who had not reported having a respiratory disease, indicating the possibility of a higher total prevalence of respiratory problems in our sample, as one would expect. A limitation of our study is that we did not ask about workplace-related respiratory complaints. This could explain the discrepancy between previous papers and ours regarding respiratory diseases.

In the present study we found a higher prevalence of back complaints among waste collectors compared to the German general population [23]. This result is in accordance with previous reports in the literature [2, 6]. Although in our study we could not establish whether the reported back complaints were workplace-related, the available evidence indicates that waste collectors may have a higher incidence of musculoskeletal complaints than other occupations, equivalent to the findings of Kujier et al. [6]. In addition, musculoskeletal

Table 4 Health problems and health-related quality of life limitations.

Health problem	EQ5D 11111 (no problems)		EQ5D other than 11111 (at least slight problems in at least one dimension)		RR (raw)	95 % CI
	Number	Percent	Number	Percent		
Back complaints	5	25.0	36	85.7	3.07	1.54-6.10
Vision problems or eye diseases	11	55.0	26	60.5	1.01	0.76-1.52
Long-term drug treatment	6	30.0	16	37.2	1.11	0.79-1.55
Allergies	7	35.0	14	32.7	0.97	0.67-1.39
Currently under medical treatment	5	25.0	14	32.6	1.12	0.79-1.57
Cardiovascular diseases	3	15.0	12	27.9	1.24	0.89-1.72
Respiratory diseases	2	10.0	11	25.6	1.32	0.97-1.80

RR: relative risk

disorders have been reported as accounting for about one fifth of sickness absence in the waste industry [24]. This is not surprising since handling waste containers represents a considerable strain for the musculoskeletal system, particularly of the back, through the combination of trunk lateral flexion, bending and torsion, as shown in ergonomic observations [25]. The waste collectors included in our study pick up two-wheeled waste containers (120 L volume) from houses and cellars (partially overcoming stairs) and also shift large four-wheeled waste containers (240 L) from storerooms to the truck. The ergonomic field study demonstrated through mobile spiroergometry (measurement of oxygen uptake) a high physical demand in the job of both refuse collectors and street cleaners [14]. The qualitative interviews also showed that the job is psychologically demanding because of time pressure, accident risks and perceived unfairness of quality control [26], which can also represent a strain related to musculoskeletal complaints. Further, we found a high prevalence of overweight in our sample. Overweight has been associated with back pain and other musculoskeletal complaints [27, 28] and may represent an additional strain for the musculoskeletal system.

Our findings indicate an impaired HRQoL among this occupational group as compared to the reference population: Whereas 47.5 % of a representative sample of the German general population (i.e. including unemployed, chronically ill, etc.) reported the ideal EQ-5D health status [29], only one third (31.7 %) of the waste collectors rated their health status as without problems in all of the 5 dimensions. Taking the VAS score, HRQoL of waste collectors is comparable to that of German population samples. In a survey in the years 2002/2003, VAS score among employees was 82.3 (SD not reported), whereas the general population had a mean VAS score of 77.4 (SD 19.0) [30]. A more recent survey (data from 2006-2008) reported a mean VAS score for the general German population of 79.8 (SD not reported) [31]. However, comparisons with published results for the general population are to be interpreted carefully since weighting for sociodemographic factors is not possible.

We found an association between back complaints and limitations in the quality of life of municipal waste collectors. After adjusting for BMI and smoking back pain remained the most important factor limiting HRQoL, although the precision of our estimate was limited by the small size of our study (95 % CI 3.4-59.0). Back pain has been described before as a limiting factor of HRQoL among industrial workers [32] and also among sedentary office workers [33]. Although our cross-sectional study design does not allow drawing conclusions on causality, the frequent limitations in the dimensions 'pain/discomfort' and 'mobility' of the EQ-5D point at back complaints as being one of the explaining factors for the limitation of overall HRQoL among the examined group of municipal waste collectors. This is also supported by the differences in VAS scores according to problems in the dimensions 'pain/discomfort' and 'mobility' of the EQ-5D. The mean VAS score among those without problems in the dimension 'pain/discomfort' indicated better health than among waste collectors with problems in this dimension (86.9 SD 7.4 vs. 77.3 SD 14.1, $p = 0.0077$). Similarly, the VAS score showed better results among those without problems in the dimension 'mobility' (83.2 SD 11.4 vs. 74.7 SD 14.8, $p = 0.026$). All in all our study shows an association between back complaints and limitations in HRQoL. Interventions addressing ergonomic handling of waste containers and street sweeping may reduce back complaints and finally contribute to improve quality of life among these workers.

To our knowledge, only few studies have been conducted on HRQoL among waste collectors and these were limited to the special group of gatherers of recyclable materials in Brazil. One study used the WHOQOL-100 instrument but reported results too briefly to draw any sound conclusions [34], another one did not report having used a validated instrument to assess HRQoL and actually was focused on personal satisfaction [35], thus not being comparable with our work.

To our knowledge ours is the first published systematic assessment of HRQoL among a group of municipal waste collectors using a validated instrument, the EQ-5D.

Besides the cross-sectional design, which lacks the temporary dimension for cause-effect relationships, another limitation of our study is the small self-selected non-random sample. Our group included workers from the household collection (including organic waste collection) and the street sweeping services. According to age, gender distribution and length of work in waste collection, the participants can be considered to be representative of the employees of the municipal waste collection services.

Recruitment of the participants by the human resources department could have introduced selection bias, i.e. through recruitment of healthier workers. Indeed all participants were active at the time of participating in the study – i. e. not on sick leave – thus a healthy worker effect could have led to underestimation of the prevalence of disease. Potential participants were approached in order to represent the broad spectrum of working conditions in the collection department and participated voluntarily. Since absolute confidentiality was warranted in our study and the health check and interview were conducted in our Institute, we do not think that reporting of symptoms and health problems has been relevantly affected by the recruitment method. Being afflicted with health problems could have been the motivation to participate in the volunteer study, which would bias our results. Since our study was only a part of a broader ergonomic study in which field observations had the prominent role, we do not think the main motive to participate was own health complaints. In the qualitative interviews of the broader ergonomic study, the reported main motivations to take part in the study were to show how hard the job of a waste collector is and to contribute to improvements in the company [26].

Conclusions

In summary, we found back complaints to be a frequent health problem among municipal waste collection workers, more frequent than in the general population. These complaints are associated with limitations in health-related quality of life and probably explain at least some of these impairments. Interventions to enhance ergonomic work processes in this occupational field are warranted in order to reduce musculoskeletal problems and should be evaluated taking HRQoL into account.

Abbreviations

BMI: Body mass index; CI: Confidence interval; COPD: Chronic obstructive pulmonary disease; HRQoL: Health related quality of life; IQR: Interquartile range; OR: Odds ratio; RR: Relative risk; SD: Standard deviation; VAS: Visual analogue scale.

Competing interests

The authors declare that they have no competing interests.

Authors' contributions

MVG conceived and designed the study, acquired, analysed and interpreted the data and wrote the manuscript; CB acquired and interpreted the data and wrote the manuscript; VH interpreted data and revised the manuscript, AP conceived and designed the study, acquired and interpreted the data and wrote the manuscript. All authors read and approved the final manuscript.

Acknowledgements

We thank all participating waste collection workers of the Hamburg municipal waste collection services. We also thank Lutz Herrmann, safety engineer, for his support in participant recruitment. We are indebted to Thomas von Münster, MD, who conducted clinical interviews and examinations during the study. Finally we also thank Sabine Bößler and Anne Winkelmann for coordinating visits, performing medical technical procedures and for data managing.

The study was funded by a grant of 'Stadtreinigung Hamburg' (municipal sanitation department). The funder was neither involved in design, nor collection, nor analysis, nor interpretation of data, nor preparation of the manuscript. The funder was either involved in the decision to submit the manuscript.

References

1. Hoornweg D, Bhada-Tata P. What a waste: A global review of solid waste management. Urban Development Series, no 15. Washington DC: World Bank; 2012.
2. Kuijer PPFM, Frings-Dresen MH. World at work: Refuse collectors. Occup Environ Med. 2004;61:282–6.
3. Poulsen OM, Breum NO, Ebbehøj N, Hansen AM, Ivens UI, van Lelieveld D, et al. Collection of domestic waste. Review of occupational health problems and their possible causes. Sci Total Environ. 1995;170:1–19.
4. Ivens UI, Lassen JH, Kaltoft BS, Skov T. Injuries among domestic waste collectors. Am J Ind Med. 1998;33:182–9.
5. Athanasiou M, Makrynos G, Dounias G. Respiratory health of municipal solid waste workers. Occup Med (Lond). 2010;60:518–23.
6. Kuijer PPFM, Sluiter JK, Frings-Dresen MH. Health and safety in waste collection: Towards evidence-based worker health surveillance. Am J Ind Med. 2010;53:1040–64.
7. Fitzpatrick R, Davey C, Buxton MJ, Jones DR. Evaluating patient-based outcome measures for use in clinical trials. Health Technol Assessment. 1998;2.
8. Karvala K, Uitti J, Luukkonen R, Nordman H. Quality of life of patients with asthma related to damp and moldy work environments. Scand J Work Environ Health. 2013;39:96–105.
9. Knoeller GE, Mazurek JM, Moorman JE. Health related quality of life among adults with work-related asthma in the United States. Qual Life Res. 2013;22:771–80.
10. Chattopadhyay K, Chattopadhyay C, Kaltenhaler E. Health related quality-of-life of coal-based sponge iron plant workers in Barjora, India: a cross-sectional study. BMJ Open. 2014. doi:10.1136/bmjopen-2014-006047.
11. Rodríguez-Romero B, Pita-Fernández S, Pertega-Díaz S, Chouza-Insua M. Health-related quality of life in women working in the fishing industry measured through the Short-Form 36 questionnaire. Gac Sanit. 2013;27:418–24.
12. Jha A, Sadhukhan SK, Velusamy S, Banarjee G, Banarje A, Saha A, et al. Exploring the quality of life (QOL) in the Indian software industry: a public health viewpoint. Int J Public Health. 2012;57:371–81.
13. Zentralinstitut für Arbeitsmedizin und Maritime Medizin, Gesellschaft für Betriebsforschung und angewandte Arbeitswissenschaft, Institut für Arbeit und Technik e.V. Arbeitswissenschaftliche Untersuchung Entsorger Sytemmüllabfuhr/Straßenreinigung. Hamburg; 2014.
14. Preisser A, Zhou L, Velasco Garrido M, Harth V. Measured by the oxygen uptake in the field, the work of refuse collectors is particularly hard work: Are the limit values for physical endurance workload too low? Int Arch Occup Environ Health. 2015. [Epub ahead of print]
15. The EuroQol Group. EuroQol –a new facility for the measurement of health-related quality of life. Health Policy. 1990;16(3):199–208.

16. Herdman M, Gudex C, Lloyd A, Janssen MF, Kind P, Parkin D, et al. Development and preliminary testing of the new five-level version of EQ-5D (EQ-5D-5L). Qual Life Res. 2011;20:1727–36.
17. van Reenen M, Janssen B. EQ-5D-5L User guide. Basic information on how to use the EQ-5D-5L instrument. Version 2.1, April 2015. http://www.euroqol.org/fileadmin/user_upload/Documenten/PDF/Folders_Flyers/EQ-5D-5L_UserGuide_2015.pdf. Accessed 06 July 2015.
18. Kearns B, Ara R, Young T, Relton C. Association between body mass index and health-related quality of life, and the impact of self-reported long-term conditions – cross-sectional study from the south Yorkshire cohort dataset. BMC Public Health. 2013. doi:10.1186/1471-2458-13-1009.
19. Rachiotis G, Behrakis PK, Vasiliou M, Yfantopoulos J. Quality of life and smoking among industrial workers in Greece. Med Lav. 2006;97:44–50.
20. Schantora AL, Casjens S, Deckert A, van kampen V, Neumann HD, Brüning T, et al. Prevalence of work-related rhino-conjunctivitis and respiratory symptoms among domestic waste collectors. Advs Exp Medicine Biology. 2014; doi: 10.1007/5584_2014_71.
21. Lampert T, von der Lippe E, Müters S. Prevalence of smoking in the adult population of Germany: results of the German Health Interview and Examination Survey for Adults (DEGS1). Bundesgesundheitsblatt Gesundheitsforschung Gesundheitsschutz. 2013;56:802–8.
22. Robert Koch Institut. Daten und Fakten: Ergebnisse der Studie „Gesundheit in Deutschland aktuell 2010". Beiträge zur Gesundheitsberichterstattung des Bundes. Berlin: Robert Koch Institut; 2010.
23. Neuhauser H, Ellert U, Ziese T. Chronic back pain in the general population in Germany 2002/2003: prevalence and highly affected population groups. Gesundheitswesen. 2005;67:685–93.
24. Holmes E. Review of sickness absence data in the waste and recycling industry. Health and Safety Executive Research Report RR750. London: Health and Safety Executive; 2009.
25. Backhaus C, Jubt KH, Post M, Ellegast R, Felten C, Hedtmann J. The musculoskeletal strain during pushing and pulling of waste containers. Z Arb Wiss. 2012;66:327–46.
26. Martiny U, Frosch A, Paulus S. Sozialwissenschaftliche Untersuchung – Subjektive Wahrnehmung und Einschätzung ihrer Arbeit durch die Entsorger. In: Zentralinstitut für Arbeitsmedizin und Maritime Medizin, Gesellschaft für Betriebsforschung und angewandte Arbeitswissenchaft, Institut für Arbeit und Technik e.V. (eds.). Arbeitswissenschaftliche Untersuchung Entsorger Sytemmüllabfuhr/ Straßenreinigung. Hamburg; 2014. p. 113-180.
27. Shiri R, Karppinen J, Leino-Arjas P, Slovieva S, Viikari-Juntura E. The association between obesity and low back pain: a meta-analysis. Am J Epidemiol. 2010;171:135–54. doi:10.1093/aje/kwp356.
28. Kortt M, Baldry J. The association between musculoskeletal disorders and obesity. Aust Health Rev. 2002;25:207–14.
29. Hinz A, Kohlmann T, Stöbek-Richter Y, Zenger M, Brähler E. The quality of life questionnaire EQ-5D-5L: psychometric properties and normative values for the general German population. Qual Life Res. 2014;23:443–7. doi:10.1007/s11136-013-0498-2.
30. König HH, Bernert S, Angermeyer MC. Health Status of the German population: results of a representative survey using the EuroQol questionnaire. Gesundheitswesen. 2005;67:173–82.
31. Mielck A, Reitmeier P, Vogelmann M, Leidl R. Impact of educational level on health-related quality of life (HRQoL): results from Germany based on the EuroQol 5D (EQ-5D). Eur J Public Health. 2013;23:45–9.
32. Morken T, Riise T, Moen B, Bergum O, Vigeland Hauge SH, Holien S, et al. Frequent musculoskeletal symptoms and reduced health-related quality of life among industrial workers. Occup Med. 2002;52:91–8.
33. del Pozo-Cruz B, Gusi N, Adsuar JC, del Pozo-Cruz J, Parraca JA, Hernandez-Mocholí M. Musculoskeletal fitness and health-related quality of life characteristics among sedentary office workers affected by sub-acute, non-specific low back pain: a cross-sectional study. Physiotherapy. 2013;99:194–200.
34. de Barros Pimenta PA, dos Reis Santos SM, Pinto de Jesis MC, Martins Borges M, de Oliveira Marques GL, Francis Abdalla JG. The municipal solid waste and the quality of life of collectors of recyclable materials in Juiz de Fora, Minas Gerais. Work. 2012;41:5681–3.
35. Rabelo Almeida J, Tavares Elias E, Alves de Magalhaes M, Dias Vieira AJ. Age effect on the life quality and health of garbage collectors of an association in Governador Valadares, Minas Gerais State, Brazil. Cien Saud Col. 2009;14:2169–80.

17

The rubber manufacturing industry: a case report and review of cutaneous exposure and sequelae

Claire Powers[1] and Heather P. Lampel[2*]

Abstract

Exposure to chemical carcinogens in rubber manufacturing remains a serious occupational health concern. Workers are exposed to these carcinogens via skin or inhalation. Rubber manufacturing work is associated with a high prevalence of dermatologic diseases such as eczema, allergic contact dermatitis and atopic dermatitis. The role that epidermal exposure plays in the development of malignancies historically associated with the rubber industry is less certain. We present a case relevant to this discussion and review the role of skin exposure in the rubber industry, providing an overview of the cutaneous and systemic manifestations of occupational exposures in modern day rubber workers.

Background

In their seminal report in 1982, the International Agency for Research on Cancer (IARC) determined the rubber industry "entailed exposures that are carcinogenic to humans [1]." During the following decades, control measures aimed at reducing exposure were instituted, such as removal of known carcinogens from the rubber production process. As a result, exposure to airborne particulate [2] and dermal exposure in rubber factories [3] has decreased drastically since the 1980s.

Rubber production has increased considerably in Asia over the past century, with fewer factories in Europe and North America. In 1989, 54,600 workers were employed in the United States rubber industry, compared to 88,300 workers in 1977 [4]. However, the majority of health data regarding the rubber industry arises from Western countries [5].

The process of rubber manufacturing is complex and continually changing, thus making the study of occupational exposures in the rubber industry difficult. Rubber workers' route and compounds of chemical exposure depend largely on the specific employee work task and environment. In 1994, the Centers for Disease Control and the National Institute for Occupational Safety and Health summarized these various exposures. Handling raw materials can give rise to considerable amounts of airborne dust particulate, while mixing, extruding, calendaring and vulcanizing (curing) rubber exposes workers to inhaled fumes. The specific carcinogens contained in these fumes have not yet been fully identified, yet studies have demonstrated the mutagenic potential of the fumes [6, 7]. Vulcanizing rubber releases N-nitrosamines and polycyclic aromatic hydrocarbons, both known carcinogens. Workers in final inspection and finishing tasks have extensive skin contact with finished rubber [4].

Case report: a tire-maker's traumatic tattoos

A 57-year-old white male patient who has worked in a tire manufacturing plant for 37 years and retired 6 years prior, presented with asymptomatic dermally-implanted rubber in the bilateral hands, forearms and upper arms (Fig. 1). The dermally implanted rubber is most pronounced on his left index finger, which is darkly discolored (Fig. 2). These "rubber tattoos" resulted from frequent trauma while cutting unvulcanized rubber implanted with sharp metal strips. His work task was specifically manipulating and hand cutting unvulcanized rubber sheets which had uniform, thin metal wires embedded. These metal wires also extended beyond the ends of the sheets, exposing the worker to repeated puncture wounds. He reported regular notice of rubber

* Correspondence: drheatherlampel@gmail.com
[2]Department of Dermatology, Duke University, Durham, North Carolina, USA
Full list of author information is available at the end of the article

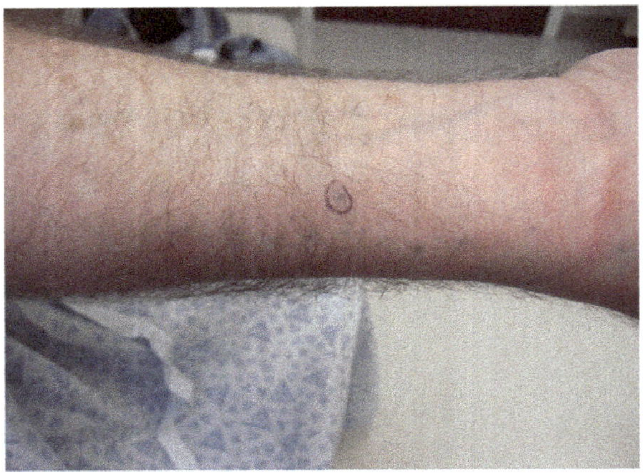

Fig. 1 Forearm demonstrating numerous blue-black macules

particulate on his hands. It is likely that these repeated wire punctures essentially "tattooed" the worker's skin over time with rubber particles by traumatic implantation. He wore forearm sleeves for over a decade, but not gloves. The patient noted that many coworkers in his department had similar skin findings. Biopsy of these lesions demonstrated perivascular pigment consistent with rubber tattoo. No systemic biomarkers were measured given his lengthy retirement. The patient expressed an understanding of the well-known link between cancer and the rubber manufacturing industry [8] but was specifically inquisitive about the increased risk of malignancies given his dermally implanted "rubber tattoos."

Skin exposure

Manufacturing jobs in general harbor the largest burden of occupational skin diseases compared with other industries [9] and dermal exposure is an important route of toxin acquisition, especially in the rubber industry.

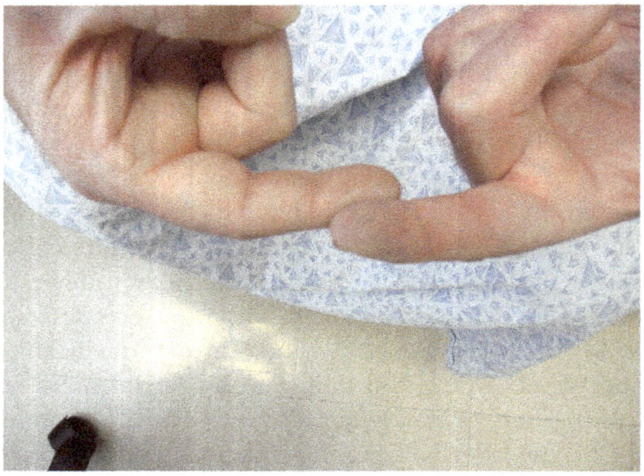

Fig. 2 Coalescent hyperpigmentation of the distal fingertip due to traumatic rubber tattoos

Repetitive skin contact with warm unfinished rubber products is thought to be the primary route for dermal contamination [10]. Depending on the factory conditions and the use of protective equipment, soluble dermal exposure may be as much as tenfold higher than inhaled amounts [3]. This may not be the case in curing departments, where exposure to large quantities of cyclohexane-soluble fumes occurs [10]. Soluble cyclohexane was adapted by the British Rubber Manufacturers association as a measure of the fraction of the fume or dust that "contains the constituents most likely to be harmful" to human health [11]. Indeed, one study of 225 Dutch rubber tire workers in 2008 demonstrated that increased levels of soluble dermal cyclohexane on the hands and wrists was correlated with increased urinary levels of polycyclic aromatic hydrocarbons but that urinary mutagenicity seemed to be more associated with inhalable dust exposure [12]. However, other studies have observed a direct relation between urinary mutagenicity and skin contamination, notably after controlling for cigarette use [13, 14]. Therefore, intake through the skin may play an important role in occupational exposure to mutagenic compounds in the rubber industry.

Cutaneous manifestations of occupational exposure in the rubber industry

Dermatitis

Frequent causes of allergic contact dermatitis, rubber additives such as accelerators, antioxidants and vulcanizers are increasingly utilized in the modern manufacturing process to improve quality, speed of production, and product durability [15, 16]. Multiple chemicals have been identified as sensitizing agents for rubber-related contact dermatitis (Table 1) [4]. The prevalence of type IV hypersensitivity reactions to rubber constituents is estimated between 3.8 % and 4.4 % [15, 17]. These allergies are often related to rubber glove use in health services and laboratory workers; however, a distinct subset of allergies due to non-glove, industrial exposure in rubber manufacturers exists. A cross-sectional survey of 999 workers in an Australian tire plant reported a prevalence rate of 37 cases of occupational contact dermatitis per 1,000 workers, highlighting the risks of dermatitis associated with the rubber industry [18].

Skin cancer

The relationship between occupational rubber exposure and skin cancer is less certain. Increased incidence of cutaneous squamous cell carcinoma among workers exposed to rubber stock and lubricating oils was found in a nested case–control study in Akron, Ohio in 1987 [19]. The distribution of these cancers on the body was similar to a sun-exposed population, with the head and neck most common, followed by the hands and arms.

Table 1 Agents reported to cause contact dermatitis in rubber product workers according to the CDC & NIOSH 1993 report (Table adapted from Reference 4)

Chemical	CAS Number	Process	Product
2-(2′-4′ dinitrophenylthio) benzothiazole	17586–89–9	All areas	Tires
4,4′-dithiodimorpholine, 1 %	103–34–4	Not specified	Tires
n-isopropyl-n- phenylparaphenylenediamine (IPPD)	101–72–4	Assembly, maintenance, compounding	Tires
n-dimethyl-1,3 butyl-n- phenylparaphenylenediamine	793–24–8	Assembly, maintenance, compounding	Tires
para-phenylenediam ne compounds	106–50–3	Handling of uncured rubber	Tires, footwear
ethylene thiourea (ETU)	96–45–7	Sewing	Non-tire
resorcinol	108–46–3	Not specified	Tires

This unexpected distribution questions whether these cancers were indeed related to an occupational exposure. Exposure to well—accepted skin carcinogens polycyclic aromatic hydrocarbons (PAHs) [1] is greatest in the mixing, milling, and assembly areas where direct handling of uncured rubber stock occurs [19]. PAHs are still very much present in the modern day rubber industry, as demonstrated by measuring higher weekday vs. weekend urinary 1-hydroxypyrene levels (a valid marker for PAH exposure) in rubber workers in 2008 [12]. The IARC acknowledged an increased risk of skin cancer in 1982, also noting that lubricating oils in uncured rubber contain known skin carcinogens [1]. However, a more recent Swedish study conducted in 2007 examined 5,745 rubber workers and failed to demonstrate increased risk of skin cancer in the rubber industry [20]. In 2012, the IARC concluded that there is insufficient evidence to determine the relationship between the rubber industry and skin cancer [5].

Cancers other than skin

In an updated 2012 report, the IARC reviewed three-decades of new data on the rubber industry. The IARC re-confirmed there is sufficient evidence of excess risk of bladder, leukemia, lung and stomach cancer in the modern rubber manufacturing industry. This recent report differed from the previous 1982 report in that the IARC acknowledged an excess risk of malignant lymphomas including multiple myeloma and esophageal cancers in rubber industry workers, while finding inconclusive evidence to link laryngeal cancer to the rubber industry. Prostate, brain, thyroid and pancreatic cancer continue to have insufficient evidence of increased risk in the rubber industry [5].

Well-documented associations of cancer in the rubber industry related to specific occupational exposures include the excess risk of leukemia with benzene exposure [20, 21], bladder cancer with 2-naphthylamine [22] and o-toluidine exposure [23], lung cancer with asbestos and carbon black [24], and nitrosamines released during vulcanization posing excess risk of pharyngeal, esophageal and cancers of the oral cavity [25]. This distinction highlights the importance of understanding worker duties and exposures when advising industrial rubber workers about cancer risk. A prospective cohort study from 1999 on 11,633 German rubber workers conducted in five different plant departments found the highest mortality in the early production stages involving mixing and weighing of uncured rubber products [24]. They hypothesized that mixing and weighing disturbs large quantities of dusts, possibly talc, asbestos or carbon black, while directly handling uncured rubber exposes to PAHs. In our case study, we report the patient worked directly with unvulcanized rubber in these early production processes, which was noted by this study of German rubber workers to be of high risk. Specific biomarkers exist for monitoring some chemical exposures (Table 2).

Conclusion

Our patient worked in a tire-manufacturing plant for more than three decades. His specific role in the manufacturing line contributed to skin exposure to unvulcanized rubber stock. He also suffered repeated puncturing of the skin from the wires in his medium and subsequent “rubber tattoos.” No studies to date address the subsequent health risks from skin-implanted rubber. Our patient did not have any current evidence of allergic contact dermatitis and no history of cancers. As mentioned above, rubber workers in early production stages working with uncured rubber and those with direct, extensive skin-contact with rubber precursors may have

Table 2 Accepted biomarkers of exposure in the rubber industry

Chemical	Biomarker
Asbestos	Lung x-rays and pulmonary function testing; others in development
Polycyclic aromatic hydrocarbons	Urine 1-hydroxypyrene
Benzene	Urine s-phenylmercapturic acid; urine t,t-muconic acid

higher rates of bladder, leukemia, lung, stomach cancers, malignant lymphomas and esophageal cancers. In alignment with the IARC, we find that there is insufficient evidence to support increased risk of skin cancer in such workers. However, rubber stock is known to contain polycyclic aromatic hydrocarbons, demonstrated skin-carcinogens that have not been eliminated from the modern rubbery industry. Therefore, evidence suggests that rubber workers with extensive skin contact, especially direct, repetitive traumatic introduction of uncured rubber into the skin may be a unique sub-group in this industry deserving further study.

It is wise to recommend personal protective equipment including gloves to prevent skin contact with uncured rubber in such employment. However, our particular patient stated that any glove use compromised his tactile ability. He did wear forearm sleeves for some of his employment, and these can be considered. In areas of fumes or dust particulate, we recommend task-specific mask filters for inhalation prevention. Enclosing processes and automating tasks when possible could decrease worker exposure.

Further research is needed to determine the risks of skin cancer in the dynamic rubber industry, as additional study could directly support safer handling practices and the further removal of carcinogens from the industry for workers.

Abbreviations

(IARC): International Agency for Research on Cancer; (PAH): Polycyclic aromatic hydrocarbon.

Competing interests

The authors declare that they have no competing interests.

Authors' contribution

CP wrote the initial manuscript, HPL is the senior author and attending, addended manuscript and revised, and performed all patient care and communication. All authors read and approved the final manuscript.

Authors' information

HPL is a practicing dermatologist board-certified in both dermatology and occupational and environmental medicine. CP is a medical student interested in a career in internal medicine.

References

1. The rubber industry. IARC Monogr Eval Carcinog Risk Chem Hum. 1982;28:1–486.
2. de Vocht F, Vermeulen R, Burstyn I, Sobala W, Dost A, Taeger D, et al. Exposure to inhalable dust and its cyclohexane soluble fraction since the 1970s in the rubber manufacturing industry in the European Union. Occup Environ Med. 2008;65(6):384–91.
3. Vermeulen R, De Hartog J, Swuste P, Kromhout H. Trends in exposure to inhalable particulate and dermal contamination in the rubber manufacturing industry: effectiveness of control measures implemented over a nine-year period. Ann Occup Hyg. 2000;44(5):343–54.
4. Publication of Special NIOSH hazard review of the rubber products manufacturing industry. MMWR Morb Mortal Wkly Rep. 1994;43(14):266.
5. Occupational exposures in the rubber manufacturing industry. IARC Monogr Eval Carcinog Risk Hum. 2102;100F:541–62.
6. Lee N, Lee BK, Jeong S, Yi GY, Shin J. Work environments and exposure to hazardous substances in Korean tire manufacturing. Saf Health Work. 2012;3(2):130–9.
7. Kim EA, Park J, Kim KH, Lee N, Kim DS, Kang SK. Outbreak of sudden cardiac deaths in a tire manufacturing facility: can it be caused by nanoparticles? Saf Health Work. 2012;3(1):58–66.
8. Kogevinas M, Sala M, Boffetta P, Kazerouni N, Kromhout H, Hoar-Zahm S. Cancer risk in the rubber industry: a review of the recent epidemiological evidence. Occup Environ Med. 1998;55(1):1–12.
9. Lushniak BD. The importance of occupational skin diseases in the United States. Int Arch Occup Environ Health. 2003;76(5):325–30.
10. Kromhout H, Swuste P, Boleij JS. Empirical modelling of chemical exposure in the rubber-manufacturing industry. Ann Occup Hyg. 1994;38(1):3–22.
11. Laboratory, H.a.S., Methods for determination of hazardous substances. Determination of rubber process dust and rubber fume (measured as cyclohexane-soluble material) in air. 1999.
12. Peters S, Talaska G, Jönsson BA, Kromhout H, Vermeulen R. Polycyclic aromatic hydrocarbon exposure, urinary mutagenicity, and DNA adducts in rubber manufacturing workers. Cancer Epidemiol Biomarkers Prev. 2008;17(6):1452–9.
13. Bos RP, Kromhout H, Ikink H, De Haan W, Koppejan J, Theuws JLG. Mutagens in urine of non-smoking and smoking workers in an aircraft tyre retreading plant. Skin exposure as a causal factor? Mutat Res. 1989;223(1):41–8.
14. Vermeulen R, Bos RP, Pertijs J, Kromhout H. Exposure related mutagens in urine of rubber workers associated with inhalable particulate and dermal exposure. Occup Environ Med. 2003;60(2):97–103.
15. von Hintzenstern VJ, Heese A, Koch HU, Peters KP, Hornstein OP. Frequency, spectrum and occupational relevance of type IV allergies to rubber chemicals. Contact Dermatitis. 1991;24(4):244–52.
16. Warburton KL, Urwin R, Carder M, Turner S, Agius R, Wilkinson SM. UK rates of occupational skin disease attributed to rubber accelerators, 1996–2012. Contact Dermatitis. 2015;72(5):305–11.
17. Chen HH, Sun CC, Tseng MP. Type IV hypersensitivity from rubber chemicals: a 15-year experience in Taiwan. Dermatology. 2004;208(4):319–25.
18. Varigos GA, Dunt DR. Occupational dermatitis. An epidemiological study in the rubber and cement industries. Contact Dermatitis. 1981;7(2):105–10.
19. Bourguet CC, Checkoway H, Hulka BS. A case–control study of skin cancer in the tire and rubber manufacturing industry. Am J Ind Med. 1987;11(4):461–73.
20. Wingren G, Axelson O. Cancer incidence and mortality in a Swedish rubber tire manufacturing plant. Am J Ind Med. 2007;50(12):901–9.
21. Hosseini SY, M.R.A, Taiefeh Rahimian R, Tavakkol E. Occupational Risk Assessment of Benzene in Rubber Tire Manufacturing Workers. Int J Occup Hygiene. 2014;6(4):220–7.
22. Veys CA. Bladder tumours in rubber workers: a factory study 1946–1995. Occup Med (Lond). 2004;54(5):322–9.
23. Carreon T, Hein MJ, Hanley KW, Viet SM, Ruder AM. Bladder cancer incidence among workers exposed to o-toluidine, aniline and nitrobenzene at a rubber chemical manufacturing plant. Occup Environ Med. 2014;71(3):175–82.
24. Straif K, Chambless L, Weiland SK, Wienke A, Bungers M, Taeger D, et al. Occupational risk factors for mortality from stomach and lung cancer among rubber workers: an analysis using internal controls and refined exposure assessment. Int J Epidemiol. 1999;28(6):1037–43.
25. Straif K, Weiland SK, Bungers M, Holthenrich D, Taeger D, Yi S, et al. Exposure to high concentrations of nitrosamines and cancer mortality among a cohort of rubber workers. Occup Environ Med. 2000;57(3):180–7.

Muscular imbalances and balance capability in dance

Eileen M. Wanke[1*], Julia Schreiter[2], David A. Groneberg[1] and Burkhard Weisser[2]

Abstract

Objective: A high unilateral load to the musculoskeletal system is specific for formation dance. Due to the lack of data the aim of this study was the side-related (right – left) analysis of strength- and balance capability subject to injuries, gender and performance standards.

Methods: $N = 51$ dancers (m: $n = 24$, f: $m = 27$) of two performance levels participated in this cross-sectional study. Double-sided tests of the isometric maximal strength of relevant muscle groups and the balance capability were carried out. The tests were supplemented by a self report questionnaire.

Results: Tests of the isometric maximal strength in the elite performance level showed significant differences between either side of the body. As to the balance capability, no significant side-related differences could be found in. Correlations between the strength capability and the injuries could be observed in either group.

Conclusion: The significant strength differences are presumably caused by the right-sided load in the dance-specific movements. The cautious conclusion that movement patterns challenge the stability of either side of the body likewise may be allowed. The increased injury frequency at the muscularly stronger side of the body primarily results from an overload. An additive muscular training should be considered as a preventive measure.

Keywords: Formation dance, Laterality, Motor skills, Injuries

Background

Dance sport is the competition- and performance-oriented variant of ballroom dancing. Within dance sport, which is one of the technical/compositional and aesthetic sports, formation dance is a further discipline in addition to single-pair dance [1]. As a result of the 1950s, formation dance sport has become established in its present form with a 5-level league system and annual national and international championships. As in single pair dancing, a distinction is made between standard and Latin American formations. The aim of formation dancing is to have the 8 couples of a team moving synchronously and precisely on the dance floor during the five Latin American dances (Samba, Rumba, Jive, Cha-Cha-Cha, Paso Doble) [2].

In contrast to the single pair dance, a performance in formation dance lasts six minutes, 4.5 min of which are allotted to the main part relevant for the evaluation with the remaining 1.5 min to the marching in and out with. The cardiovascular stress extends in the fast Latin American dances (e. g. Jive) into the maximum stress range, with high demands being conductive to injuries [3, 4]. In contrast to single pair dance, there are formation dance-characteristic elements of movement in Latin American formation dance that go beyond the dance steps, the gender-specific tasks and movement and posture characteristics which are either more frequent (e. g. the *Lankenau* pirouette, *Cha-Cha-s-pins*) or they are found exclusively in the Latin American formation dance (e. g. *round-about, potstirrer*) (Fig. 1). These steps are often key elements in the rating during a competition for they require a high strength capability and major coordination skills [5]. In addition to their high movement dynamics, these characteristic elements are associated with a one-sided right-sided load on the movement and support system of either dance partner and characteristically initiated and terminated by the male partner in each case as well as predominantly presented unilaterally (on the right) [6, 7]. In combination with the already

* Correspondence: wanke@med.uni-frankfurt.de
[1]Institute of Occupational, Social and Environmental Medicine, Goethe-University Frankfurt Main, Theodor-Stern-Kai 7, 60590 Frankfurt am Main, Germany

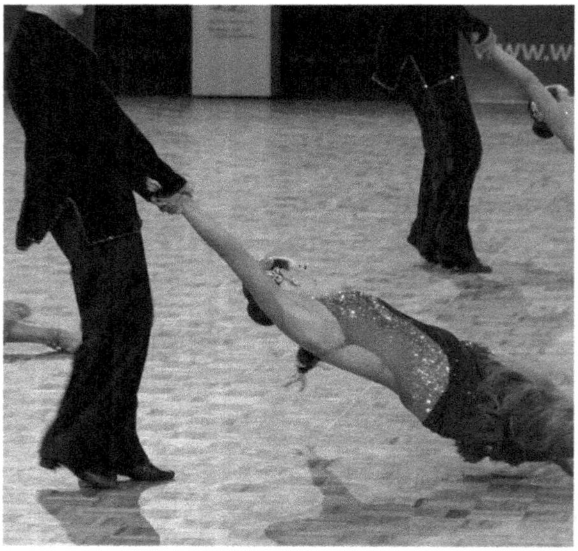

Fig. 1 "slingshot" as a characteristic element of movement in Latin American formation dance with one side loaded (Photo: Oldenbüttel)

open dance posture performed on the right, this results in a laterality of movements in favor of the right side.

In the last few years the formation dance has changed a lot [7]. Speed and dynamics have increased [8]. Numerous flowing position changes without a complete standstill as well as the trend towards a direct line-up of several extreme difficulties have further increased the demands on dance technique, the musculoskeletal as well as the cardiovascular system. This development seems to be necessary in order to remain competitive both on nationally and internationally. In addition to the high, often one-sided, loads, this results in a training time of up to 15 h weekly combined with only occasional professionalism and a not to be underestimated subordination of individual physical prerequisites to the benefit of group performance [9].

Objective of the present study

There are characteristic stylistic elements in formation dance associated with unilateral loads on the body. While there are studies on other dance directions indicating a morphological laterality according to a higher right-sided force level [10–12]. As a consequence of the gender-specific and dance direction-specific movement contents, there have been no studies on dance sport in this respect. Hitherto, it is largely unclear to what extent these asymmetric loads lead to morphological and/or functional adjustments [13]. At that, a correlation with the frequency of injuries on a certain side of the body has not yet been sufficiently investigated. Studies on the side-related balance capability of the body, as well as the relation to develop the strength capability of either side of the body have also been lacking. However, it cannot be ruled out that the named factors favor the occurrence of traumatic (acute) injuries as well as the inappropriate loads and overloads of the musculoskeletal system [14]. Mergenthaler [15] and Strauss [16, 17] have already ranked formation dancing as the discipline with the highest injury risk within the various dance sports disciplines. Wanke et al. [9] observed a possible correlation between gender-specific movement elements and injuries or chronic sports injuries in formation dance and pointed to a further need for research in this discipline.

The aim of the present study is therefore to analyze the balance as well as the maximal isometric strength capability (hamstrings, quadriceps, triceps, biceps, shoulder elevators) in formation dancers regarding body sides, injury frequency, gender and performance standard (performance class: EPL; junior level: JL).

Methods

Subjects

Table 1 shows the descriptive data of the participants. The study included a total of $n = 51$ formation dancers with an average age of 21.6 (± 4.0) years and an average height of 174.5 (±10.3) cm. The mean body mass index (BMI) and body weight (kg) were 21.8 (±2.1) and 66.6 (±11.1) kg, respectively. Only significant differences were found between the male and female dancers but not between the JL and EPL level groups. The junior level dancers (JL, regional league or lower) consisted of $n = 29$ dancers with the performance level dancers (EPL, highest national league) consisting of $n = 22$ dancers. All participants were healthy at the time of the examination and took part in competitions as members of a dance formation.

Balance measurement

The MFT S3-Check device (measurement of stability and sensorimotor index, symmetry ratio) was used to measure the balance capability and body stability. This measuring device consists of an unstable disc, equipped with sensors that detect all movements of the subjects. As soon as the centre of gravity was removed from the center of the disc, the measuring plate tilted to a maximum of 12° towards the pre-determined direction. The test subject's task was to re-stabilize the standing base as quickly as possible and to keep it as immobilized as possible for a period of 30 s. Deviations from the so-called optimum state (parallel to the ground) were registered by means of acceleration and inclination sensors. The measuring plate was connected to computer software via an USB interface and could be evaluated. The better the sensorimotor regulation capability, the better the sensorimotor index was assessed. The balance of the movement deviations to the different directions was given with the symmetry ratio. The stability index was

Table 1 Descriptive data of the group of test subjects

Test subjects (n)	Age in years M(SD)	Height in cm M(SD)	Weight in kg M(SD)	Body Mass Index (BMI) M(SD)
All ($n = 24$) Male	22.8 (±5.0)	182.8 (±7.6)	74.6 (±9.7)	22.3 (±2.0)
All ($n = 27$) Female	20.5 (±2.4)	167.2 (±5.6)	59.5 (±6.5)	21.3 (±2.0)
EPL all ($n = 22$)	21.7 (±2.2)	175.4 (±11.5)	67.4 (±12.4)	21.8 (±2.0)
EPL ($n = 11$) Male	22.2 (±2.2)	184.5 (±8.4)	75.2 (±1[illegible].5)	22.0 (±2.1)
EPL ($n = 11$) Female	21.3 (±2.2)	166.2 (±4.6)	59.7 (±7.5)	21.6 (±2.0)
JL all ($n = 29$)	21.5 (±5.0)	173.9 (±9.4)	65.9 (±10.2)	21.7 (±2.1)
JL ($n = 13$) Male	23.4 (±6.6)	181.4 (±6.8)	74.1 (±8.3)	22.5 (±2.0)
JL ($n = 16$) Female	19.9 (±2.4)	167.8 (±6.3)	59.4 (±6.0)	21.1 (±2.1)

Mean value (M) and standard deviation (SD)

composed of the two values described above and evaluated the body stability while standing on an unstable base. Within the scope of this study, the following measurements were carried out (2 in each case with the better one evaluated):

- Right - left - right (R-L, sagittal plane, double-legged)
- Forward and backward (F-B, frontal plane, double-legged).

For bipedal measurements, validated reference values were available [18].

Measurement of the isometric maximum force

The measurements were carried out with the device "*m3 Diagnosis professional*" whose use corresponds to scientific quality criteria [19, 20] from *SCHNELL Trainingsgeräte GmbH*. After correct individualized adjustment of the device, the test subject was instructed to reach the individual maximum force within a period of 5 s. Alternately, the right and left sides were tested three times and the best value was recorded. The following relevant muscles or muscle groups were examined:

- Upper extremity and shoulder: M. biceps, M. triceps, shoulder elevators
- Lower extremity and pelvis: *M. quadriceps*, ischiocrural muscles (hamstrings)

Five muscle groups were chosen for the specific movements in formation dance in order not to overstrain the subjects. The selection was made according to relevance and feasibility to ensure a comparison of the results.

Questionnaire

The questionnaire was used to collect anthropometric data, as well as acute injuries and chronic complaints (including behavior, localization, type, presumed cause, therapy or form of treatment, respectively) according to de Marees [21] by comparing both body sides over a period of 24 months as recommended by Liederbach et al. [22]· and modified according to Wanke et al. [23]. These data were correlated with the force values and the results of the muscle function tests. All data have been collected in strictly pseudonymized form.

Data analysis

The evaluation was carried out with SPSS (IBM SPSS Statistics 21). Frequency distributions were recorded on the basis of descriptive statistics and graphically displayed. Difference hypotheses were verified by t-tests for dependent or independent samples (right-left). The Levene test was used to check the mean values for variance homogeneity. The calculation for correlations of force differences in lateral comparison and injury patterns was carried out as a bivariate correlation according to Pearson. The significance level was determined at $p < 0.05$. For the simultaneous observation of a laterality of the parameter, the respective difference (right - left) of the variable was calculated using the data with the corresponding sign (− = left-sided).

In the calculation of the correlations between strength capability and injuries, injuries with different force variables (type of the examined musculature as difference between the right and left side of the body) were carried out.

A positive ethics vote of the ethical committee of the university had been obtained before the studies began. All volunteers gave informed consent to the tests.

Results

Table 2 shows the differences in the isometric maximum force between the right and left side of the examined musculature. Significant force differences were found almost exclusively in the area of the upper extremity (UE) as well as in the dancers of the EPL (all examined muscle groups of the UE) and the JL (2 out of 3 examined muscle groups of the UE). For the male dancers, only the differences in the area of the M. triceps were significant. There were hardly any significant differences in the lower extremity. With one exception, a dominance of the right side of the body could be observed.

Balance capability

Although the female dancers in both groups (achieved a better value in the bipedal balance measurement than the male test subjects of the respective grouping, the differences in the EPL group were not significant (All: R-L: $p < 0.001$, F-B: $p = 0.024$; EPL: R-L: $p = 0.14$, F-B: $p = 0.76$; NL: R-L: $p = 0.002$, F-B: $p < 0.001$).

Injuries

A total of 114 injuries could be identified in 51 subjects on the basis of the questionnaire. Chronic injuries (44.7%) were less frequent than acute injuries (55.3%). The diseases and injuries were relatively evenly distributed between EPL ($n = 61$) and JL ($n = 53$), but all female dancers reported more injuries than their male counterparts. Chronic injuries were predominant in the EPL with acute injuries (Table 3) in the JL.

Within the JL, no significant differences regarding the injury frequency (chronic and acute as a whole) could be found in comparing the right and left side of the body. In the EPL, on the other hand, differences were found between the two sexes compared to the JL (acute: $p = 0.038$), chronic: $p = 0.015$). From a gender-specific point of view, however, these differences were significant only in the male dancers.

As a whole, the lower extremity was most frequently affected with 20.2% of ankle joint injuries. This was followed by hand and wrist injuries with 19.2% and by foot and shoulder injuries with 11.7% each. The localizations significantly differed between female and male dancers particularly at the right side of the hand (m > f, $p = 0.013$), the shoulder (m > f, $p = 0.017$) and hip (f > m, $p = 0.032$) being higher on the right side (m vs. f, $p = 0.009$). Taking into account gender and level of performance, the right shoulder of the EPL male dancers was injured more often ($p < 0.025$) than the right shoulder of the JL male dancers. The same was observed with the right hand (EPL male and female) in relation to the JL ($p = 0.021$). All further calculations did not result in any significant differences with respect to a preferred side for certain

Table 2 Differences in maximum isometric strength between the right and left side of the body ($n = 51$)

Muscle (group)		Test group	Number (n)	*t*-value	*p*-value	Dominating side
Upper extremity	M. biceps	EPL male	11	−1.22	0.256	
		EPL female	11	−7.4	< 0.001**	right
		JL male	13	−0.32	0.753	
		JL female	16	−5.84	< 0.001**	right
	M. triceps	EPL male	11	−2.95	0.014*	right
		EPL female	11	−3.82	0.003*	right
		JL male	13	−1.2	0.255	
		JL female	16	−1.23	0.239	
	Shoulder elevators	EPL male	11	−0.20	0.844	
		EPL female	11	2.471	0.033*	right
		JL male	13	1.38	0.193	
		JL female	16	2.83	0.013*	right
Lower extremity	*M. quadriceps*	EPL male	11	1.93	0.083	
		EPL female	11	1.10	0.297	
		JL male	13	−2.52	0.027*	left
		JL female	16	1.28	0.219	
	Ischiocrural muscle group	EPL male	11	1.93	0.082	
		EPL female	11	−1.45	0.177	
		JL male	13	0.74	0.473	
		JL female	16	0.90	0.403	

* $p < 0.05$, ** $P < 0.001$

Table 3 Differences in injury frequency between the right and left side of the body

Test group	Type of injury Acute (n)	Chronic (n)	Total (n)	Side differences Acute (side)	Chronic (side)	Total (side)
EPL male	14	12	26	0.031* (r)	0.026* (r)	0.015* (r)
EPL female	14	21	35	0.553	0.211	0.255
JL male	11	4	15	0.436	0.082	0.753
JL female	24	14	38	0.270	0.669	0.453
Total	63	51	114			

* $p < 0.05$, right: r, left: l

injury localizations. Therefore, no significant gender- or performance-related differences within the JL dancers were found.

Correlation between balance capability and injury frequency subject to the body side

In the EPL, no correlations between injuries and balance could be calculated. In the JL, it turned out that a poorer capability to balance was associated with the development of chronic overload damage on the right side ($p = 0.028$; $r = 0.605$). The same was valid for the female dancers of the JL ($p = 0.045$ and $r = 0.507$).

Correlation between strength capability and injury frequency subject to the body side

Numerous significant correlations were observed with the injuries.

EPL males: There were clear, mostly negative correlations. Thus, the greater right-sided maximum strength of the hamstrings of the EPL male dancers correlated with an increased injury frequency on the contra lateral, weaker side (with injuries overall: $p = 0.028$, $r = -0.656$; acute injuries: $p = 0.025$, $r = -0.667$; injuries to the lower extremities: $p < 0.001$, $r = -0.878$). Furthermore, the same group showed a significant correlation between the stronger right side muscle strength in the M. biceps region and the number of injuries on the left, weaker, side of the body ($p = 0.027$, r = – 0.66).

EPL females: Here, too, there was a clear correlation between the stronger (mostly right-sided) muscle strength on the one hand and the occurrence of injuries on the weaker, contra lateral left side of the body as negative correlations on the other (Table 4).

For the JL, positive correlations between force and injury were calculated: With the male dancers of the JL, the higher right-sided strength in the shoulder elevators correlated with the higher total number of injuries on the right side ($p = 0.033$, $r = 0.592$) and also with a higher number of injuries of the lower extremities on the right side of the body ($p = 0.011$, $r = 0.677$).

Similarly, the higher strength of the right ischio-crural musculature positively correlated with the higher number of acute injuries on the right side of the body ($p = 0.043$, $r = 0.567$). The only negative correlation of the JL with the male dancers was between the higher maximum strength of the M. biceps on the right and the increased number of injuries on the left side of the body. No significant correlations could be calculated for the female dancers of the JL in this respect. On the other hand, comparing the JL to the EPL, there was predominantly an increased susceptibility to injury on the ipsi lateral - actually stronger – side, possibly resulting from inappropriate - or over- loading.

Discussion

The Latin American formation dance sport has enjoyed great popularity for years. This sport discipline is associated with considerable psycho-physical - including asymmetric – loads on both sides of the body [1, 9, 16, 24, 25]. The influence of this movement characteristic on motor skills - as well as the highest risk of injury within the dance sport disciplines - have not been assessed to date. The aim of this study was therefore to analyze the side-related strength and balance capability subject to injuries, gender and performance standards. The results are supposed to better understand the effects of the specific movement elements and to reduce the injury risk.

Isometric maximum strength and balance capability

In formation dance, the upper extremity is loaded via the right side of the body during guidance or contact, as well as the execution of the specific maximum difficulties. In this study, a significant strength difference was determined in favor of the right side of the body, especially at the upper extremity. This scientifically confirms the assumption of a functional and morphological adaptation in terms of laterality. This would coincide with the results in other dance styles - albeit the professional dance [10–12]. However, the influence of right-handedness (82%) is neglected here, which may possibly reduce the significance [26, 27]. This influence should be taken into account in future investigations.

Table 4 Correlations between balance, isometric maximum strength of selected muscle groups and injuries/chronic damages/complaints of the EPL ($n = 22$)

		Vtotal		Vacute		Vchron		Vuex		Vtor	Vlex	
		m p (r)	f p (r)	m p (r)	f p (r)	m p (r)	f p (r)	m p (r)	f p (r)	m p (r)	m p (r)	f p (r)
Balance	Stability r – l	0.810	0.419	0.497	0.837	0.682	0.133	0.183	0.177	0.845	0.561	0.986
	Stability forward – backward	0.884	0.847	0.515	0.790	0.571	0.592	0.263	0.595	0.781	0.264	0.813
	Stability total	0.945	0.440	0.959	0.692	0.943	0.101	0.111	0.129	0.968	0.288	0.839
Strength	M. biceps	0.066	0.397	.084	0.801	0.186	0.270	0.521	0.384	0.573	0.027* (r = −0.67)	0.732
	M. triceps	0.996	0.146	0.668	0.633	0.559	0.059	0.432	0.053	0.748	0.620	0.980
	Shoulder elevators	0.438	0.036* (r = – 0.63)	0.480	0.198	0.537	0.044* (r = – 0.62)	0.545	0.581	0.292	0.742	0.116
	M. quadriceps	0.844	0.034* (r = 0.64)	0.716	0.076	0.368	0.111	0.481	0.061	0.962	0.808	0.352
	Ischiocrural muscle group	0.028 (r = −0.656)	0.0135	0.025* (r = – 0.67)	0.808	0.179	0.024 * (r = – 0.62)	0.863	0.002* (r = – 0.83)	0.701	0.00** (r = – 0.88)	0.663
	Upper extremity	0.302	0.132	0.181	0.635	0.741	0.047* (r = 0.61)	0.833	0.048* (r = 0.61)	0.912	0.095	0.916
	Torso	0.438	0.036* (r = – 0.63)	0.480	0.198	0.537	0.044* (r = – 0.62)	0.545	0.581	0.292	0.742	0.116
	Lower extremity	0.547	0.029* (r = – 0.65)	0.251	0.265		0.018* (r = – 0.69)	0.572	0.001** (r = 0.83)	0.885	0.183	0.789

*: $p < 0,05$
**: $p < 0,001$
Vtotal total injuries, *Vacute* acute injuries, *Vchron* chronic damages/complaints, *Vuex* Injuries/damages/complaints at the upper extremity, *Vlex* Injuries/damages/complaints at the lower extremity, *Vtor* Injuries/damages/complaints at the torso

The lower extremities are less (*M. quadriceps*) or not at all (hamstrings) affected by the rather accidental differences, which again would suggest a more even load on the lower extremities -, compared to the upper extremities - and which is supported by the results of the balance measurement. Simultaneously, it should be considered that there is a methodological limitation, influence of which on the results remains unclear.

Injuries

Although there were only minor differences as to number of performance groups, there were even more significant differences in the further differentiation (chronic-acute, JL-EPL and m - f). In contrast to the EPL, no evidence of laterality within the JL was accounted for. The right side of the body was more frequently affected in the EPL, which can be interpreted as a consequence of the higher asymmetric load in this group. The fact that an injury risk rises with the performance level, as already described in dance medicine literature e. g. [28–30], could be confirmed with this study.

In order to cause chronic complaints, the loads must affect the body over a certain period of time. This may serve as an explanation why the dancers of the EPL suffer from chronic complaints more often than those of the JL. This has already been described by other authors investigating the dance sport [23]. The same applies to the localizations. Various studies have shown that, not only in Latin American dance, especially the lower extremities show an increased susceptibility to injury [24, 31–36]. In addition, the extreme difficulties in Latin American formation dance have to be added that comprise an increased risk of injury to shoulder, spine, pelvis and hip as demonstrated in this study [6, 17, 29].

A high susceptibility to injury of the hand and wrist was found, too. This may also be explained by the excessive guiding of the male partner and contact of the dance couple via hand. While fatigue processes favor injuries in dancing [37], it is still unclear to date - at least in formation dance - to what extent other aspects, such as anthropometric aspects (e. g. also the size/weight ratio between male and female dancers are involved [6, 38]. These could be potential issues to be addressed in future, because the dance couples of a formation have been assembled more according to aesthetic and less according to functional-preventive aspects, which can result in an increased risk of health damage if the matching of the couples is not optimal. The lack of coordination within the couple is also a major cause of injury in single couples [7].

Balance - isometric maximum strength - injuries/chronic complaints

There was no evidence of any correlation between the balance and injuries in the EPL. In the JL, however, injuries were localized on the less well-balanced side. The technical overload in the JL could serve as an explanation due to an overload and fatigue processes of the heavily loaded right side in the young dancers [37]. In the EPL, injuries were significantly more frequent at the muscularly weaker side, which could in turn indicate a lack of compensatory capacity, e. g. in the form of a balancing training. This could be a good argument for an accompanying strength training of the upper extremity not yet included in the standard training program. The strength training would have the function of preparing for maximum difficulty in the JL and the function of compensating in the EPL. However, particular care must be taken to ensure that the aesthetic ideal image of both sexes is not endangered. In addition, further studies with larger groups of test subjects are necessary in order to support the results described in this pilot project.

Limitations

The test subjects were recruited from one dance club which guaranteed a certain degree of homogenity. On the one hand, a cautious generalization of the results can be justified by the fact that the clubs in a national league system take part in competitions several times a year. On the other hand, an excessive differentiation of groups can have an adverse effect as calculations on a random basis may contain inaccuracies or result in fictitious earnings.

The force measurement with the power chair "m3 Diagnosis professional" offers many advantages. Due to the fixed construction of the device, the degrees of freedom during the movement are limited to a minimum and thus ensure an easy handling with a low risk of injury. Repeated runs can therefore provide a higher guarantee to achieve the same results. In the isometric measurement of torque, disturbing variables, such as the change in muscle length and the individual speed of joint movements, are largely eliminated by immobile resistance. The superiority of a better lever length can be prevented by the torque and allows to compare subjects of any body size. However, force measurements should be interpreted with caution, as the required maximum force values can be influenced by factors such as compliance, fatigue and the subject's motivation. The influence of the strength-enhancing auxiliary musculature could be reduced by a strictly given and continuously controlled measuring position and thus a quite exact estimation of the desired musculature could be achieved.

A questionnaire with self-assessment covering a period of 24 months is critically evaluated in science [39]. In addition, dancers tend to minimize physical discomfort. Therefore, it cannot be ruled out that the results may be influenced by lacking injury data [31].

Another weak point is the small group which limits the informative value. Larger subject groups seem to increase the informative value and are suggested for future research.

Conclusion

The partly asymmetrical, one-sided and gender-specific movement elements of the Latin American formation dance partly lead to morphological and functional asymmetric adaptations depending on the performance standard and gender. These adjustments are closely related to acute injuries and chronic complaints. This must be taken into account with the derived preventive measures. In addition to the implementation of prevention measures, further studies in the field of dance sports with larger numbers of cases and styles are required.

Acknowledgements
Not applicable.

Funding
This research did not receive any specific grant from funding agencies in the public, commercial, or not-for-profit sectors.

Medical ethics
A positive ethics vote of the ethical committee of the university had been obtained before the studies began. All volunteers gave informed consent to the tests.

Prior presentation
No

Authors´ contributions
EMW drafted the manuscript and has made substantial intellectual contributions to the interpretation of data. JS did the tests and statistical evaluation. DG has been involved in revising the manuscript critically for important intellectual content. BW has made substantial contributions to conception and design of this study and has given final approval of the version to be published. All authors read and approved the final manuscript.

Competing interest
The authors declare that they have no competing interests.

Author details
[1]Institute of Occupational, Social and Environmental Medicine, Goethe-University Frankfurt Main, Theodor-Stern-Kai 7, 60590 Frankfurt am Main, Germany. [2]Department Sports Medicine and Training Science, Christian-Albrechts-Universität Kiel, Institute of Sports Science, Olshausenstrasse 74, 24098 Kiel, Germany.

References

1. Kummer B. Grundelemente der Biomechanik für Tänze. In: C. Burgauner, Tanzen in Deutschland. München: Kastell; 1986. p. 79–81.
2. Deutscher Tanzsportverband e.V. (DTV) (Hrsg.). Rahmentrainingsplan (2. Aufl.). Frankfurt a. M.: Tanzwelt; 2003.
3. Liiv H, Jurimae T, Klonova A, Cicchella A. Performance and recovery: stress profiles in professional ballroom dancers. Med Probl Perform Art. 2013;28(2):65–9.
4. McCabe TR, Wyon M, Ambegaonkar JP, Redding E. a bibliographic review of medicine and science research in dancesport. Med Probl Perform Art. 2013; 28(2):70–9.
5. Kattenstroth JC, Kalisch T, Kolankowska I, Dinse HR. Balance, sensorimotor, and cognitive performance in long-year expert senior ballroom dancers. J Aging Res. 2011;2011:176709.
6. Liiv H, Wyon MA, Jürimäe T, Saar M, Mäestu J, Jürimäe J. Anthropometry, somatotypes, and aerobic power in ballet, contemporary dance, and dancesport. Med Probl Perform Art. 2013;28(4):207–11.
7. Wanke EM. Choreografie und Trainingsinhalte. In: Wanke EM. (Hrsg.). TanzSportMedizin. Köln: Sportbuch Strauß; 2011. p. 105–9.
8. Oldörp T. Tanzen – gesunder Breitensport mit Hochleistungsspitzen. TW Sport und Medizin. 1992;4:425–9.
9. Wanke EM, Fischer T, Pieper HG, Tanzsport GDA. Verletzungsprofil im lateinamerikanischen Formationstanz. Sportverletz Sportschaden. 2014 Sep; 28(3):132–8.
10. Gupta A, Fernihough B, Bailey G, Bombeck P, Clarke A, Hopper D. An evaluation of differences in hip external rotation strength and range of motion between female dancers and non-dancers. Br J Sports Med. 2004; 38(6):778–83.
11. Hamilton WG, Hamilton LH, Marshall P. Molnar M. a profile of the musculoskeletal characteristics of elite professional ballet dancers. Am J Sports Med. 1992;20(3):267–73.
12. Mostardi P, Porterfield J, Greenberg B, Goldberg D, Lea M. Musculoskeletal and cardiopulmonary characteristics of the professional ballet dancers. Physician Sportsmed. 1983;11(12):53–61.
13. Borges EG, Cader SA, Vale RG, et al. The effect of ballroom dance on balance and functional autonomy among the isolated elderly. Arch Gerontol Geriatr. 2012;55(2):492–6.
14. Berndt C, Strahler J, Kirschbaum C, Rohleder N. Lower stress system activity and higher peripheral inflammation in competitive ballroom dancers. Biol Psychol. 2012 Dec;91(3):357–64.
15. Mergenthaler K. Tanzen: Wenn selbst das Lächeln Stress ist. TW Sport und Medizin. 1992;4:401.
16. Strauß B. Sportverletzungen und Sportschäden im Tanzsport [Dissertation]. Lübeck: Med. Hochsch; 1993.
17. Strauß B, von Salis-Soglio G. Sportverletzungen und Sportschäden im Tanzsport. Sportorthopädie – Sporttraumatologie. 1997;13(3):173–6.
18. Raschner C, Lembert S, Platzer HP, et al. S3-Check - Evaluierung und Normwerteerhebung eines Tests zur Erfassung der Gleichgewichtsfähigkeit und Körperstabilität. Sportverletzt Sportschaden. 2008;22(2):100–5.
19. Bula PU. M3 Diagnos + Normwertstudie. Isometrische Maximalkraft als maximale Drehmomente im Bereich der Armbeuge- und Kniestreckmuskulatur. [Dissertation]. In: Ludwig-Maximilians-Universität zu München; 2007.
20. Dorstewitz B. Normwertstudie M3 Diagnos System. Maximalkraft als maximale Drehmomente bei gesunden Probanden im Bereich der Armbeuge und Kniestreckmuskulatur. [Dissertation]. In: Ludwig-Maximilian-Universität München; 2008.
21. de Marées H. Sportphysiologie. 9. Aufl. Köln: Sportverlag Strauß; 2009. p. 16.
22. Liederbach MJ, Hagins M, Gamboa JM, Welsh TM. Assessing and reporting dancer capacities, risk factors, and injuries. Recommendations from the IADMS standard measures consensus initiative. J Dance Med Sci. 2006;16(4): 139–53.
23. Wanke EM, Borchardt M, Fischer A, Groneberg DA. Injury profile in competitive senior ballroom dancers. Sportverletz Sportschaden. 2014; 28(4):204–10.
24. Kapp A, Böhmer D. Tanzsport. In: W. Pförringer, B. Rosemeyer & H.-W. Bär (Hrsg.), Sport-Trauma und Belastung. Erlangen: Perimed, 1985: 437–439.
25. Pieper HG, Groneberg DA, Wanke EM. Chronische Schulterschmerzen bei einer lateinamerikanischen Formationstänzerin von Weltrang. Eine Fallbeschreibung SOT. 2014;30(1):33–6.
26. Golomer E, Rosey F, Dizac H, Mertz C, Fagard J. The influence of classical dance training on preferred supporting leg and whole body turning bias. Laterality. 2009 Mar;14(2):165–77.
27. Kimmerle M. Lateral bias, functional asymmetry, dance training and dance injuries. J Dance Med Sci. 2010;14(2):58–66.
28. Campoy FA, Coelho LR, Bastos FN, Netto Júnior J, Vanderlei LC, Monteiro HL, Padovani CR, Pastre CM. Investigation of risk factors and characteristics of dance injuries. Clin J Sport Med. 2011;21(6):493–8.
29. Vetter RE, Symonds ML. Correlations between injury, training intensity, and physical and mental exhaustion among college athletes. J Strength Cond Res. 2010;24(3):587–96.
30. Young A, Lorna P. Incidence of Achilles tendon injuries in competitive Highland dancers. J Dance Med Sci. 2002;2:46–9.
31. Arendt YD, Kerschbaumer F. Verletzungen und Überlastungserscheinungen im professionellen Ballett. Z Orthop. 2003;141:349–56.
32. Echegoyen S, Acuña E, Rodríguez C. Injuries in students of three different dance techniques. Med Probl Perform Art. 2010 Jun;25(2):72–4.
33. Evans RW, Evans RI. Varvaja S. a survey of injuries among Broadway performers: types of injuries, treatments and perceptions of performers. Med Probl Perform Art. 1996;11:15–9.
34. Evans RW, Evans RI, Carvajal S. Survey of injuries among west end performers. Occup Environ Med. 1998 Sep;55(9):585–93.
35. Kapp A. Tanzen und Gesundheit: Tänzerschmerz. In: C. Burgauner (Hrsg.), editor. Tanzen in Deutschland. München: Kastell; 1986. p. 7–16.
36. Miletic A, Miletic D, Males B. Morphological differences and pain status monitoring in dance training. Facta Univ Phys Educ Sport. 2008;6(2):159–68.
37. McCabe TR, Hopkins JT, Vehrs P, Draper DO. Contributions of muscle fatigue to a neuromuscular neck injury in female ballroom dancers. Med Probl Perform Art. 2013;28(2):84–90.
38. Liiv H, Wyon M, Jürimäe T, et al. Anthropometry and somato types of competitive dance sport participants: a comparison of three different styles. Homo. 2014;65(2):155–60.
39. Begg D, Langley L, Williams S. Validity of self reported crashes and injuries in a longitudinal study of young adults. Injury Prevention. 1999;5(2):142–4.

Holi colours contain PM10 and can induce pro-inflammatory responses

Katrin Bossmann[1*], Sabine Bach[1], Conny Höflich[1], Kerttu Valtanen[2], Rita Heinze[3], Anett Neumann[1], Wolfgang Straff[1] and Katrin Süring[1]

Abstract

Background: At Holi festivals, originally celebrated in India but more recently all over the world, people throw coloured powder (Holi powder, Holi colour, Gulal powder) at each other. Adverse health effects, i.e. skin and ocular irritations as well as respiratory problems may be the consequences. The aim of this study was to uncover some of the underlying mechanisms.

Methods: We analysed four different Holi colours regarding particle size using an Electric field cell counting system. In addition, we incubated native human cells with different Holi colours and determined their potential to induce a pro-inflammatory response by quantifying the resulting cytokine production by means of ELISA (Enzyme Linked Immunosorbent Assay) and the resulting leukocyte oxidative burst by flow cytometric analysis. Moreover, we performed the XTT (2,3-Bis-(2-methoxy-4-nitro-5-sulfophenyl)-2H-tetrazolium-5-carboxanilide) and Propidium iodide cytotoxicity tests and we measured the endotoxin content of the Holi colour samples by means of the Limulus Amebocyte Lysate test (LAL test).

Results: We show here that all tested Holi colours consist to more than 40 % of particles with an aerodynamic diameter smaller than 10 μm, so called PM10 particles (PM, particulate matter). Two of the analysed Holi powders contained even more than 75 % of PM10 particles.
Furthermore we demonstrate in cell culture experiments that Holi colours can induce the production of the pro-inflammatory cytokines TNF-α (Tumor necrosis factor-α), IL-6 (Interleukine-6) and IL-1β (Interleukine-1β). Three out of the four analysed colours induced a significantly higher cytokine response in human PBMCs (Peripheral Blood Mononuclear Cells) and whole blood than corn starch, which is often used as carrier substance for Holi colours. Moreover we show that corn starch and two Holi colours contain endotoxin and that certain Holi colours display concentration dependent cytotoxic effects in higher concentration. Furthermore we reveal that in principle Holi colours and corn starch are able to generate an oxidative burst in human granulocytes and monocytes. In Holi colour 1 we detected a fungal contamination.

Conclusions: Some of the observed unwanted health effects of Holi colours might be explained by the high content of PM10 particles in conjunction with the possible induction of a pro-inflammatory response and an oxidative leukocyte burst.

Keywords: Holi colours, PM10, Pro-inflammatory response, TNF-α, IL-6, IL-1β, Oxidative burst

Abbreviations: BSA, Bovine Serum Albumin; E.coli, Escherichia coli; ELISA, Enzyme Linked Immunosorbent Assay; EU, Endotoxin Units; FCS, Fetal Calf Serum; IL-1β, Interleukine-1β; IL-6, Interleukine-6; IL-8, Interleukine-8; LAL, Limulus Amebocyte Lysate; LPS, Lipopolysaccharide; PBMCs, Peripheral Blood Mononuclear Cells; PBS, Phosphate buffered saline; PM, Particulate matter; SD, Standard deviation; TNF-α, Tumor necrosis factor α; VLE, Very low endotoxin; XTT, (2,3-Bis-(2-methoxy-4-nitro-5-sulfophenyl)-2H-tetrazolium-5-carboxanilide)

* Correspondence: katrin.bossmann@uba.de
[1]Environmental Medicine and Health Effects Assessment, Federal Environment Agency, Corrensplatz 1, 14195 Berlin, Germany
Full list of author information is available at the end of the article

Background

Holi is a traditional Hindu festival originated in India. Lasting for several days in spring and celebrating the victory of good over evil it is a very colourful event. Differences in people's caste, age, sex and status seem to be abrogated by throwing Gulal, a special coloured powder, at each other to make everybody and everything look equal. About 3 years ago, the traditional Indian festival was transferred to Europe and adapted to a commercial party event. Meanwhile it takes place in many different cities all over the world: people listen to music, dance and throw coloured powder. This so called Holi powder/Holi colour/Gulal powder or Micro Confetti is distributed by different companies. The quality and the amount of information given on the outer packaging about the ingredients of the particular Holi colour are mostly very poor. So far, there is no European or US regulation about Holi colours and it is not clear whether they should be categorised for instance as cosmetic products or general consumer products. Although many manufacturers claim that their products are harmless to health and environment, organisers of Holi festivals often recommend wearing eye and respiratory protection (like goggles and face masks) and advise people with respiratory disorders not to participate. There are several reports of adverse health effects probably caused by the use of Holi powder: various forms of cutaneous diseases [1] as well as ocular irritations [1, 2] and a case of periorbital necrotizing fasciitis [3] have been described after exposure to Holi colours. In addition, high total suspended particulate concentrations occurred during Holi events [4] that may also cause or aggravate adverse health effects like respiratory irritations.

To assess possible hazards to human health, we ordered four different Holi powder products of three different distributors via the internet and analysed them regarding particle size and their potential to induce pro-inflammatory responses in cell culture systems. Cell-based in vitro assays have been used widely to imitate in vivo situations [5, 6]. For example the whole blood assay was used to describe pro-inflammatory activity of dust sample extracts [7]. Moreover, we tested the cytotoxic potential of corn starch and the different Holi colours, analysed the endotoxin and mould content of corn starch and the Holi colours and screened for corn starch-/Holi colour-leukocyte interactions in vitro.

Methods

Holi colours

Four different Holi colour products were ordered via a renowned internet retailer. General information like producing country, ingredients or indications relevant for impacts on health either given on the internet or on the outer packaging of the product are shown in Table 1. As corn starch is often used as carrier substance for Holi colours, commercially available corn starch (RUF Lebensmittelwerk KG, Quakenbrück, Germany) designated as food ingredient was purchased to serve as a control.

Electric field cell counting system (CASY®) of corn starch and Holi particles

We used a CASY® cell counter (Schärfe System GmbH, CASY Cell Counter + Analyser System, Model TTC) with a 60 µm measuring capillary to determine particle size and number of (i) BD Cytometer Setup and Tracking beads of 2 and 3 µm diameter (Becton Dickinson,

Table 1 Available information on the different Holi colours, either communicated with the product itself or online

Holi Colour Number	1	2	3	4
Shade/ characterisation of colour	black/ Holi colour, perfumed natural colour, Holi powder Gulal	pink/ Holi powder (Holi gulal Holi colour), used at Holi Festivals	orange/ "Effect colour powder", optically like Holi powder/ Holi colours	green/ Holi colour, Gulal festival
Produced in	India	Germany	n.s.	n.s.
MSDS available	n.s.	yes	n.s.	n.s.
EU Regulation	n.s.	according to Art. 19 EU regulation of cosmetic products	n.s.	n.s.
Ingredients	natural colour, plant based	corn starch, water, hydrated silica, sodium chloride, sodium sulphate, E127	n.s.	flour powder, dyed
Recommended application	Holi open air festivals, creative areas	Holi festivals, for throwing up into the air, sprinkle powder onto hands and throw up into air (away from body) for adult use only	for decor use or throwing up into the air	for decor use or throwing up into the air
Warning	environmental friendly, mild on skin, nontoxic	don't use with a history of asthma and allergies, avoid contact with mucus membranes, wear mouth, nose and eye protection, not edible	don't use at festivals or on skin, not classified as cosmetic product	don't use at festivals or on skin, not classified as cosmetic product

n.s. not specified, *MSDS* material safety data sheet, *number 2 and 3* same distributor

Lot: 22680), (ii) blank calibration particles (BD Biosciences, Lot: 63100) of 6.0–6.4 μm diameter, (iii) corn starch and (iiii) four different Holi colours. Respective particles were suspended in PBS (Phosphate buffered saline) (Biochrom, Berlin, Germany) and diluted with CASY® ton (La Roche Diagnostics GmbH, Basel, Switzerland) according to the manufacturer's instructions for measuring. Particle count was evaluated in a size range between 0.7 and 30 μm.

Stimulation of PBMCs

Blood was withdrawn under authorised supervision from six healthy donors who had given their informed consent. PBMCs were isolated from lithium heparin anti-coagulated blood by Ficoll-Paque™ Plus (GE Healthcare Bio-Sciences AB, Uppsala, Sweden) density gradient centrifugation and resuspended in VLE RPMI 1640 (Very Low Endotoxin) media (Biochrom AG, Berlin, Germany) supplemented with 10 % (v/v) FCS (Fetal Calf Serum), 2 mM L-glutamine (Sigma Aldrich, Chemie GmbH, München, Germany) and 1 % (v/v) penicillin/streptomycin (Biochrom AG, Berlin, Germany). 500 μl of a suspension of PBMCs (2×10^6 cells/ml) were incubated in sterile 24-well plates (Multiwell™, Falcon®, Becton Dickinson Labware, NJ, USA) for 4 h at 37 °C and 5 % CO_2 with corn starch and the four different Holi colours (see above), respectively, each at 1.5×10^6 particles/ml. The utilised concentration of the Holi colours and corn starch arose from dose-effect experiments that we performed with ambient dust (data not shown). Cells treated with PBS only (7.5 % v/v) served as negative control. Cells treated with LPS (Lipopolysaccharide) (Enzo Life Sciences, NY, USA) at 100 ng/ml served as positive control. Samples were centrifuged for five minutes at 300 g and supernatants were transferred to fresh cell culture plates and frozen at −20 °C until further analysed.

Stimulation of whole blood

Blood was withdrawn under authorised supervision from six healthy donors who had given their informed consent. 100 μl of a PBS suspension containing corn starch, the four different Holi colours or LPS respectively was mixed with 1 ml of a 0.9 % NaCl solution (Fresenius Kabi Deutschland GmbH, Bad Homburg, Germany). Subsequently 100 μl of lithium heparin anti-coagulated whole blood was added, samples were mixed carefully and stimulated in sterile 1.5 ml safe-lock tubes (Biopur, Eppendorf AG, Hamburg, Germany) overnight at 37 °C and 5 % CO_2. The final concentration of corn starch and the four different Holi colours was 6.8×10^5 particles/ml and for LPS it was 45.45 ng/ml. PBS only served as negative control. Samples were then mixed carefully and centrifuged for 5 min at 300 g and supernatants were transferred to fresh Eppendorf tubes and frozen at −20 ° C until further analysed.

Analysis of cytokine production by ELISA

The concentration of the cytokines TNF-α, IL-6 and IL-1β in the supernatant was determined using commercially available ELISA kits (R&D Systems, Minneapolis, USA) following the manufacturer's instructions. PBMC samples were blocked with 300 μl 1 % BSA (Bovine Serum Albumin) (Sigma Aldrich, St. Louis, USA) in PBS and whole blood with 300 μl 3 % BSA in PBS.

ELISA data are presented as mean ± SD (standard deviation) values from six independent experiments. Statistical analysis was performed using SPSS software version 18 (SPSS Inc., Chicago, USA). The Wilcoxon matched pairs signed-ranked test was used to test for group differences. P-values < 0.05 (two-tailed) were considered as significant.

Analysis of endotoxin content of samples by Limulus Amebocyte Lysate test (LAL test)

The endotoxin content of an unstimulated control, Holi colours 1–4, corn starch and LPS was determined using a commercially available Limulus Amebocyte Lysate test kit (Pierce® LAL Chromogenic Endotoxin Quantitation Kit, Pierce Biotechnology, Rockford, USA) as described by the manufacturer. Corn starch and Holi colour samples were applied in duplicate at 1.5×10^6 particles/ml, LPS at 100 ng/ml.

XTT test

100 μl HepG2 cells ($c = 2.5 \times 10^5$ cells/ml, Leibniz Institut, DSMZ, Braunschweig, Germany) were disseminated in RPMI 1640 media (Sigma-Aldrich Chemie GmbH, München, Germany) supplemented with 10 % (v/v) FCS (Sigma-Aldrich Chemie GmbH, München, Germany) in a 96 well plate (Cellstar, Greiner Bio One International GmbH, Leipzig, Germany) and incubated over night at 37 °C and 5 % CO_2 for adherence. Then media was discarded and replaced by 100 μl RPMI 1640 supplemented with 1 % (v/v) FCS. Subsequently 100 μl of a single Holi colour or corn starch suspension in PBS were added at a final concentration of 1.7×10^6, 2.5×10^6, 5×10^5 and 1×10^7 particles/ml, each in quadruplicate. After 4 h of incubation cells were washed with PBS and supplemented with 100 μl of fresh RPMI 1640 containing 1 % (v/v) FCS. Then 50 μl of XTT reagent was added according to the manufacturer's instructions (Cell Proliferation Kit II (XTT), product number 11465015001, Sigma-Aldrich Chemie GmbH, München, Germany). After 3 h of incubation at 37 °C and 5 % CO_2 samples were mixed thoroughly and measured on a microplate reader (Anthos Zenyth 200RT, Biochrom, Cambridge, UK) at 490 nm (reference wavelength 690 nm). Vitality of cells was calculated in percent in relation to an unstimulated control sample.

Propidium iodide test

500 µl Jurkat cells (c = 1 × 10^6 cells/ml, Leibniz Institut, DSMZ, Braunschweig, Germany) in RPMI 1640 media supplemented with 10 % (v/v) FCS were disseminated in a 24 well plate (Cellstar, Greiner Bio One International GmbH, Leipzig, Germany). Then 500 µl of single Holi colour or corn starch suspension in PBS were added to reach a final concentration of 1.7 × 10^6, 2.5 × 10^6, 5 × 10^6 and 1 × 10^7 particles/ml, respectively. Samples were incubated for 4 h and for 20 h at 37 °C and 5 % CO_2. After washing with 1 ml PBS cells were suspended in 1 ml fresh media without FCS and phenol red (RPMI 1640, Sigma-Aldrich Chemie GmbH, München, Germany), incubated for 15 min with 8 µg/ml propidium iodide (Sigma-Aldrich Chemie GmbH, München, Germany) in the dark at room temperature and analysed by Flow Cytometry (FACS Calibur, BD Biosciences). Vitality of cells was calculated in percent in relation to an unstimulated control sample.

Light Microscopy of corn starch and Holi colours together with human leukocytes

Blood was withdrawn under authorised supervision from two healthy donors who had given their informed consent. Cells were treated as described for the stimulation of PBMCs and stimulation of whole blood. After the 4 h, respectively overnight incubation, 20 µl of the cell-corn starch or cell-Holi colour mixture was pipetted onto an object slide, covered with a cover slip and immediately analysed under a light microscope (Axio Vert A1 with Axiovision Rel.4.8.2 software, Zeiss, Jena, Germany). Some of the whole blood samples were also stained with Syto 9 (Life Technologies, USA,) for 10 min as described by the manufacturer and analysed under the microscope in the green fluorescence channel.

Phagoburst Assay

Blood was withdrawn under authorised supervision from four healthy donors who had given their informed consent. Phagoburst™ reagent Kit (Glycotope Biotechnology, Germany) was used to measure the oxidative burst activity of monocytes and granulocytes in human whole blood as described by the manufacturer except for the incubation time at 37 °C which was reduced to overall 12 min instead of 20 min due to a reduced cell viability observed at the longer incubation time. Additionally to the reagents in the kit, corn starch and Holi colour 1 were incubated with the heparinised human whole blood. The concentrations of corn starch and Holi colour 1 corresponded to the E.coli (Escherichia coli) concentration of 2 × 10^9 particles/ml. Samples remaining on ice served as negative control.

Analysis of mould content

100 µl of each Holi colour and corn starch suspension (c = 1.5 × 10^6 particles/ml) was inoculated under sterile conditions on malt extract agar (MEA, OXOID GmbH, Wesel, Germany) and Dichloran 18 % Glycerol agar (DG18, heipha Dr. Müller GmbH, Eppelheim, Germany). The agar plates were incubated at 25 °C and 36 °C for 10 days, respectively. The micro-morphology of selected colonies was analysed by optical microscopy (Axioskop 40 FL, Carl Zeiss MicroImaging GmbH, Göttingen, Germany) at 200× and 1000× magnification and subsequently photographed with a digital camera (Canon PowerShot Gs, Canon Deutschland, Krefeld, Germany).

Results

The tested Holi colours consist of more than 40 % PM10 particles

We analysed commercially available particles of known size, corn starch - often used as Holi colour carrier substance - and four different Holi powders regarding particle size and number by use of a CASY® Cell Counter (Fig. 1). BD Cytometer Setup and Tracking beads of 2 and 3 µm diameters mixed with blank calibration particles of 6.0–6.4 µm diameter show precise peaks at the respective sizes (Fig. 2a), thus confirming CASY® Technology as an accurate method regarding particle size characterisation. To identify the inhalable fraction of the analysed particles the percentage of counts <10 µm in diameter was determined. Because of background artefacts the range from 0 to 0.7 µm was excluded. This resulted in a gate set between 0.7 and 10 µm ($P_{0.7-10\mu m}$ in Fig. 1). The content of particles between 0.7 and 10 µm in diameter varied between the analysed powders: corn starch consisted to 51 % of particles >0.7 µm and <10 µm (Fig. 1b) while the content of particles between 0.7 and 10 µm in the Holi colours ranged from 43 to 80 % (Fig. 1c–f). Thus all four Holi powders consisted of more than 40 % potentially inhalable particles that might reach the lower respiratory tract.

Holi colours can induce the production of TNF-α, IL-6 and IL-1β

To assess the pro-inflammatory capacity of the different Holi colours, we tested their potential to induce the production of the pro-inflammatory cytokines TNF-α, IL-6 and IL-1β. We used two different cell culture systems and two different incubation times: human PBMCs were incubated for 4 h and human whole blood was incubated overnight with corn starch and four different Holi colours. The resulting cytokine production was analysed by ELISA. Cells treated with PBS only served as unstimulated control and cells treated with LPS served as positive control.

In both cell culture systems, cells incubated with corn starch or Holi colours showed a higher production

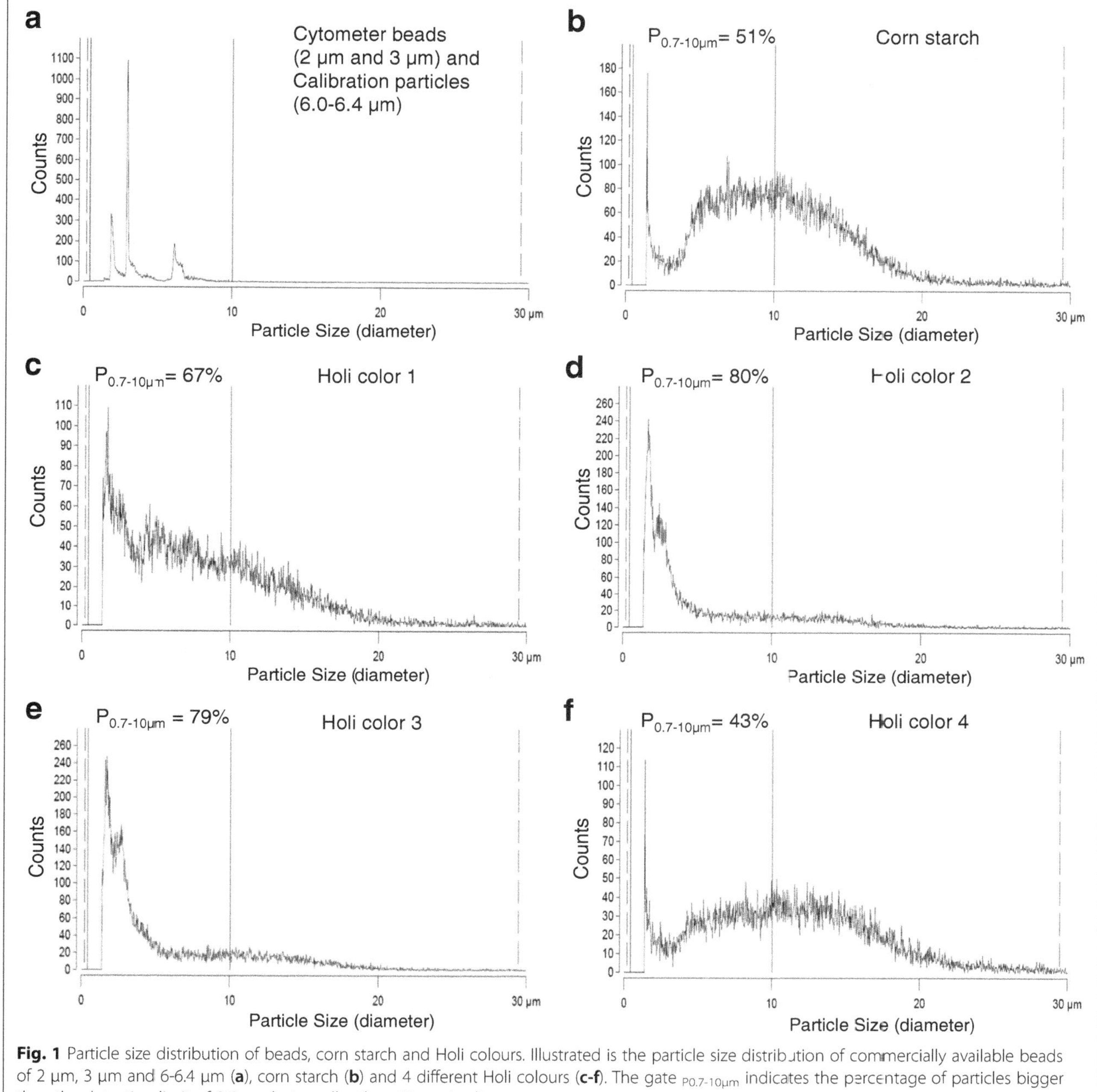

Fig. 1 Particle size distribution of beads, corn starch and Holi colours. Illustrated is the particle size distribution of commercially available beads of 2 µm, 3 µm and 6-6.4 µm (**a**), corn starch (**b**) and 4 different Holi colours (**c-f**). The gate $P_{0.7\text{-}10\mu m}$ indicates the percentage of particles bigger than the detection limit of 0.7 µm but smaller than 10 µm in diameter

of TNF-α, IL-6 and IL-1β than unstimulated cells (Fig. 2). This increase was significant ($p < 0.05$) for all analysed cytokines and all Holi samples except for Holi colour 2. Holi colours 1, 3 and 4 induced a significantly higher cytokine production than corn starch ($p < 0.05$ for TNF-α, IL-6 and IL-1β). Corn starch also slightly increased the production of TNF-α, IL-6 and IL-1β when compared to the cells treated with PBS only (Fig. 2). This increase was significant ($p < 0.05$) for TNF-α, IL-6 and IL-1β in PBMCs and for IL-6 and IL-1β in the whole blood experiments.

Corn starch and Holi colours 3 and 4 contain endotoxin

As endotoxin is a potent inducer of pro-inflammatory cytokines [8], an endotoxin quantification test was performed to determine the endotoxin content of corn starch and the different Holi colours. Hereby, the same particle and LPS concentration was used as for the stimulation of PBMCs. In the unstimulated control and

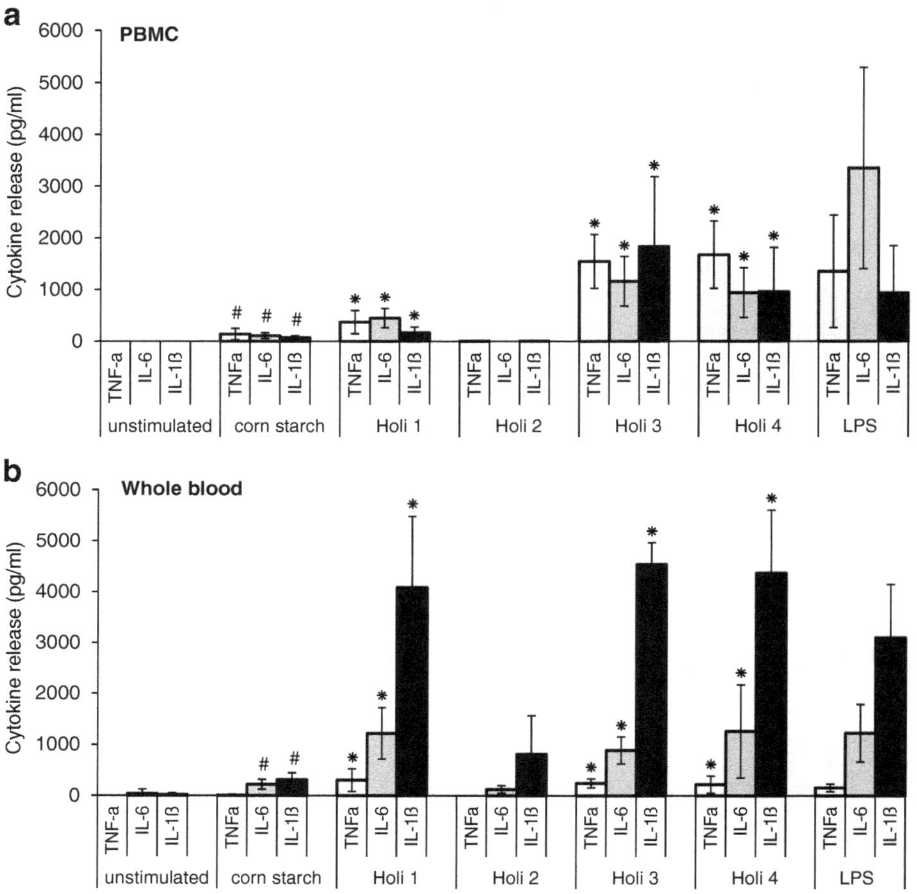

Fig. 2 Induction of pro-inflammatory cytokines by corn starch and Holi colours. Shown is the production of TNF-α, IL-6 and IL-1β induced by corn starch and Holi colours 1-4 in (**a**) PBMCs and (**b**) whole blood. PBS served as negative and LPS as positive control. Each bar represents the mean value of six independent experiments representing 6 different probands. The standard deviation is depicted by the error bars. # significant ($p < 0.05$) when compared to unstimulated cells. * significant ($p < 0.05$) when compared to unstimulated cells and cells treated with corn starch

in Holi colours 1 and 2 no endotoxin was detectable, while corn starch exhibited an endotoxin level of 0.11 EU/ml (Endotoxin Units/ml), Holi colour 3 of 0.23 EU/ml, Holi colour 4 of 1.99 EU/ml and the positive control LPS of 9 EU/ml (Fig. 3).

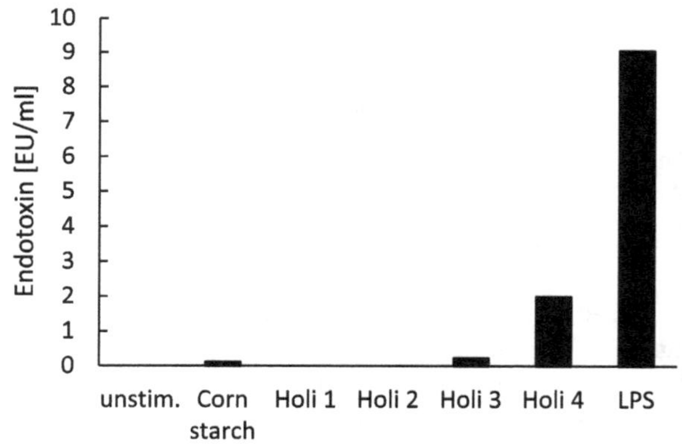

Fig. 3 Endotoxin content of corn starch and Holi colours 1–4. The endotoxin content of corn starch and Holi colours 1–4 was determined by LAL test. The resulting endotoxin amount was measured in Endotoxin Units per ml (EU/ml). Samples were applied in the same concentration as used for stimulation of PBMCs (corn starch and Holi colours 1–4: $c = 1.5 \times 10^6$ particles/ml, LPS: 100 ng/ml)

Holi colour 2 and 3 show cytotoxicity with increasing particle concentration

To determine possible cytotoxic effects of Holi colours and corn starch we performed two different cytotoxicity tests: the XTT test and the Propidium iodide test. The XTT test revealed that neither corn starch nor Holi colours 1, 3 or 4 exhibited cytotoxicity towards HepG2 cells in the concentration range tested. Holi colour 2 showed no cytotoxicity in the lowest concentration (1.7×10^6 particles/ml) but cytotoxicity increased with raising particle concentration (data not shown). In the Propidium iodide test corn starch and Holi colours 1, 2 and 4 did not show any cytotoxic effects. Holi colour 3 displayed increasing cytotoxicity with increasing particle concentration (data not shown). But due to interferences with the fluorescence of the Holi colours and the fluorescence to be measured by flow cytometry, the evaluation of the Propidium iodide test was very difficult and the data should be considered preliminary.

Holi colour particles are associated with human leukocytes in the microscopic image

Human PBMCs and human whole blood were incubated for 4 h and overnight with corn starch and four different Holi colours to determine the fate of the particles when administered to cells and to test for possible cell-particle-interactions.

Light Microscopy of human PBMCs together with Holi colours and corn starch demonstrated the irregular shape of the bigger particles (radius of about 3 to 10 μm) and showed an even distribution of cells and particles (Fig. 4a–e). Due to the autofluorescence of Holi colours 2, 3 and 4, Holi particles could be visualised by Fluorescence Microscopy. When cells were stained with the nucleic acid dye Syto 9, this revealed a close particle-cell-association of the smaller Holi particles with human leukocytes as shown in Fig. 4f for Holi colour 3.

Holi colour 1 and corn starch can induce an oxidative burst in human granulocytes and monocytes

We incubated human whole blood ($n = 4$) with corn starch and the different Holi colours and determined the resulting leukocyte oxidative burst by flow cytometric analysis. Due to interference of the autofluorescence of Holi colours 2, 3 and 4 with the fluorescence measured as a result of the oxidative burst, only corn starch and Holi colour 1 could be tested. Preliminary data revealed that 29.5–39.3 % of human granulocytes and 11.4–25.7 % of human monocytes produced reactive oxidants after incubation with corn starch. Holi colour 1 induced an oxidative burst in 16–24.1 % of human granulocytes and 2.7–4.3 % of human monocytes (Fig. 5).

Holi colour 1 contains mould fungi

Agar plates inoculated with Holi colour 1 exhibited fungal growth of several macromorphologically different colonies (Fig. 6a). Fungal growth was not observed on

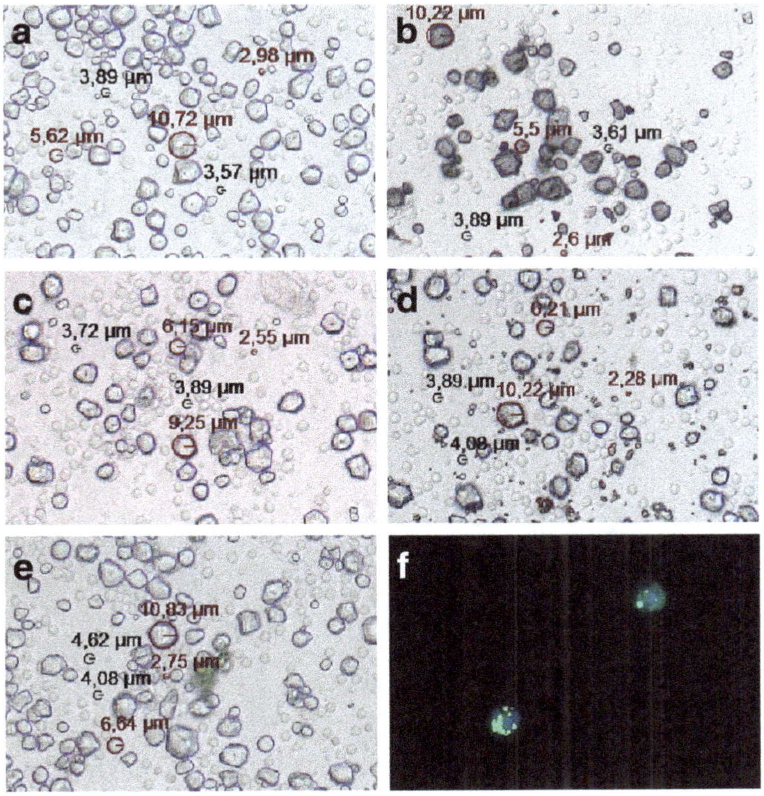

Fig. 4 Light Microscopic images of human PBMCs together with Holi colours or corn starch. **a**–**e** shows 200 fold magnifications of native preparations of human PBMCs incubated for 4 h together with corn starch (**a**), Holi colour 1 (**b**), Holi colour 2 (**c**), Holi colour 3 (**d**) and Holi colour 4 (**e**). Cell sizes are indicated in black and particle sizes in red and the respective radiuses are stated. (Note that very small particles could not be indexed.) **f** displays a 400 fold magnification of cells incubated overnight with Holi colour 3, then stained with the nucleic acid dye Syto 9 and analysed in the green fluorescence channel

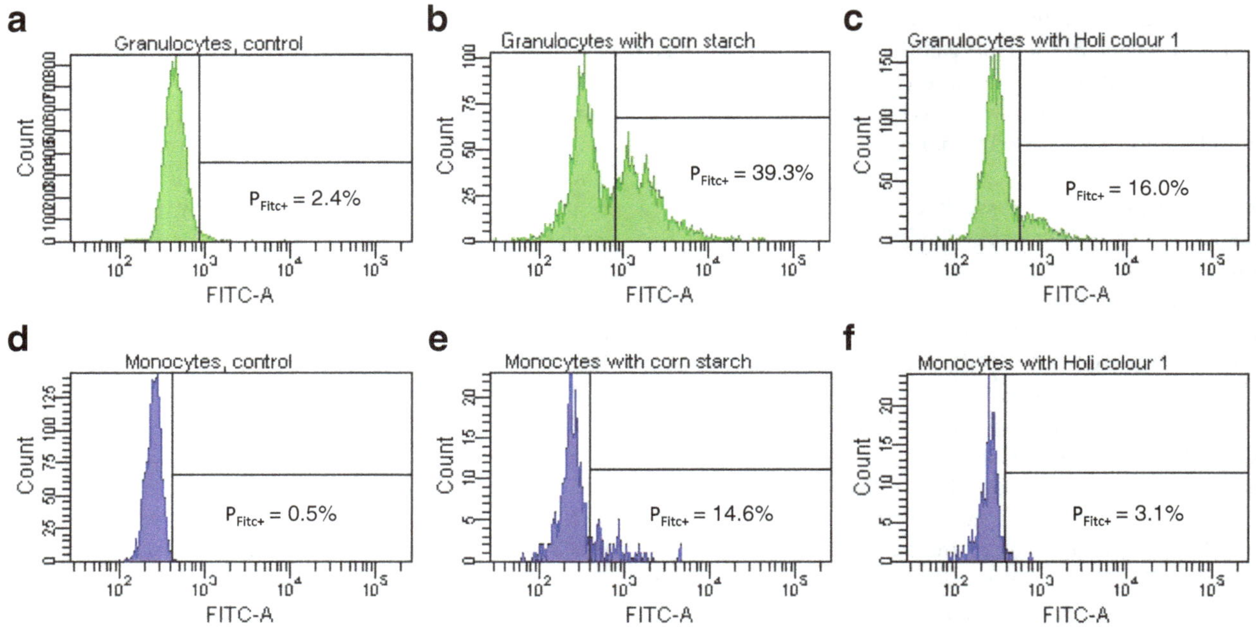

Fig. 5 Induction of leukocyte oxidative burst by corn starch and Holi colour1. Exemplified is the illustration of the percentage of granulocytes (**a-c**) and monocytes (**d-f**) which produce reactive oxidants in one proband after **a** and **d**: incubation with corn starch at 0 °C (negative control); **b** and **e**: incubation with corn starch at 37 °C; **c** and **f**: incubation with Holi colour 1 at 37 °C. The gate P_{FITC+} displays the particles considered FITC positive and respective percentages are given

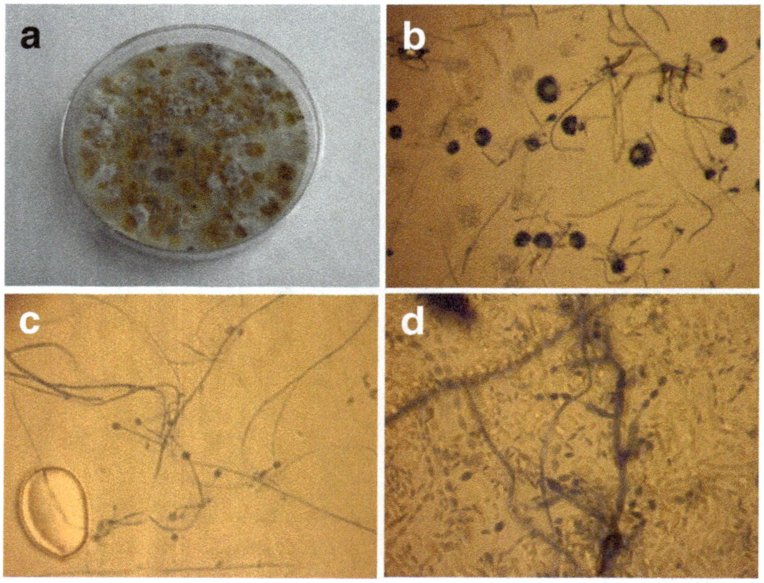

Fig. 6 Holi colour 1 contains mould. **a** exhibits a photograph of a DG18 agar plate after inoculation with Holi colour 1 and incubation for 10 days at 25 °C. **b–d** displays microscopic images of different isolates of mould fungi (**b** *Aspergillus sp.*, **c** unidentified *Zygomycete* species, **d** unidentified *Paecilomyces/Bossychlamus* species) found in Holi colour 1 (Magnification: 200×)

plates inoculated with Holi colours 2–4 and corn starch (data not shown).

By micromorphological analysis different isolates of *Aspergillus spp.*; unidentified *Zygomycete* species and unidentified *Paecilomyces/Bossychlamus* species were detected (Fig. 6b–d).

Discussion

Holi colours can potentially be harmful to human health: they contain a considerable amount of particles with an aerodynamic diameter smaller than 10 μm and at least in vitro they show a close association with human leukocytes, a pro-inflammatory potential, they can have cytotoxic effects in higher concentration and can induce an oxidative burst in human granulocytes and monocytes.

Extensive use of Holi powder at Holi festivals will result in a considerable increase in PM10 concentrations in ambient air. Adverse health effects due to long-term exposure to high PM10 concentrations are widely known: increasing concentrations of particulate matter are related to a higher cardiovascular and respiratory morbidity and mortality [9–13]. Also, there is evidence for short-term effects of air pollutants: increased PM10 concentrations were also associated with an increase in daily mortality [14, 15]. In addition, a positive association of dust storms with mild asthma manifestations in children, as indicated by medication purchases, could be shown recently [16].

In this study the particle size of the examined Holi colours differed (Fig. 1). While Holi colours 2 and 3 consisted of about 80 % of particles smaller than 10 μm in diameter - with the majority of particles being even smaller than 5 μm (Fig. 1d–e) -, the particle size of Holi colours 1 (Fig. 1c) and 4 (Fig. 1f) ranged between 0.7 and 20 μm with a PM10 content of 67 and 43 %, respectively.

The size resolution in the CASY® analysis confirmed approximately the average particle size of corn starch (Fig. 1b) stated in the literature: 15 μm in diameter [17]. But except for Holi colour 4 the other colours contained a greater number of smaller particles. Thus, the corn starch used for Holi colour production might be somehow modified during the colour production process or mixed with other substances. For the Holi colours 1, 3 and 4 it is also possible that they comprise another carrier substance, e.g. rice flour or other anticaking agents.

It is difficult to compare the specific exposure at/or in the vicinity of Holi festivals with the "normal" ambient PM10 exposure i.e. caused by road traffic or combustion processes. The composition of the particulate matter seems to have a great influence on the biological effects as i.e. assessed by cytokine induction [18]. Also epidemiological data show that not only the particle size but furthermore the chemical composition accounts for harmful health effects [19, 20].

In this study, the four different Holi colours induced diverging amounts of pro-inflammatory cytokines as shown in the cell culture experiments (Fig. 2). Differences in the proportion of particle size alone cannot account for the different levels of pro-inflammatory potential: although Holi colours 2 and 3 had nearly the same amount of particles >0.7 μm and <10 μm (about 80 %), they induced significantly diverging amounts of TNF-α, IL-6 and IL-1β.

In general as compared to PBMCs, which were stimulated for 4 h, (Fig. 2a) we found a decrease in TNF-α production and an increase in IL-1β production in the whole blood experiments (Fig. 2b), where cells were incubated with the respective substances overnight. This corresponds well with the kinetics of release of TNF-α and IL-1β in whole blood and PBMCs: TNF-α reaches maximal levels within 6 h of stimulation, whereas IL-1β reaches maximal levels between 12 and 16 h [21, 22].

The release of the pro-inflammatory cytokines TNF-α, IL-6 and IL-1β by human cells stimulated in vitro with particulate matter PM10 or nanoparticles has been shown in various studies [18, 23–27]. The fact that exposure to swine dust in vivo also leads to an increase of TNF-α, IL-6 and IL-1β in peripheral blood of healthy volunteers [28] suggests, that these cytokines might also be able to mediate this kind of inflammatory response in vivo.

Endotoxin is a potent inducer of various pro-inflammatory cytokines [8]. To elucidate the role of endotoxin in the cytokine induction of the Holi colours, we measured the amount of endotoxin in the different Holi samples by means of the LAL test. We did not detect any endotoxin in Holi colours 1 and 2, but discovered endotoxin in corn starch as well as in Holi colours 3 and 4, albeit these amounts of endotoxin are much below the endotoxin level measured in LPS (Fig. 3). But since already very low amounts of endotoxin in the picogramme range (which represent Endotoxin units of 1 EU/ml or even below according to the manufacturer's product guide of the LAL test used here) can be responsible for considerable cytokine secretions the observed cytokine induction of Holi colours 3 and 4 might be caused by endotoxin. (We performed dose response tests for endotoxin levels and cytokines of interest. The results will be subject of a separate publication.) Nevertheless as Holi colour 1 contains no endotoxin and Holi colours 3 and 4 contained lesser endotoxin than LPS but induced a stronger cytokine release, we argue that also other factors than endotoxin might drive the cytokine answer.

Hansen et al. have shown that the potency of endotoxin from different Gram-negative bacteria in the LAL-assay is not closely correlated with the potency of the endotoxin to induce IL-8 (Interleukine-8) secretion from pulmonary epithelial cells [29]. This observation might be true for other pro-inflammatory cytokines as well. Hence the results of the LAL-test do not necessarily have to correlate with the cell culture data. This would also explain why corn starch, which contained endotoxin, only induces a very low cytokine release.

The XTT test and Propidium iodide test showed possible cytotoxic effects of Holi colours 2 and 3 with increasing Holi colour concentration, while corn starch and Holi colours 1 and 4 did not display any cytotoxicity thus underlying the heterogeneity of Holi colours. Since the observed cytotoxicity occurs only at higher concentrations or is rather less pronounced in the lowest concentration tested, respectively, their relevance to health regarding a real Holi festival situation would need further investigation.

Although fluorescence microscopy (Fig. 4f) showed a close particle-cell-association the nature of this association remains unclear: are the particles bound to the cell surface and if so through what kind of receptor or are the particles phagocytosed by the cell? Due to the impossibility of quenching the autofluorescent signal of the Holi colours in the flow cytometric analysis an exact discrimination of particles bound to the cell surface and particles phagocytosed by the cell was not feasible and we were not able to show an internalisation of Holi particles directly (data not shown). But as corn starch and to a lesser extent also Holi colour 1 induced an oxidative burst in human granulocytes and monocytes (Fig. 5), one can speculate that these cells might engulf the particles. However, the limitation remains, that the Phagoburst assay is an in vitro setup that is very different from the situation in vivo regarding i.e. time of exposure and particle concentration. Still, phagocytosis and processing of particulate matter by the macrophages in the lung is an established phenomenon which leads to diverse immunological responses and cytokine release [30].

Aspergillus spp. as well as other filamentous fungi could be detected in Holi colour 1 (Fig. 6). Moulds in general pose a risk to human health, can be involved in disorders of the respiratory tract and may contribute to the manifestation of asthma and allergies [31]. As Kawakami et al. [32] and Wykoff et al. [33] reported, *Aspergillus* and *Paecilomyces* species can play a role in ocular infections with soft contact lens use as one predisposing factor. In the context of numerous ocular irritations reported by medical services on Holi festivals (Becker et al., *submitted*) this detection of fungi may be of clinical relevance. Deeper insights in the microbiological contamination profile of Holi colours might be of interest for future investigations.

Not much is known about the ingredients of the Holi colours (see Table 1). Even the carrier substance often remains unknown. As the composition (carrier substance, colour pigments, anticaking agents, etc.) varies from colour to colour, also the observed in vitro effects differ. Similarly, underlying mechanisms as well as the generation of possible health effects might be diverse and dependent on the specific colour. However, these various modes of action might also work in an additive or synergistic fashion as i.e. endotoxin, fungal contamination and leukocyte oxidative bursts might potentially lead to the observed induction of pro-inflammatory cytokines. Further experiments are needed to elucidate the distinct underlying mechanisms in more detail.

Conclusion

Holi festivals - with intense throwing of Holi powder in the air - are becoming popular all over the world. Although adverse health effects like skin, ocular or respiratory irritations may be the consequence, the hazard of Holi powder and possible underlying mechanisms of harmful effects have not been studied so far. We show here that the composition and the observed in vitro effects differ from colour to colour: Holi colours can contain up to 80 % of PM10 particles, they can have a pro-inflammatory and a cytotoxic potential, they can induce a leukocyte oxidative burst and they might be contaminated with mold fungi. These facts may account for some of the observed adverse health effects described by participants of Holi festivals and may improve the risk assessment of Holi colours.

Acknowledgements
Not applicable.

Funding
This study has no external funding.

Authors' contributions
KB designed the study and carried out the data analysis together with SB. CH performed the statistical analysis. KS drafted the manuscript. RH performed various toxicological tests and KV analysed the mycological aspects. AN and WS advised on particulate matter health effects issues and revised the manuscript. All authors participated in the study conception and coordination and read and approved the final manuscript.

Competing interests
The authors declare that they have no competing interests.

Author details
[1]Environmental Medicine and Health Effects Assessment, Federal Environment Agency, Corrensplatz 1, 14195 Berlin, Germany. [2]Microbiological Risk Assessment, Federal Environment Agency, Corrensplatz 1, 14195 Berlin,

Germany. [3]Toxicology of drinking water, Federal Environment Agency, Heinrich-Heine-Str. 12, 08645 Bad Elster, Germany.

References

1. Ghosh SK, Bandyopadhyay D, Chatterjee G, Saha D. The 'holi' dermatoses: annual spate of skin diseases following the spring festival in India. Indian J Dermatol. 2009;54(3):240–2.
2. Velpandian T, Saha K, Ravi AK, Kumari SS, Biswas NR, Ghose S. Ocular hazards of the colors used during the festival-of-colors (Holi) in India–malachite green toxicity. J Hazard Mater. 2007;139(2):204–8.
3. Chauhan D, Arora R, Das S, Shroff D, Narula R. Bilateral periorbital necrotizing fasciitis following exposure to Holi colors: a case report. Indian J Ophthalmol. 2007;55(5):373–4.
4. Pachauri T, Singla V, Satsangi A, Lakhani A, Kumari KM. Characterization of major pollution events (dust, haze, and two festival events) at Agra, India. Environ Sci Pollut Res Int. 2013;20(8):5737–52.
5. Hessle CC, Andersson B, Wold AE. Gram-positive and Gram-negative bacteria elicit different patterns of pro-inflammatory cytokines in human monocytes. Cytokine. 2005;30(5):311–8.
6. Schindler S, Spreitzer I, Loschner B, Hoffmann S, Hennes K, Halder M, et al. International validation of pyrogen tests based on cryopreserved human primary blood cells. J Immunol Methods. 2006;316(1-2):42–51.
7. Liebers V, Stubel H, Duser M, Bruning T, Raulf-Heimsoth M. Standardization of whole blood assay for determination of pyrogenic activity in organic dust samples. Int J Hyg Environ Health. 2009;212(5):547–56.
8. Moller W, Heimbeck I, Hofer TP, Khadem Saba G, Neiswirth M, Frankenberger M, et al. Differential inflammatory response to inhaled lipopolysaccharide targeted either to the airways or the alveoli in man. PLoS One. 2012; 7(4):e33505.
9. Anderson JO, Thundiyil JG, Stolbach A. Clearing the air: a review of the effects of particulate matter air pollution on human health. J Med Toxicol. 2012;8(2):166–75.
10. Chen H, Goldberg MS, Villeneuve PJ. A systematic review of the relation between long-term exposure to ambient air pollution and chronic diseases. Rev Environ Health. 2008;23(4):243–97.
11. Adam M, Schikowski T, Carsin AE, Cai Y, Jacquemin B, Sanchez M, et al. Adult lung function and long-term air pollution exposure. ESCAPE: a multicentre cohort study and meta-analysis. Eur Respir J. 2015;45(1):38–50.
12. Adar SD, Filigrana PA, Clements N, Peel JL. Ambient coarse particulate matter and human health: a systematic review and meta-analysis. Curr Environ Health Rep. 2014;1:258–74.
13. Schwartz J. Air pollution and daily mortality: a review and meta analysis. Environ Res. 1994;64(1):36–52.
14. Faustini A, Stafoggia M, Colais P, Berti G, Bisanti L, Cadum E, et al. Air pollution and multiple acute respiratory outcomes. Eur Respir J. 2013;42(2):304–13.
15. Zeka A, Zanobetti A, Schwartz J. Short term effects of particulate matter on cause specific mortality: effects of lags and modification by city characteristics. Occup Environ Med. 2005;62(10):718–25.
16. Yitshak-Sade M, Novack V, Katra I, Gorodischer R, Tal A, Novack L. Non-anthropogenic dust exposure and asthma medication purchase in children. Eur Respir J. 2015:45:652–60.
17. Jane J, Shen L, Wang L, Maningat CC. Preparation and properties of small-particle corn starch. Cereal Chem. 1992;69:280–3.
18. Monn C, Becker S. Cytotoxicity and induction of proinflammatory cytokines from human monocytes exposed to fine (PM2.5) and coarse particles (PM10-2.5) in outdoor and indoor air. Toxicol Appl Pharmacol. 1999; 155(3):245–52.
19. Pun VC, Yu IT, Qiu H, Ho KF, Sun Z, Louie PK, et al. Short-term associations of cause-specific emergency hospitalizations and particulate matter chemical components in Hong Kong. Am J Epidemiol. 2014;179(9):1086–95.
20. Bell ML, Ebisu K, Leaderer BP, Gent JF, Lee HJ, Koutrakis P, et al. Associations of PM(2). (5) constituents and sources with hospital admissions: analysis of four counties in Connecticut and Massachusetts (USA) for persons >/= 65 years of age. Environ Health Perspect. 2014;122(2):138–44.
21. Mathiak G, Kabir K, Grass G, Keller H, Steinringer E, Minor T, et al. Lipopolysaccharides from different bacterial sources elicit disparate cytokine responses in whole blood assays. Int J Mol Med. 2003;11(1):41–4.
22. Lonnemann G, Endres S, Van der Meer JW, Cannon JG, Koch KM, Dinarello CA. Differences in the synthesis and kinetics of release of interleukin 1 alpha, interleukin 1 beta and tumor necrosis factor from human mononuclear cells. Eur J Immunol. 1989;19(9):1531–6.
23. Brown DM, Donaldson K, Borm PJ, Schins RP, Dehnhardt M, Gilmour P, et al. Calcium and ROS-mediated activation of transcription factors and TNF-alpha cytokine gene expression in macrophages exposed to ultrafine particles. Am J Physiol Lung Cell Mol Physiol. 2004;286(2):L344–53.
24. Brown DM, Donaldson K, Stone V. Effects of PM10 in human peripheral blood monocytes and J774 macrophages. Respir Res. 2004;5:29.
25. Bengalli R, Molteni E, Longhin E, Refsnes M, Camatini M, Gualtieri M. Release of IL-1 beta triggered by Milan summer PM10: molecular pathways involved in the cytokine release. Biomed Res Int. 2013;2013:158093.
26. Yazdi AS, Guarda G, Riteau N, Drexler SK, Tardivel A, Couillin I, et al. Nanoparticles activate the NLR pyrin domain containing 3 (Nlrp3) inflammasome and cause pulmonary inflammation through release of IL-1alpha and IL-1beta. Proc Natl Acad Sci U S A. 2010;107(45):19449–54.
27. Yang EJ, Kim S, Kim JS, Choi IH. Inflammasome formation and IL-1beta release by human blood monocytes in response to silver nanoparticles. Biomaterials. 2012;33(28):6858–67.
28. Wang Z, Manninen A, Malmberg P, Larsson K. Inhalation of swine-house dust increases the concentrations of interleukin-1 beta (IL-1 beta) and interleukin-1 receptor antagonist (IL-1ra) in peripheral blood. Respir Med. 1998;92(8):1022–7.
29. Hansen LA, Poulsen OM, Wurtz H. Endotoxin potency in the A549 lung epithelial cell bioassay and the limulus amebocyte lysate assay. J Immunol Methods. 1999;226(1-2):49–58.
30. Miyata R, van Eeden SF. The innate and adaptive immune response induced by alveolar macrophages exposed to ambient particulate matter. Toxicol Appl Pharmacol. 2011;257(2):209–26.
31. Bush RK, Portnoy JM, Saxon A, Terr AI, Wood RA. The medical effects of mold exposure. J Allergy Clin Immunol. 2006;117(2):326–33.
32. Kawakami H, Inuzuka H, Mochizuki K, Takahashi N, Muto T, Ohkusu K, et al. Clinical manifestations, treatment and outcome of ocular infections caused by Paecilomyces species. Nippon Ganka Gakkai Zasshi. 2012;116(7):613–22.
33. Wykoff CC, Flynn Jr HW, Miller D, Scott IU, Alfonso EC. Exogenous Fungal Endophthalmitis: Microbiology and Clinical Outcomes. Ophthalmology. 2008;115(9):1501–7.e2.

20

Migrating pleural plaque in a patient with asbestos induced pleural disease

Christian Eisenhawer[1*], Michael K. Felten[1], Thomas Hager[2], Mikhail Gronostayskiy[3], Philipp Bruners[4], Andrea Tannapfel[5] and Thomas Kraus[1]

Abstract

Background: Health surveillance of formerly asbestos exposed individuals focus on early detection of asbestos related diseases, such as lung fibrosis (asbestosis), pleural plaques, mesothelioma and lung cancer in particular. One main concern is the early and clear identification of lesions with a high risk of malignant changes and their undelayed clinical work-up. False positive results may lead to unnecessary and often painful diagnostic interventions, which create high costs when applied to a large cohort and also may discredit the whole program. We describe an unusual presentation of a common lesion among asbestos exposed individuals, which has to our knowledge never been described before. Being aware of this pathological pathway may prevent inadequate clinical decisions with disadvantages for the patient. Underlying implications regarding health surveillance and the reading of CT-scans of the thorax are important for the management of formerly asbestos exposed individuals.

Case presentation: During follow-up of an asbestos exposed 72 year old former power plant worker with known pleural changes, a nodule located next to the left costophrenic angle was newly discovered on CT-scan. As the previous scan 1 year before did not show any changes in that area, a fast growing tumour was suspected and an immediate biopsy performed. The tissue showed the characteristics of a pleural plaque with no signs of malignancy. After carefully reviewing all previous radiographs a rounded opacity attached to the mediastinal pleura close to the oesophagus and slightly cranial to the position of the removed nodule could be discerned. That nodule had increased in size over several years and was no longer visible on the latest scan. It appeared that the originally slow growing plaque had migrated to the costophrenic angle some time before it was discovered in the latest scan thus imposing as a fast growing tumour.

Conclusions: We concluded that asbestos related pleural plaques can under special circumstances get separated from the pleura and migrate to another position in the pleural cavity. The case provides new insights in the development and properties of pleural lesions and may offer new options for the management of formerly asbestos exposed patients.

Keywords: Asbestos, Plaques, CT-scan, Surveillance, Tumour

* Correspondence: ceisenhawer@ukaachen.de
[1]Institute of Occupational and Social Medicine, RWTH Aachen University, Pauwelsstraße 30, 52074 Aachen, Germany
Full list of author information is available at the end of the article

Background

In formerly asbestos exposed individuals non-malignant changes of the pleura are usually developing over years in the form of plaques or diffuse pleural thickening, which do not require specific clinical work-up or intervention. As recommended in the Helsinki criteria for diagnosis and attribution for asbestos related diseases atypical changes on radiography related to the pleura call for immediate diagnostic work-up with biopsy to rule out early malignant mesothelioma and other malignancies [1–4]. While low-dose CT-scans are currently the most effective method of detecting asbestos related diseases, conventional chest X-ray and possibly ultrasonography of the chest are alternative techniques particularly suitable for low-risk groups [5].

In our surveillance program of formerly highly asbestos exposed employees with a diagnosis of non-malignant asbestos related disease of lung or pleura are invited for medical examinations annually or every other year. These examinations include a physical status, lung function testing and a CT-scan of the thorax. For CT examination a standard lowdose MDCT protocol is used (SOMATOM Sensation 16, Siemens Medical Solutions, Forchheim, Germany): 120 kV, individuals weighing less than 80 kg with 10mAseff/individuals weighing 80 kg and more with 20mAseff, 16 × 0.75 mm collimation, a rotation time of 0.5 s, and a table feed/rotation of 18 mm. The CT-scans are routinely read by a radiologist and an experienced occupational health specialist. In cases of disagreement an expert opinion can be obtained from an external specialist with particular experience in the field of asbestos related radiological changes. The examinations are mainly intended for early detection of mesothelioma, lung cancer and restrictive lung disease caused by proceeding lung fibrosis or pleural plaques. Such a diagnosis would entitle the patient for immediate clinical treatment, rehabilitation and possibly compensation payments by the Statutory Accident Insurance System. In addition to the medical diagnosis, proof of a significant cumulative asbestos exposure of 25 fibre-years or more is an important precondition for compensation. The early diagnosis of plaques and their differentiation from other pathological changes can be complicated and even “typical” results misleading [6–8].

Case presentation

In the year 2014 a 72 year old formerly asbestos exposed power plant worker (welder, fitter) presented for routine medical examination as participant of the surveillance program for patients with non-malignant asbestos related diseases. He had been registered for the program years earlier when bilateral partially calcified pleural plaques had been discovered (Fig. 1).

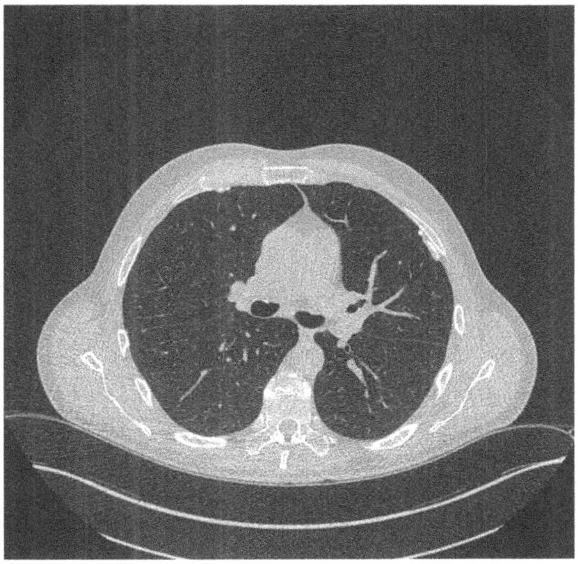

Fig. 1 CT-scan of the thorax of 2014 with partially calcified plaque

In comparison to the previous examination in 2013 the asbestos related changes showed no signs of progression. The patient could not recall any significant symptoms especially shortness of breath, coughing with or without sputum or chest pain. In the years 1959 to 1960 he had smoked about 10 cigarettes per day. Other than symptomatic treatment for prostatic hyperplasia, he took no oral medication. The physical status, including auscultation of heart and lungs, was unremarkable and consistent with his age. The bodyplethysmographic lung function test showed no signs of restrictive or obstructive lung disease, and no indication of emphysema. The results of capillary blood gas analysis and single breath carbon monoxide diffusion before and during standardised cycle ergometry (100 W for 4 min) showed no signs of impaired ventilation.

The direct comparison of CT-scans without contrast material of 2013 and 2014 revealed a newly appeared large (21 × 13 mm) nodule with a central calcification located in the left costophrenic angle and attached to the paravertebral chest wall (Fig. 2).

Based on the tentative diagnosis of a fast growing tumour with no radiological signs of malignancy and the urgent need of further diagnostic clarification, a left sided antero-axillary thoracotomy with atypical wedge resection of segment S10, removal of lymph nodes and ablation of the tumorous mass attached to the pleura was carried out. Figure 3 shows the situation of the parietal pleura close to the left costophrenic angle during the operation with a spherical smooth mass (3a) and multiple hyaline plaques located in the same area (3b). The nodule could be easily removed from the diaphragmatic pleura. After histological analysis the removed

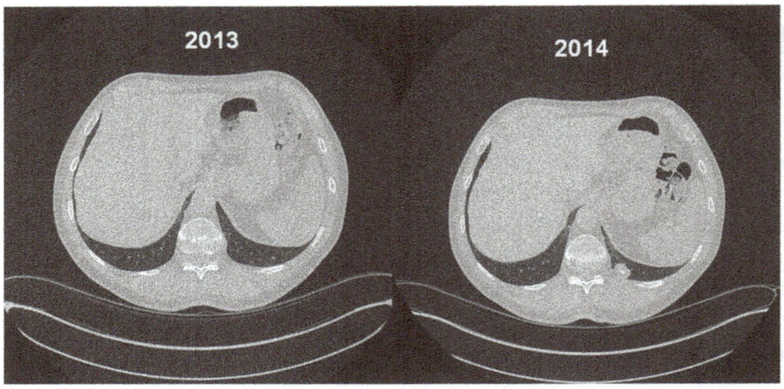

Fig. 2 CT-scans of the thorax (*left*: 2013, *right*: 2014) showing identical levels of the costophrenic sinus, with a newly emerged large, smooth nodule paravertebral attached to the *left* chest wall (dimensions 21 × 13 mm, central calcification, no contrast material)

tissue was described as a hyaline pleural plaque with central calcification and no signs of asbestos bodies or malignancy (Fig. 4). The postoperative rehabilitation of the patient was uneventful. One year later lung function testing showed normal results for FEV1 and VC max. The described nodule was no longer visible on CT-scan.

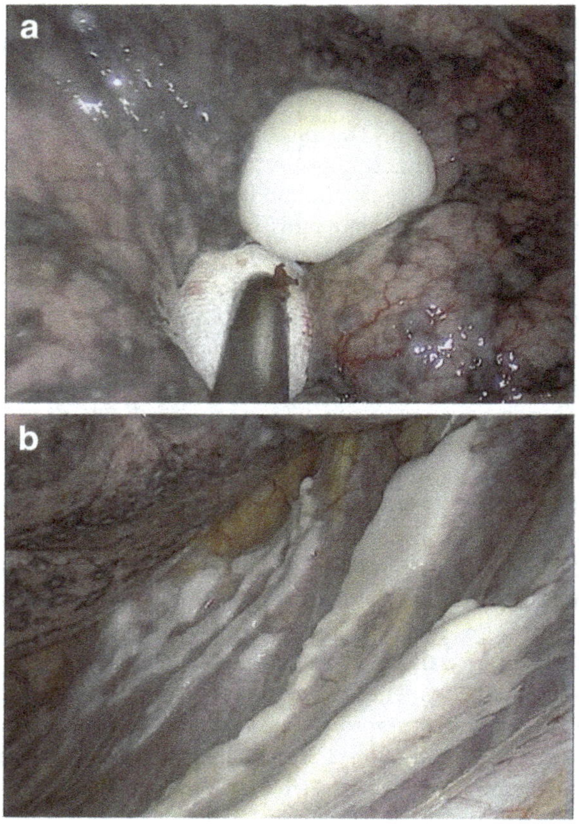

Fig. 3 Situation of the parietal pleura close to the *left* costophrenic angle during operation with a spherical smooth mass (**a**) and multiple hyaline plaques (**b**)

At that time the patient felt a slight discomfort in the left chest wall when taking a deep breath.

An extensive review of all available previous CT-scans of the patient going back to the year 2005 revealed a rounded opacity with central calcification which had been attached to the mediastinal pleura close to the oesophagus and slightly cranial to the position of the removed nodule (Fig. 5). That opacity started as a small nodule hardly discernible from the surrounding tissue and slowly increased in size until the year 2014 when it emerged lower down in the costophrenic sinus and was described for the first time (Figs. 5 and 6). The other asbestos related changes of the chest wall and the diaphragmatic pleura showed no progress during the observation period.

The re-examination of the tissue in a second pathological laboratory confirmed the original result describing the nodule as a typical asbestos associated pleural plaque with the special feature of a pedunculated fixation point to the pleura. This was consistent with the

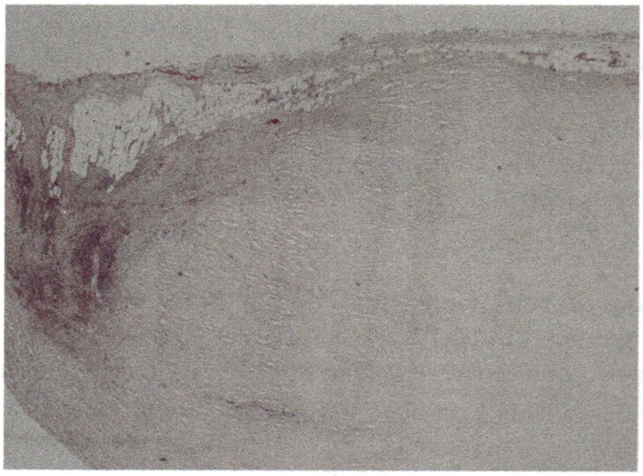

Fig. 4 Histological image of the parietal pleura showing typical signs of a pleural plaque (fat tissue in the border area)

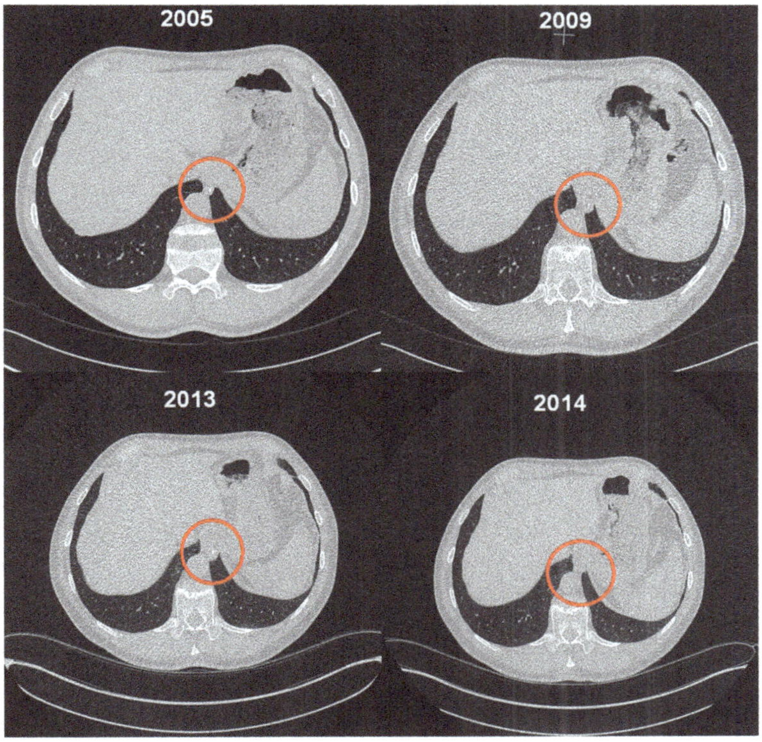

Fig. 5 CT-scans taken between 2005 and 2013 showing the growing nodule attached to the mediastinal pleura next to the oesophageal hiatus. The discovery of the presumably same nodule further down the sinus in 2014 triggered further diagnostic interventions

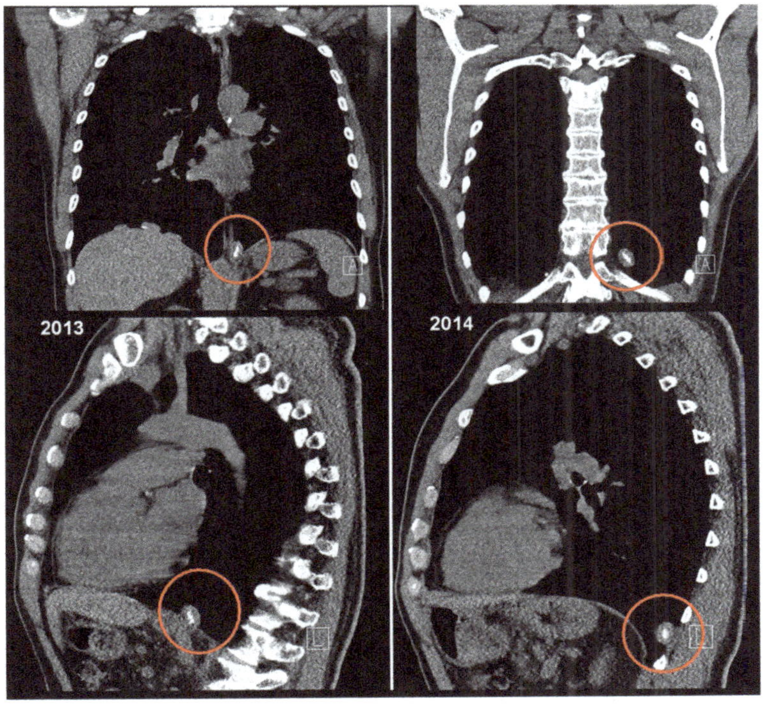

Fig. 6 Location of a partly calcified nodule shown in lateral projection and comparing the situation in the years 2013 (*left*) and 2014 (*right*). It can be assumed that the dislocation of the nodule, later identified as a pleural plaque, took place sometime between the two scans. The dislocation was probably caused by physical exertions during a mountain hike and marked by an episode of thoracic pain shortly after the hike

observation that the plaque was not firmly adherent, which is atypical for plaques on the diaphragm [9].

The patient recalled participating in an extensive mountain hike over several weeks involving great physical exertions, which took place few weeks before the medical examination in the year 2014 when the nodule attached to the pleura was discovered. About 2 weeks after returning from the hike the patient developed massive pain in the thorax with dyspnoea at rest, which lasted for several hours. Other symptoms were not observed and he did not see a doctor at that time.

Discussion and Conclusions

In this case of a formerly asbestos exposed patient with massive asbestos related changes of the pleura the clinical work up was complicated by a combination of two rather unusual features: the inconspicuous original location of the plaque and its detachment and migration within the pleural cavity, which lead to the tentative diagnosis of fast growing tumour. Despite repeated medical examinations over several years, the plaque developed unnoticed in an unusual location and continued to increase in size. The steady growth which could not be observed in any of the other plaques may be partly explained by its location on the diaphragm next to the oesophageal hiatus. One could speculate that the extreme motility in this area created an additional stimulus for growth or that the proximity to the oesophagus may have led to the accumulation of swallowed fibres creating a "hot spot" of plaque development. Alternative mechanisms such as the absorption of a foreign body through the oesophageal wall and its subsequent wandering or some kind of tumorous growth have been effectively ruled out by the results of the histological analysis [9–11].

When reviewing the series of CT-scans taken over a period of 10 years, it seems evident that the discovered nodule, after a phase of steady growth unnoticed by the CT-readers, had somehow migrated to the spot where it was eventually discovered. Although its location, structure, size and partial calcification, as well as the lack of any related symptoms, did not support the tentative diagnosis of fast growing tumour, it was difficult to identify the nodule as a dislocated pleural plaque at that time without taking the results of the previous CT-scans into consideration. We found no report in the literature indicating the possibility of migrating plaques or a hypothesis of the mechanism involved. For our case we propose the explanation that the physical exertion during a mountain hike somehow started the separation of the plaque. The wandering along the pleural cavity was probably facilitated by the continuous motions of diaphragm and lung combined with the effect of gravity.

It is important to note that even with the early discovery of the plaque at its original location, the operation with removal of the nodule and its careful examination would have been unavoidable. As the diagnosis of "migrating plaque" was unlikely, a CT-guided biopsy was considered too risky and tumorous growth could not be ruled out, the operation would still have been the recommended strategy.

The correct identification of pleural plaques is complicated by their similarity with other structures often leading to over-diagnosis, but they can also be overlooked through extended periods of time when developing in unusual locations. The possibility of migrating plaques mimicking fast growing tumours should be taken into consideration, particularly in patients with known asbestos related pleural changes.

Abbreviations

CT: Computed tomography; FEV1: Forced expiratory volume in 1 s; VC max: Maximum vital capacity

Acknowledgements

Not applicable.

Funding

This project was funded by the Institution for Statutory Accident Insurance and Prevention in the Energy, Textile, Electrical, and Media Industry (BGETEM), Cologne, Germany (grant number 360057) and RWE Power AG (grant number 370221) with unrestricted grants to the Medical Faculty, RWTH Aachen University.

Authors' contributions

CE examined the patient, reviewed all CT-scans and drafted the manuscript. MF extracted the history and patient reports on biopsies and CT-scans. TH examined the tissue specimen after surgery. MG operated the patient and reported the findings. PB re-read the CT-scans in the light of the biopsy results and the surgical report. AT re-examined the tissue specimen with a view to the previous history and CT-results. TK organized the surveillance of the patient and designed the health program. All authors read and approved the final manuscript.

Authors' information

The authors are medical doctors attached to the Institute of Occupational and Social Medicine, RWTH Aachen University (CE, TK are specialists in occupational medicine, MF is a research fellow), the Department of Diagnostic Radiology, RWTH Aachen University (PB is a radiologist), and the Division of Thoracic Surgery, West German Lung Center, Ruhrlandklinik, University Hospital Essen (MG is a thoracic surgeon). TH and AT are pathologists attached to the Institute of Pathology, University Hospital of Essen and the Department of Pathology, Ruhr-University Bochum.

Competing interests

The authors declare that they have no competing interests.

Author details
[1]Institute of Occupational and Social Medicine, RWTH Aachen University, Pauwelsstraße 30, 52074 Aachen, Germany. [2]Institute of Pathology, University Hospital of Essen, University of Duisburg-Essen, Hufelandstraße 55, 45147 Essen, Germany. [3]Division of Thoracic Surgery, West German Lung Center, Ruhrlandklinik, University Hospital Essen, Tüschener Weg 40, 45239 Essen, Germany. [4]Department of Diagnostic Radiology, RWTH Aachen University, Pauwelsstraße 30, 52074 Aachen, Germany. [5]Department of Pathology, Ruhr-University Bochum, Bürkle de la Camp-Platz 1, 44789 Bochum, Germany.

References

1. Wolff H, et al. Asbestos, asbestosis, and cancer, the Helsinki criteria for diagnosis and attribution 2014: Recommendations. Scand J Work Environ Health. 2015;41:5–15.
2. AmericanThoracicSociety. Diagnosis and initial management of nonmalignant diseases related to asbestos. Am J Respir Crit Care Med. 2004; 170:691–715.
3. Eisenhawer C, Felten MK, Tamm M, Das M, Kraus T. Radiological surveillance of formerly asbestos exposed power industry workers: rates and risk factors of benign changes on chest x-ray and MDCT. Journal of Occupational Medicine and Toxicology. 2014;9:18.
4. Hagemeyer O, Otten H, Kraus T. Asbestos consumption, asbestos exposure and asbestos-related occupational diseases in Germany. Int Arch Occup Environ Health. 2006;79:613–20. doi:https://doi.org/10.1007/s00420-006-0091-x.
5. Smargiassi A, et al. Chest ultrasonography in health surveillance of asbestos-related lung diseases. Toxicol Ind Health. 2017;33:537–46.
6. Alfudhili KM, et al. Focal pleural thickening mimicking pleural plaques on chest computed tomography: tips and tricks. Br J Radiol. 2016;89:20150792.
7. Kim YK, et al. Multidetector CT findings and differential diagnoses of malignant pleural mesothelioma and metastatic pleural diseases in Korea. Korean J Radiol. 2016;17:545–53.
8. Zhanlong M, et al. Variable solitary fibrous tumor locations: CT and MR imaging features. Medicine. 2016;13:1–7.
9. Roberts GH. The pathology of parietal pleural plaques. J Clin Pathol. 1971;24:348–53.
10. Papadopoulos A, et al. A rare clinical case - solitary fibrous tumor of the pleura. Respiratory Medicine Case Reports. 2015;16:117–9.
11. Sulu E, et al. Castleman's disease presenting as a pleural mass in the thoracic cavity. Monaldi Arch Chest Dis. 2012;77:139–40.

21

Associations of physical activity, fitness, and body composition with heart rate variability–based indicators of stress and recovery on workdays

Tiina Teisala[1*], Sara Mutikainen[1], Asko Tolvanen[2], Mirva Rottensteiner[1], Tuija Leskinen[3], Jaakko Kaprio[4,7,8], Marjukka Kolehmainen[5], Heikki Rusko[6] and Urho M Kujala[1]

Abstract

Background: The purpose of this study was to investigate how physical activity (PA), cardiorespiratory fitness (CRF), and body composition are associated with heart rate variability (HRV)-based indicators of stress and recovery on workdays. Additionally, we evaluated the association of objectively measured stress with self-reported burnout symptoms.

Methods: Participants of this cross-sectional study were 81 healthy males (age range 26–40 y). Stress and recovery on workdays were measured objectively based on HRV recordings. CRF and anthropometry were assessed in laboratory conditions. The level of PA was based on a detailed PA interview (MET index [MET-h/d]) and self-reported activity class.

Results: PA, CRF, and body composition were significantly associated with levels of stress and recovery on workdays. MET index ($P < 0.001$), activity class ($P = 0.001$), and CRF ($P = 0.019$) were negatively associated with stress during working hours whereas body fat percentage ($P = 0.005$) was positively associated. Overall, 27.5% of the variance of total stress on workdays ($P = 0.001$) was accounted for by PA, CRF, and body composition. Body fat percentage and body mass index were negatively associated with night-time recovery whereas CRF was positively associated. Objective work stress was associated ($P = 0.003$) with subjective burnout symptoms.

Conclusions: PA, CRF, and body composition are associated with HRV-based stress and recovery levels, which needs to be taken into account in the measurement, prevention, and treatment of work-related stress. The HRV-based method used to determine work-related stress and recovery was associated with self-reported burnout symptoms, but more research on the clinical importance of the methodology is needed.

Keywords: Body composition, Body fat percentage, BMI, Cardiorespiratory fitness, HRV, Physical activity, Recovery, Working hours, Work stress

Background

Physical activity (PA) is one of the factors that protects against stress [1]. Exercise and psychological stress have similar acute physiological effects because both result in potent increases in cardiovascular, sympathetic, and hypothalamic pituitary adrenocortical responses and decreases in parasympathetic responses [2]. Repeated bouts of exercise lead to physiological adaptations, including decreased resting heart rate (HR) and blood pressure and increased parasympathetic activity [3]. The theory of "cross-stressor adaptation" suggests that regular PA and good fitness lead to adaptations in response to both exercise and psychological stressors [2,4].

The assessment of heart rate variability (HRV) has gained importance as a technique to explore the function of the autonomic nervous system (ANS) and has been widely used to diagnose both psychological and physiological disorders [5]. HRV is the beat-to-beat variation in time of consecutive heartbeats expressed in normal sinus rhythm on an electrocardiogram [6,7]. The separate rhythmic

* Correspondence: tiina.teisala@jyu.fi
[1]Department of Health Sciences, University of Jyväskylä, P.O. Box 35, Jyväskylä FIN-40014, Finland
Full list of author information is available at the end of the article

contributions from sympathetic and parasympathetic autonomic activity modulate the heart's R wave to R wave intervals (RR intervals) of the QRS complex at distinct frequencies [8]. Both sympathetic and parasympathetic activity have been suggested to be associated with the low frequency (LF) range (0.04–0.15 Hz) because parasympathetic activity is a major contributor to the high frequency (HF) range (0.15–0.4 Hz) component in modulation of frequencies of the HR [9,10]. Higher HRV characterizes a healthy person with efficient autonomic mechanisms and good adaptation ability while lower HRV is an indicator of abnormal and insufficient adaptation of the ANS [7,11]. Reduced HRV is suggested to be associated with harmful events in health [12].

A greater amount of reported stress is suggested to be associated with lower HRV [13]. Also, the effects of PA, cardiorespiratory fitness (CRF), and adiposity on HRV profile have been of interest. Chronic exercise increases HRV [14-16], and favorable HRV profiles are associated with higher levels of PA [17] and better CRF [18]. Additionally, obesity has been associated with altered ANS activity [19]. Some studies have found HRV profiles to be relatively poor among obese subjects [20,21] and to improve with weight loss [22].

Work-related stress and physical inactivity are major concerns in society today. The current interest is in reducing both work-related stress and inactivity, and objective methods, such as the HRV-based approach, are needed to diagnose stress symptoms. To make recording of HRV a practical tool for field measurements, new approaches for HRV analysis are needed. For instance, age is an important determinant of HRV, which also has a large inter-individual variability [9,23]. Firstbeat Technologies Ltd. has been developing this kind of diagnostic tool to measure and define stress and recovery based on individual values for HR and HRV (for more information, see the company's web page [24]). Some stress and recovery variables, calculated with this tool, are suggested to be related to chronic work stress and emotions at work [25]. Using this tool, we investigated how different indicators of PA, CRF, and body composition, which are related to each other, are associated with HRV-based indicators of stress and recovery on workdays among healthy young men. The secondary aim was to evaluate the association between objectively measured stress and self-reported burnout symptoms.

Methods

Subjects

The population of this cross-sectional study consisted of groups from two separate studies, the FitFatTwin study (FFT study) and the Body & Future Health study (BFH study). The identical measurements of the cross-sectional FFT study and the baseline measurements of the BHF were pooled for this analysis. In total, 46 men (23 monozygotic twin pairs) participated in the FFT study. The BFH study included 37 men, two of whom were excluded from this study because their HRV recordings included only days off from work. Altogether, 81 healthy males (age range 26–40 y) who were not on regular medication were included in the present study. The twin study was enriched with pairs having within-pair differences in their PA habits. Because the BFH study was originally planned to investigate overweight and physically inactive individuals, it involved the following inclusion criteria: BMI 25.0–35.0 kg/m^2, waist circumference ≥94 cm, no vigorous exercise (>20 min/session) more than twice a week, and no smoking; for more information, see the registered controlled trial protocol [26]. Levels of HRV-based stress and recovery did not differ between the participants of these two studies. However, the participants from the FFT study had more favorable body composition, better CRF, and a higher self-rated activity class. The characteristics of the participants of the present study are presented in Table 1.

Both studies were conducted according to the ethical rules stated in the Declaration of Helsinki. All participants were informed about the study, and they signed written informed consent prior to any measurements. The study

Table 1 Characteristics of the study population

	Mean	Range
Age (y)	34	26–40
Weight (kg)	83.5	51.3–123.2
Height (cm)	179.1	156.5–198.0
BMI (kg/[m]^2)	26.0	19.8–35.0
Body fat%	24.5	7.6–41.8
VO_{2max}[a] (ml/kg/min)	39.6	23.3–72.6
MET index[b]	3.5	0.1–27.7
Activity class (0–10)	4.4	0.0–9.5
Working time (h)	8.4	2.8–16.0
Sleeping time (h)	7.7	4.7–10.3
Bergen burnout inventory total scores[c]	36	16–74
Firstbeat variables		
Work stress (%)	72.8	14.5–99.2
Total stress (%)	49.9	12.6–79.1
Stress index	122.3	80.5–193.3
RMSSD (sleep)	56.78	22.6–150.6
Stress balance (−1 to 1)	0.69	−0.43–1.00
Total recovery (%)	29.3	4.6–67.0
Recovery index (24 h)	92.2	74.0–112.2
Recovery index (sleep)	111.4	45.8–246.9

(n = 81).
[a]n = 78 [b]MET-h/day, based on retrospective PA interview [c]n = 80.

protocols were approved by the ethics committee of the Central Finland Health Care District.

Measurements

The stress and recovery variables were calculated objectively from the HR and HRV recordings, which were executed over three days using Bodyguard, a measurement device developed by Firstbeat Technologies Ltd. (Jyväskylä, Finland). The HRV recordings from these three days were downloaded with Firstbeat Health Software (version 3.1.1.0.). The Firstbeat Health Software first scans the recorded ambulatory RR interval data through an artifact detection filter to perform an initial correction of falsely detected, missed, and premature heart beats [27]. The data were transferred to the Matlab environment (R2007B), where the analyses of physiological variables describing stress and recovery were performed with the Firstbeat Analysis Server program (version 5.3.0.4). This program calculates HRV indices second-by-second using the short-time Fourier transform method and HR- and HRV-derived variables of respiration rate and oxygen consumption using neural network modeling of data [27-29] (for more details, see the white paper by Firstbeat Technologies Ltd. [30]). The program also calculates second-by-second indices of recovery and stress, reflecting activities of the sympathetic (absolute stress vector, ASV) and parasympathetic (absolute recovery vector, ARV) nervous systems. The ASV is calculated from the HR, HF, and LF components and respiratory variables. The ASV is high when HR is elevated, HRV is reduced, and the frequency distribution of HRV is inconsistent because of changes in respiratory period. The ARV, which is calculated from the HR and HF components, is high when HR is close to the basic resting level and HRV is high and regular. The program takes into account individual basic resting HR and HRV values in the determination of the physiological states of the body, including PA, stress state, recovery state, or unrecognized state, and detected based on the above-mentioned variables. The stress and recovery variables used in the present study are based on Firstbeat Analysis Server analyses and are described in Table 2. These variables included the traditional HRV variable RMSSD (root mean square of successive differences), which is a time domain measure of HRV, and plots HRV as the change in normal RR intervals over time [31].

The HRV data consisted of successfully recorded (RR intervals corrected max 25 percentages) workdays. The stress and recovery values were the mean values of the workdays with the number of days being one (n = 10), two (n = 70), or three (n = 1). The stress and recovery variables were determined from the whole recording day (24 h) or only from working hours or sleeping hours. Working hours, sleeping time, and alcohol consumption were determined from the participants' measurement diaries, which they were advised to keep over the measurement period. Alcohol consumption was reported daily in standard units of approximately 12 g of ethanol (one unit: 33 centiliter [cl] beer or 12 cl red or white wine or 8 cl fortified wine or 4 cl liquor).

The Bergen Burnout Inventory (BBI) was used in the assessment of occupational burnout. This inventory is employed in some Finnish occupational health services to monitor and screen stress levels [32] and includes 15 questions concerning three subcategories of burnout: exhaustive fatigue, cynicism, and impaired occupational self-respect. Answers to the 15 questions were given using a Likert-type response scale, which was scored from 1 (totally disagree) to 6 (totally agree), and the total scores were between 15 and 90 [33].

Body weight and height were measured in the morning. The body mass index (BMI) is computed as weight/height^2 (kg/m^2). The whole body fat percentage was evaluated after fasting 10–12 h using dual-energy X-ray absorptiometry (GE Lunar Prodigy Advance, GE Healthcare). The software used for picture handling and analysis was enCORE™ 2009, version 13.20 (GE Healthcare).

The volume of PA (MET index) was retrospectively inferred using a modified version [34] of the Kuopio Ischemic Heart Disease Risk Factor Study Questionnaire [35], which included questions on leisure-time PA and PA during journeys to and from work, as well as daily activities such as gardening and berry picking. Monthly frequency, mean duration, and mean intensity of each form of activity were evaluated. A multiple of the resting metabolic rate (MET) was assigned for each activity to describe the intensity of the form of PA. The 3-month (BFH study) and 12-month (FFT study) MET indexes for each form of PA were calculated by multiplying the intensity (MET), duration (h), and monthly frequency of the activity, and the MET index was expressed as the sum score of different activities (MET-h/d).

The other method used to estimate PA level was self-reported activity class using a 0–10 scale to represent the activity level of the previous 2–3 months. The values from 0 to 7 were modified from Ross and Jackson's [36] scale. The values from 7.5 to 10 were added by Firstbeat to include more seriously training individuals and athletes in the scale (for more details, see the white paper by Firstbeat Technologies Ltd. [37]).

CRF was assessed using the cycle ergometer test and a slightly modified World Health Organization protocol [38] with 2-min stages and 25 W/stage increases in workload. The test was submaximal in the BHF study and maximal with breath-by-breath respiratory gas-exchange analysis in the FFT study. The submaximal cycle ergometer test was ended after the workload during which the tested person achieved the submaximal HR level (85–88% from the maximal HR), which was defined from maximal

Table 2 The description of variables of stress and recovery based on firstbeat analysis server

Stress variables For non-exercise data segments, continuous indices of stress are used to identify the time when the body is in a stress state. Stress state is defined as an increased activation in the body when sympathetic nervous system activity is dominating and parasympathetic activation is decreased. Stress can be induced by external and internal stress factors, and the definition of the stress state does not take into account the nature of the stress response, i.e., whether it is positive or negative.	
Work stress	The percentage of stress time during working hours
Total stress	The percentage of stress time in a workday (including leisure time and night)
Stress index	Absolute value characterizing the magnitude of stress processes on a workday (including leisure time and night)
Recovery variables, 24 hours Continuous indices of recovery are used to identify the time when the body is in a recovery state. Recovery state is defined as a decreased activation in the body during recovery, rest, and/or peaceful working. This state is related to the lack of external and internal stress factors, and parasympathetic activation is dominating.	
Total recovery	The percentage of recovery time in a workday (including leisure time and night)
Recovery index	Absolute value characterizing the magnitude of recovery processes in a workday (including leisure time and night)
Recovery variables, sleep time	
RMSSD	Average of the RMSSD (root mean square of successive differences) vector values during sleep periods. High RMSSD values are associated with increased parasympathetic activity and good recovery while low values during rest indicate poor recovery. The RMSSD value should be over 20 during sleep in a normal situation.
Stress balance	Indicates proportion of time of stress and recovery reactions during sleep periods in the measurement period; the used values are from −1 to 1. Values from 0.5 to 1 indicate good recovery; values from 0 to 0.5 indicate moderate recovery; and values from 0 to −1 indicate weak recovery.
Recovery index	The recovery index gives an estimate of a person's recovery during sleep time. The 4-h window for determining the recovery index is set to start 30 min after going to bed. The index summarizes several factors, including RMSSD and other HRV variables, and takes into account the other functions of ANS while determining the value for the index.

HR based on the participant's age (210 − (0.65 × age)). In the FFT study, three people did not participate in the maximal cycle ergometer test, and in the case of seven participants, a submaximal test was performed instead of the maximal test for health or motivational reasons. In the analyses, the values used for the maximal oxygen consumption (VO_{2max}) are the results of submaximal workload-based calculations for all participants. VO_{2max} was calculated from the submaximal test values of the maximal cycle ergometer test (n = 36). The correlation between this calculation from submaximal workloads and the value from the maximal oxygen consumption test was significant ($P < 0.001$).

Statistical analysis

Statistical analyses were performed using Mplus version 7 [39]. The statistical significance was set at $P \leq 0.05$. The estimator used was maximum likelihood with robust standard errors that are robust against non-normality. The effect of clustered data (twins) was controlled using the type complex definition in Mplus. A few missing values (VO_{2max} n = 3 and BBI n = 1) were inferred to be missing at random. Because the variables under interest are known to be related to each other, structural equation modeling was used to investigate how PA, fitness, and body composition are associated with HRV-based indicators of stress and recovery. In the first stage, estimates of each independent variable (body fat percentage, BMI, VO_{2max}, MET index, and activity class) were determined to explain the dependent stress and recovery variables. In the second stage, to investigate how much of the variance of the stress and recovery variables is explained by PA, fitness, and body composition together, a latent factor variable was formed from the MET index, activity class, VO_{2max}, body fat percentage, and BMI. In addition, structural equation modeling was used to investigate the association of the HRV-based stress and recovery variables with the BBI total scores.

The model fit was evaluated using the χ^2 test, comparative fit index (CFI), Tucker Lewis Index (TLI), root mean square error of approximation (RMSEA), and standardized root mean square residual (SRMR). For a good-fitting model, the χ^2 test is non-significant; CFI and TLI are at least 0.95; RMSEA is no more than 0.06; and SRMR no more than 0.08 [40].

Results

Body fat percentage was positively associated ($\beta = 0.306$, $P = 0.005$) whereas VO_{2max} ($\beta = -0.311$, $P = 0.019$), MET index ($\beta = -0.304$, $P < 0.001$), and activity class ($\beta = -0.326$, $P = 0.001$) were negatively associated with HRV-based work stress. Similarly to works stress, the other HRV-based stress variables were associated with body composition, CRF, and PA. However, BMI was positively associated with total stress ($\beta = 0.272$, $P = 0.003$) and stress index ($\beta = 0.478$, $P < 0.001$). MET index was not associated with stress index ($P = 0.440$).

The indicators of recovery during night-time sleep (RMSSD, stress balance, recovery index) were negatively associated with body fat percentage and BMI and positively associated with VO_{2max}. Activity class was positively associated with stress balance value ($\beta = 0.237$, $P = 0.025$).

Body fat percentage ($\beta = -0.445$, $P < 0.001$) and BMI ($\beta = -0.355$, $P < 0.001$) were negatively associated whereas VO_{2max} ($\beta = 0.465$, $P < 0.001$), MET index ($\beta = 0.356$, $P < 0.001$), and activity class ($\beta = 0.418$, $P < 0.001$) were positively associated with total recovery. Body fat percentage ($\beta = -0.343$, $P = 0.002$) and BMI ($\beta = -0.309$, $P = 0.001$) were negatively associated whereas VO_{2max} was positively associated with 24-h recovery index ($\beta = 0.331$, $P = 0.010$). MET index ($P = 0.414$) and activity class ($P = 0.151$) were not associated with 24-h recovery index.

Because the age range of the participants was relatively small and adjustment for age changed the results very minimally, the age-adjusted results are not shown. Adjustments for alcohol consumption, working time, or sleeping time influenced the results only minimally or modestly (Table 3). Adjustments for alcohol most influenced the associations of VO_{2max} with the stress and recovery variables. The results are presented in greater detail in Table 3.

A latent factor variable (Figure 1) was formed from body fat percentage, BMI, VO_{2max}, MET index, and activity class because these variables correlated significantly. The latent variable was a significant explanatory variable for all of the stress and recovery variables except RMSSD. It explained total recovery best at 30.1% of its variance. Among stress variables, the variance of total stress was best explained (27.5%) by the latent factor, which also explained 14.1% of the variance of work stress. The estimated model fit to the data well (χ^2 (35) = 41.09, $P = 0.22$, CFI = 0.99, TLI = 0.98, RMSEA = 0.046, SRMR = 0.06), and all the modification indices were lower than 4, which indicated that were no additional parameters that would have increased the fit of the model for the analysis.

In addition, objectively and subjectively measured stress levels were significantly associated (Table 4). HRV-based work stress ($\beta = 0.272$, $P = 0.003$) and total stress ($\beta = 0.304$, $P = 0.001$) explained the variation in total score of the BBI questionnaire. Adjustment for age changed the results only minimally, but after adjustment for body fat percentage, associations between work stress and the BBI total score did not persist.

Discussion

The results of this study showed that there were significant associations among PA, CRF, body composition, and novel HRV-based levels of stress and recovery in real life on workdays. Greater PA level, better CRF, and more favorable body composition were associated with lower stress levels during working hours as well as with lower stress levels and higher recovery levels throughout the whole day. Better recovery at night was associated with better CRF and a more favorable body composition. Additionally, the relationship between objectively measured stress and self-reported burnout symptoms was significant, and further analysis showed that body composition explained it in part.

The results of the present study are mainly in line with those of earlier studies that used traditional HRV measures. Favorable HRV profiles may be related to PA and CRF [15,16] while stress appears to be linked with reduced leisure-time PA [41] and lower physical fitness [2,42]. Earlier studies have proposed that fit individuals would show attenuated physiological reactivity to psychological stressors compared with sedentary individuals [43,44]. A more recent meta-analytic review by Forcier et al. [2] also provided support for the cross-adaptation hypothesis and suggested that fitness training may increase the ability of cardiovascular systems to control responses to acute stressors and also speed cardiovascular recovery from stress.

The present study found that among men, unfavorable body composition was associated with higher objective stress and lower recovery. According to previous studies that have examined stress as a subjective experience, the association between mental stress and body composition has been inconsistent because evidence both supports [45-49] and refutes [50-53] it. Additionally, the results suggested that body fat percentage explained part of the association between objectively and subjectively measured levels of stress, indicating that body fat percentage affects both physiological stress and subjective experience of stress among men. However, a previous study by Nyberg et al. [46] found that the relationship between stress and unfavorable body composition may not be linear. In an analysis of pooled European data (n = 161,746), both weight gain and weight loss were associated with the onset of job strain so that the cross-sectional association between job strain and BMI formed a 'U'-shaped curve [46].

The results showed that PA level was not associated with night-time recovery, although regular PA has consistently been associated with better sleep [54]. However, previous findings indicate that PA in the evening may delay the beginning of recovery. Physical fitness may have a role in recovery of HR and HRV after exercise, as could be seen even between trained and highly trained subjects, so that the recovery takes 60–90 min longer in trained subjects [55]. Recovery of HRV also depends on type, intensity, and duration of exercise [56]. In the study of Myllymäki et al. [57], a late-night exercise caused higher HR during the first three sleeping hours of an exercise day compared to a control day. Mischler et al. [58] reported that prolonged exercise had similar effects on HR during sleep. In addition to these effects of exercise on HR, HRV might decrease during the activity and, for instance, high-intensity exercises reduce HRV for 30–60 min afterward in trained and highly trained subjects [55,56]. Hynynen et al. [59] found that both moderate and heavy endurance exercise even in the daytime has an increasing effect

Table 3 The association of body composition, cardiorespiratory fitness, and physical activity with stress and recovery

	No adjustments			Alcohol adjusted			Working time adjusted			Sleeping time adjusted		
	β	S.E.	*P*	β	S.E.	*P*	β	S.E.	*P*	β	S.E.	*P*
Body fat%												
WS	0.306	0.108	0.005	0.288	0.114	0.012	0.315	0.114	0.006	0.313	0.115	0.006
TS	0.442	0.101	<0.001	0.405	0.107	<0.001	0.242	0.070	0.001	0.429	0.111	<0.001
SI	0.422	0.115	<0.001	0.395	0.108	<0.001	0.426	0.107	<0.001	0.425	0.107	<0.001
TR	−0.445	0.088	<0.001	−0.409	0.087	<0.001	−0.443	0.090	<0.001	−0.419	0.086	<0.001
RI	−0.343	0.113	0.002	−0.325	0.111	0.003	−0.338	0.103	0.001	−0.330	0.111	0.003
RMSSD	−0.293	0.123	0.017	−0.267	0.115	0.020	−0.285	0.109	0.009	−0.233	0.116	0.015
SB	−0.400	0.083	<0.001	−0.377	0.084	<0.001	−0.408	0.076	<0.001	−0.403	0.077	<0.001
RIS	−0.359	0.130	0.006	−0.328	0.127	0.010	−0.348	0.114	0.002	−0.351	0.125	<0.001
BMI												
WS	0.162	0.086	0.060	0.139	0.085	0.101	0.176	0.083	0.033	0.171	0.086	0.047
TS	0.272	0.093	0.003	0.210	0.090	0.020	0.268	0.086	0.002	0.251	0.095	0.009
SI	0.478	0.102	<0.001	0.447	0.105	<0.001	0.458	0.091	<0.001	0.482	0.097	<0.001
TR	−0.355	0.084	<0.001	−0.297	0.078	<0.001	−0.351	0.084	<0.001	−0.309	0.084	<0.001
RI	−0.309	0.093	0.001	−0.287	0.094	0.002	−0.298	0.087	0.001	−0.239	0.092	0.002
RMSSD	−0.304	0.106	0.004	−0.274	0.106	0.009	−0.290	0.097	0.003	−0.239	0.107	0.007
SB	−0.379	0.095	<0.001	−0.325	0.101	0.001	−0.395	0.087	<0.001	−0.334	0.092	<0.001
RIS	−0.395	0.102	<0.001	−0.358	0.105	0.001	−0.373	0.095	<0.001	−0.332	0.104	<0.001
VO_{2max}												
WS	−0.311	0.132	0.019	−0.282	0.147	0.055	−0.316	0.147	0.031	−0.317	0.145	0.029
TS	−0.416	0.126	0.001	−0.349	0.155	0.025	−0.411	0.145	0.004	−0.396	0.150	0.008
SI	−0.379	0.096	<0.001	−0.334	0.098	0.001	−0.377	0.094	<0.001	−0.375	0.095	<0.001
TR	0.465	0.111	<0.001	0.405	0.122	0.001	0.469	0.110	<0.001	0.429	0.107	<0.001
RI	0.331	0.128	0.01	0.302	0.139	0.030	0.319	0.133	0.016	0.307	0.143	0.032
RMSSD	0.262	0.125	0.037	0.222	0.125	0.076	0.247	0.123	0.045	0.242	0.130	0.062
SB	0.270	0.073	<0.001	0.145	0.091	0.113	0.283	0.073	<0.001	0.274	0.072	<0.001
RIS	0.294	0.125	0.019	0.243	0.131	0.063	0.275	0.121	0.023	0.276	0.136	0.042
MET index												
WS	−0.304	0.113	<0.001	−0.287	0.087	0.001	−0.308	0.087	<0.001	−0.311	0.086	<0.001
TS	−0.385	0.145	0.008	−0.349	0.084	<0.001	−0.384	0.083	<0.001	−0.368	0.086	<0.001
SI	−0.096	0.124	0.440	−0.065	0.105	0.535	−0.098	0.107	0.360	−0.099	0.105	0.343
TR	0.356	0.131	<0.001	0.316	0.102	0.002	0.355	0.095	<0.001	0.321	0.097	0.001
RI	0.138	0.173	0.414	0.120	0.140	0.390	0.135	0.136	0.319	0.122	0.141	0.389
RMSSD	0.058	0.165	0.723	0.032	0.152	0.834	0.054	0.147	0.713	0.046	0.151	0.761
SB	0.097	0.089	0.255	−0.017	0.081	0.835	0.102	0.074	0.172	0.101	0.069	0.141
RIS	0.074	0.173	0.670	0.038	0.159	0.810	0.067	0.150	0.654	0.063	0.158	0.690
Activity class												
WS	−0.326	0.102	0.001	−0.298	0.104	0.004	−0.330	0.107	0.002	−0.331	0.109	0.002
TS	−0.434	0.096	<0.001	−0.362	0.102	<0.001	−0.433	0.105	<0.001	−0.424	0.108	<0.001
SI	−0.222	0.113	0.048	−0.175	0.115	0.128	−0.224	0.115	0.051	−0.225	0.114	0.049
TR	0.418	0.097	<0.001	0.336	0.090	<0.001	0.417	0.098	<0.001	0.400	0.101	<0.001
RI	0.175	0.122	0.151	0.146	0.119	0.221	0.172	0.121	0.154	0.164	0.126	0.191

Table 3 The association of body composition, cardiorespiratory fitness, and physical activity with stress and recovery *(Continued)*

RMSSD	0.090	0.120	0.453	0.047	0.116	0.684	0.086	0.116	0.459	0.082	0.112	0.505
SB	0.237	0.106	0.025	0.082	0.095	0.390	0.241	0.107	0.024	0.239	0.106	0.024
RIS	0.132	0.129	0.305	0.076	0.125	0.544	0.127	0.125	0.311	0.125	0.132	0.343

Standardized estimate (β), standard error (S.E.), and *P* value for body fat%, BMI, VO_{2max}, MET index, and activity class in relation to Firstbeat stress and recovery variables (work stress [WS], total stress [TS], stress index [SI], total recovery [TR], recovery index 24 h [RI], RMSSD, stress balance [SB], and recovery index sleep [RIS]).

on HR and decreasing effect on HRV during sleep in a dose–response manner.

Subjective methods were used to assess the level of PA. The MET index was based on a detailed retrospective interview. This index correlated significantly with measured VO_{2max} values, supporting its validity to assess the level of PA. Subjective assessment may include some reporting bias; however, although the method undertaken was not objective, it had the advantage of taking several months of subjective data into account. The other method was self-reported activity class, which is regularly reported before the HRV measurement by Bodyguard.

One limitation of the present study is that the effect of different intensities of PA was not investigated; however, both light and moderate to vigorous leisure-time activity are related to lower likelihood of burnout [41]. Another limitation is that fat distribution was not taken into account, even though, according to earlier studies, it may have a role in relation to the HRV profile [19,60]. The nature of work in today's society is rather complex, including inexact and variable working hours and a lack of precise division between work time and leisure time, which causes difficulties in determining the level of HRV-based stress during exact working hours.

The current results cannot be generalized to women because the study population consisted of both physically inactive and active young male employees, who were not heavy drinkers or on regular medication. This population was ideal for this study because alcohol intake, diseases, and medications influence ANS [8]. The effect of possible alcohol intake on HRV was taken into account in the analyses. The fact that our study population consisted of young employees who are still establishing their careers highlights the importance of the findings.

Stress can be explained through several biological processes, such as the inflammatory, dopaminergic, and neuroendocrine systems [61]. However, in the present study, the measurement method for stress and recovery

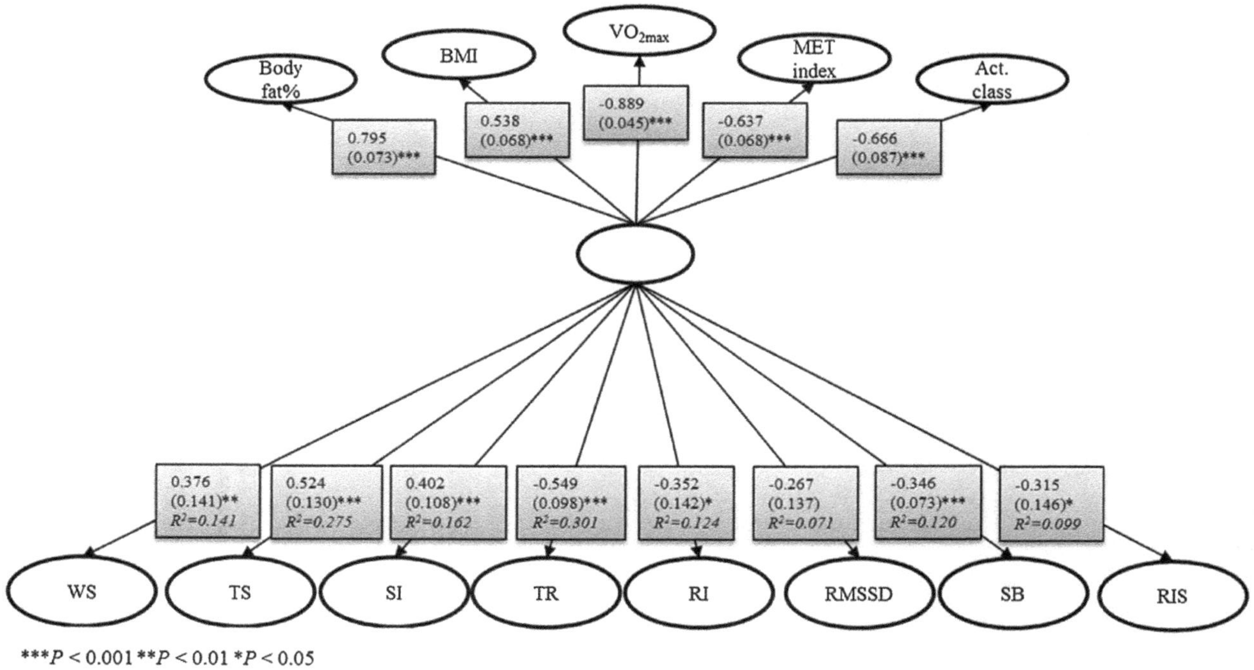

Figure 1 The variance of stress and recovery accounted for by physical activity, cardiorespiratory fitness, and body composition. The factor loadings (standardized estimate and S.E.) of body fat%, BMI, VO_{2max}, MET index, activity class, and the factor loadings (including R^2) for Firstbeat variables: work stress (WS), total stress (TS), stress index (SI), total recovery (TR), recovery index 24 h (RI), RMSSD, stress balance (SB), and recovery index sleep (RIS).

Table 4 Stress and recovery in relation to the Bergen Burnout Inventory total scores

	β	S.E.	*P*
Work stress	0.272	0.091	0.003
Total stress	0.304	0.095	0.001
Stress index	−0.080	0.118	0.500
Total recovery	−0.170	0.092	0.065
Recovery index (24 h)	−0.036	0.109	0.741
RMSSD	−0.009	0.101	0.925
Stress balance	−0.006	0.092	0.947
Recovery index (sleep)	−0.014	0.112	0.898

Standardized estimate (β), standard error (S.E.) and *P*-value.

was based on HR and HRV, which are affected by the ANS. Stressful situations result in accentuated sympatho-vagal antagonism, which may be explained by the interaction of acetylcholine and norepinephrine; consequently, HR may become remarkably unstable [62]. The findings of Tulppo et al. [62] suggest that traditional measures of HRV are not specific for measurement of accentuated sympatho-vagal interaction. The Firstbeat Analysis Server program connects information from these traditional measures of HRV, HR, and respiratory variables in the determination of stress and recovery states from individual HR and HRV values, but it does not separate eustress from distress.

Conclusions

This study used special HR- and HRV-based indicators of stress and recovery and found that PA, CRF, and body composition were associated with these indicators on workdays. On one hand, detailed interview-based MET index and self-reported activity class, and on the other hand, body fat percentage and BMI, associated rather similarly with the indicators of stress and recovery. This suggests that easily collected self-reported activity class and BMI can be used as indicators of PA and body composition in clinical work. The current findings support the usability of the objective indicators of stress (work stress and total stress) as they were associated with self-reported occupational burnout symptoms. Overall, the results support the usability of this HRV-based method in the evaluation of stress and recovery in line with some previous findings supporting its validity and reliability [25,63].

Competing interests

Rusko H. is a stockowner in Firstbeat Technologies Ltd. He did not contribute to writing the conclusions of the study. The other authors declare that they have no competing interests.

Authors' contributions

Study conception and design: TT, SM, AT, MR, JK, MK, UK. Acquisition of data: TT, SM, MR, TL, UK. Analysis and interpretation of data: TT, SM, AT, MR, TL, JK, MK, HR, UK. Statistical analysis: TT, AT. Drafting the manuscript: TT. Critical revision of the manuscript for important intellectual content: TT, SM, AT, MR, TL, JK, MK, HR, UK. Final approval of the version to be published: TT, SM, AT, MR, TL, JK, MK, HR, UK. Obtained funding: TT, JK, MK, UK. Administrative, technical, or material support: MK, UK.

Acknowledgements

The Body & Future Health study was supported by the SalWe Research Program for Mind and Body (Tekes - the Finnish Funding Agency for Technology and Innovation grant 1104/10). The FitFatTwin study was supported by the Finnish Ministry of Education and Culture. Kaprio J. and the Finnish twin studies have been supported by the Academy of Finland (grants # 265240, 263278, 264146). T. Teisala's work was supported by a personal grant from the Juho Vainio Foundation

Author details

[1]Department of Health Sciences, University of Jyväskylä, P.O. Box 35, Jyväskylä FIN-40014, Finland. [2]Methodology Centre for Human Sciences, Faculty of Social Sciences, University of Jyväskylä, P.O. Box 35 (Y 33), Jyväskylä FI-40014, Finland. [3]Turku PET Centre, University of Turku, Kiinamyllynkatu 4-8, Turku FIN-20520, Finland. [4]Hjelt Institute, Department of Public Health, University of Helsinki, P.O. Box 41, Helsinki FI-00014, Finland. [5]Institute of Public Health and Clinical Nutrition, Clinical Nutrition, University of Eastern Finland, Kuopio Campus, P.O. Box 1627, Joensuu FIN-70211, Finland. [6]Department of Biology of Physical Activity, University of Jyväskylä, P.O. Box 35, Jyväskylä FIN-40014, Finland. [7]Department of Mental Health and Substance Abuse Services, National Institute for Health and Welfare, P.O. Box 30, Helsinki FI-00300, Finland. [8]Institute for Molecular Medicine (FIMM), University of Helsinki, P.O. Box 20, Helsinki FI-00014, Finland.

References

1. Gerber M, Pühse U: **Do exercise and fitness protect against stress-induced health complaints? A review of the literature.** *Scand J Public Health* 2009, **37**(Suppl 8):801–819.
2. Forcier K, Stroud LR, Papandonatos GD, Hitsman B, Reiches M, Krishnamoorthy J, Niaura R: **Links between physical fitness and cardiovascular reactivity and recovery to psychological stressors: a meta-analysis.** *Health Psychol* 2006, **25**(Suppl 6):723–739.
3. Tulppo MP, Hautala AJ, Mäkikallio TH, Laukkanen RT, Nissilä S, Hughson RL, Huikuri HV: **Effects of aerobic training on heart rate dynamics in sedentary subjects.** *J Appl Physiol* 2003, **95**(Suppl 1):364–372.
4. Sothmann MS, Buckworth J, Claytor RP, Cox RH, White-Welkley JE, Dishman RK: **Exercise training and the cross-stressor adaptation hypothesis.** *Exerc Sport Sci Rev* 1996, **24**(Suppl 1):267–288.
5. Dishman RK, Nakamura Y, Garcia ME, Thompson RW, Dunn AL, Blair SN: **Heart rate variability, trait anxiety, and perceived stress among physically fit men and women.** *Int J Psychophysiol* 2000, **37**(Suppl 2):121–133.
6. Reed MJ, Robertson CE, Addison PS: **Heart rate variability measurements and the prediction of ventricular arrhythmias.** *QJM* 2005, **98**(Suppl 2):87–95.
7. McMillan DE: **Interpreting heart rate variability sleep/wake patterns in cardiac patients.** *J Cardiovasc Nurs* 2002, **17**(Suppl 1):69–81.
8. Acharya UR, Joseph KP, Kannathal N, Lim CM, Suri JS: **Heart rate variability: a review.** *Med Bio Eng Comput* 2006, **44**:1031–1051.
9. Task Force of the European Society of Cardiology and the North American Society of Pacing and Electrophysiology: **Heart rate variability: standards of measurement, physiological interpretation and clinical use.** *Circulation* 1996, **93**(Suppl 5):1043–1065.
10. Malliani A, Pagani M, Lombardi F, Gerutti S: **Cardiovascular neural regulation explored in the frequency domain.** *Circulation* 1991, **84**(Suppl 2):482–492.
11. Vanderlei LCM, Pastre CM, Hoshi RA, Carvalho TD, Godoy MF: **Basic notions of heart rate variability and its clinical applicability.** *Rev Bras Cir Cardiovasc* 2009, **24**(Suppl 2):205–217.
12. Pumprla J, Howorka K, Groves D, Chester M, Nolan J: **Functional assessment of heart rate variability: physiological basis and practical applications.** *Int J Cardiol* 2002, **84**(Suppl 1):1–14.
13. Chandola T, Heraclides A, Kumari M: **Psychophysiological biomarkers of workplace stressors.** *Neurosci Biobehav Rev* 2010, **35**(Suppl 1):51–57.
14. Pichot V, Roche F, Denis C, Garet M, Duverney D, Costes F, Barthélémy J-C: **Interval training in elderly men increases both heart rate variability and baroreflex activity.** *Clin Auton Res* 2005, **15**(Suppl 2):107–115.

15. Jurca R, Church TS, Morss GM, Jordan AN, Earnest CP: **Eight weeks of moderate-intensity exercise training increases heart rate variability in sedentary postmenopausal women.** *Am Heart J* 2004, **147**(Suppl 5):8–15.
16. Pober DM, Braun B, Freedson PS: **Effects of a single bout of exercise on resting heart rate variability.** *Med Sci Sports Exerc* 2004, **36**(Suppl 7):1140–1148.
17. Rennie KL, Hemingway H, Kumari M, Brunner E, Malik M, Marmot M: **Effects of moderate and vigorous physical activity on heart rate variability in a British study of civil servants.** *Am J Epidemiol* 2003, **158**(Suppl 2):135–143.
18. Buchheit M, Gindre C: **Cardiac parasympathetic regulation: respective associations with cardiorespiratory fitness and training load.** *Am J Physiol Heart Circ Physiol* 2006, **291**:451–458.
19. Gao YY, Lovejoy JC, Sparti A, Bray GA, Keys LK, Partington C: **Autonomic activity assessed by heart rate spectral analysis varies with fat distribution in obese women.** *Obes Res* 2012, **4**(Suppl 1):55–63.
20. Jeong AK, Yong-Gyu P, Kyung-Hwan C, Myung-Ho H, Hee-Chul H, Youn-Seon C, Dokyung Y: **Heart rate variability and obesity indices: emphasis on the response to noise and standing.** *J Am Board Fam Pract* 2005, **18**(Suppl 2):97–103.
21. Zahorska-Markiewicz B, Kuagowska E, Kucio C, Klin M: **Heart rate variability in obesity.** *Int J Obes* 1993, **17**(Suppl 1):21–23.
22. Rissanen P, Franssila-Kallunki A, Rissanen A: **Cardiac parasympathetic activity is increased by weight loss in healthy obese women.** *Obes Res* 2001, **9**(Suppl 10):637–643.
23. Martinmäki K, Rusko H, Kooistra L, Kettunen J, Saalasti S: **Intraindividual validation of heart rate variability indexes to measure vagal effects on hearts.** *Am J Physiol Heart Circ Physiol* 2006, **290**:640–647.
24. **Firstbeat Technologies Ltd.** www.firstbeat.com.
25. Uusitalo A, Mets T, Martinmäki K, Mauno S, Kinnunen U, Rusko H: **Heart rate variability related to effort at work.** *Appl Ergonomics* 2011, **42**(Suppl 6):830–838.
26. **International standard randomized controlled trial number register.** www.controlled-trials.com/ISRCTN92130721/kujala.
27. Saalasti S: **Neural networks for heart rate time series analysis.** In *PhD Thesis.* Finland, Jyväskylä Studies in Computing 33, Jyväskylä: Department of Mathematical Information Technology; University of Jyväskylä; 2003.
28. Kettunen J, Saalasti S, inventors; Firstbeat Technologies Ltd, assignee: *Procedure for Deriving Reliable Information on Respiratory Activity from Heart Period Measurement.*: United States patent US 20050209521A1; 2005.
29. Kettunen J, Saalasti S, inventors; Firstbeat Technologies Ltd, assignee: *Procedure for Detection of Stress by Segmentation and Analyzing Heart Beat Signal*: United States patent US 007330752B2; 2008.
30. **White papers.** http://www.firstbeat.com/physiology/white-papers.
31. Achten J, Jeukendrup AE: **Heart rate monitoring.** *Sports Med* 2003, **33**(Suppl 7):517–538.
32. Salmela-Aro K, Näätänen P, Nurmi J-E: **The role of work-related personal projects during two burnout interventions: a longitudinal study.** *Work Stress* 2004, **18**(Suppl 3):208–230.
33. Näätänen P, Aro A, Matthiesen S, Salmela-Aro K: *Bergen Burnout Indicator 15.* Helsinki: Edita; 2003.
34. Waller K, Kaprio J, Kujala UM: **Associations between long-term physical activity, waist circumference and weight gain: a 30-year longitudinal twin study.** *Int J Obes* 2007, **32**(Suppl 2):353–361.
35. Lakka TA, Salonen JT, The physical activity questionnaires of the Kuopio Ischemic Heart Disease Study (KIHD): **A collection of physical activity questionnaires for health related research.** *Med Sci Sports Exerc* 1997, **29:**46–58.
36. Ross RM, Jackson AS: *Exercise Concepts, Calculations, and Computer Applications.* Carmel, Indiana: Benchmark press; 1990.
37. **EPOC based training effect assessment.** www.firstbeat.fi/userData/firstbeat/download/white_paper_training_effect.pdf.
38. Andersen KL, Shephard RJ, Denolin H, Varnauskas E, Masironi R: *Fundamentals of Exercise Testing.* Geneva: World Health Organization; 1971.
39. Muthén LK, Muthén BO: *Mplus User's Guide.* 7th edition. Los Angeles: CA: Muthén & Muthén; 1998–2012.
40. Hu LT, Bentler PM: **Cutoff criteria for fit indexes in covariance structure analysis: conventional criteria versus new alternatives.** *Struct Equation Modeling* 1999, **6**(Suppl 1):1–55.
41. Jonsdottir IH, Rödjer L, Hadzibajramovic E, Börjesson M, Ahlborg G: **A prospective study of leisure-time physical activity and mental health in Swedish health care workers and social insurance officers.** *Prev Med* 2010, **51**(Suppl 5):373–377.
42. Holtermann A, Mortensen OS, Burr H, Søgaard K, Gyntelberg F, Suadicani P: **Physical fitness and perceived psychological pressure at work: 30-year ischemic heart disease and all-cause mortality in the copenhagen male study.** *J Occup Env Med* 2011, **53**(Suppl 7):743–750.
43. Anshel MH: **Effect of chronic aerobic exercise and progressive relaxation on motor performance and affect following acute stress.** *Behav Med* 1996, **21**(Suppl 4):186–196.
44. van Doornen LJ, de Geus EJ: **Aerobic fitness and the cardiovascular response to stress.** *Psychophysiol* 1989, **26**(Suppl 1):17–28.
45. Kitaoka-Higashiguchi K, Morikawa Y, Miura K, Sakurai M, Ishizaki M, Kido T, Naruse Y, Nakagawa H: **Burnout and risk factors for arteriosclerotic disease: follow-up study.** *J Occup Health* 2009, **51**(Suppl 2):123–131.
46. Nyberg ST, Heikkilä K, Fransson EI, Alfredsson L, De Bacquer D, Bjorner JB, Bonenfant S, Borritz M, Burr H, Casini A, Clays E, Dragano N, Erbel R, Geuskens GA, Goldberg M, Hooftman WE, Houtman IL, Jöckel KH, Kittel F, Knutsson A, Koskenvuo M, Leineweber C, Lunau T, Madsen IEH, Magnusson Hanson LL, Marmot MG, Nielsen ML, Nordin M, Oksanen T, Pentti J, *et al*: **Job strain in relation to body mass index: pooled analysis of 160 000 adults from 13 cohort studies.** *J Intern Med* 2012, **272:**65–73.
47. Block JP, He Y, Zaslavsky AM, Ding L: **Psychosocial stress and change in weight among US adults.** *Am J Epidemiol* 2009, **170**(Suppl 2):181–192.
48. Brunner EJ, Chandola T, Marmot MG: **Prospective effect of job strain on general and central obesity in the Whitehall II Study.** *Am J Epidemiol* 2007, **165**(Suppl 7):828–837.
49. Hannerz H, Albertsen K, Nielsen ML, Tüchsen F, Burr H: **Occupational factors and 5-year weight change among men in a danish national cohort.** *Health Psychol* 2004, **23**(Suppl 3):283–288.
50. Armon G, Shirom A, Berliner S, Shapira I, Melamed S: **A prospective study of the association between obesity and burnout among apparently healthy men and women.** *J Occup Health Psychol* 2008, **13**(1):43–57.
51. Ostry AS, Radi S, Louie AM, LaMontagne AD: **Psychosocial and other working conditions in relation to body mass index in a representative sample of Australian workers.** *BMC Public Health* 2006, **6**(Suppl 1):53–61.
52. Overgaard D, Gyntelberg F, Heitmann BL: **Psychological workload and body weight: is there an association? A review of the literature.** *Occup Med* 2004, **54**(Suppl 1):35–41.
53. Niedhammer I, Goldberg M, Leclerc A, David S, Bugel I, Landre M-F: **Psychosocial work environment and cardiovascular risk factors in an occupational cohort in France.** *J Epidemiol Community Health* 1998, **52**(Suppl 2):93–100.
54. Driver HS, Taylor SR: **Exercise and sleep.** *Sleep Med Rev* 2000, **4**(Suppl 4):387–402.
55. Seiler S, Haugen O, Kuffel E: **Autonomic recovery after exercise in trained athletes: intensity and duration effects.** *Med Sci Sports Exerc* 2007, **39** (Suppl 8):1366–1373.
56. Kaikkonen P, Rusko H, Martinmäki K: **Post-exercise heart rate variability of endurance athletes after different high-intensity exercise interventions.** *Scand J Med Sci Sports* 2008, **18**(Suppl 4):511–519.
57. Myllymäki T, Kyröläinen H, Savolainen K, Hokka L, Jakonen R, Juuti T, Martinmäki K, Kaartinen J, Kinnunen M-L, Rusko H: **Effects of vigorous late-night exercise on sleep quality and cardiac autonomic activity.** *J Sleep Res* 2011, **20:**146–53.
58. Mischler I, Vermorel M, Montaurier C, Mounier R, Pialoux V, Péquignot J-M, Cottet-Emard J-M, Coudert J, Fellmann N: **Prolonged daytime exercise repeated over 4 days increases sleeping heart rate and metabolic rate.** *Can J Appl Physiol* 2003, **28**(Suppl 4):616–629.
59. Hynynen E, Vesterinen V, Rusko H, Nummela A: **Effects of moderate and heavy endurance exercise on nocturnal HRV.** *Int J Sports Med* 2010, **31** (Suppl 6):428–432.
60. Grassi G, Dell'Oro R, Facchini A, Trevano FQ, Bolla GB, Mancia G: **Effect of central and peripheral body fat distribution on sympathetic and baroreflex function in obese normotensives.** *J Hypertens* 2004, **22**(Suppl 12):2363–2369.
61. Hamer M: **Psychosocial stress and cardiovascular disease risk: the role of physical activity.** *Psychosom Med* 2012, **74**(Suppl 9):896–903.
62. Tulppo MP, Mäkikallio TH, Seppänen T, Airaksinen JK, Huikuri HV: **Heart rate dynamics during accentuated sympathovagal interaction.** *AJP* 1998, **274**(Suppl 3):H810–H816.
63. Hynynen E, Konttinen N, Kinnunen U, Kyröläinen H, Rusko H: **The incidence of stress symptoms and heart rate variability during sleep and orthostatic test.** *Eup J Appl Physiol* 2011, **111**(Suppl 5):733–741.

Cotton dust exposure and self-reported respiratory symptoms among textile factory workers in Northwest Ethiopia

Sintayehu Daba Wami*, Daniel Haile Chercos, Awrajaw Dessie, Zemichael Gizaw, Atalay Getachew, Tesfaye Hambisa, Tadese Guadu, Dawit Getachew and Bikes Destaw

Abstract

Background: Cotton dust induced respiratory disorders are dramatically increased over the globe, especially the problem is serious in developing countries. Respiratory symptoms, such as cough, phlegm, wheezing, shortness of breath, chest tightness, chronic bronchitis, and byssinosis are common among workers exposed to cotton dust. However, in Ethiopia, the magnitude of the problem is not well known and information is limited about the risk factors. Therefore, this study was aimed to assess the prevalence of respiratory symptoms and associated factors.

Methods: A Comparative cross-sectional study design was employed. A total of 413 (276 exposed and 137 unexposed) participants were included in the study. Stratified and simple random sampling techniques were used to select exposed and unexposed groups to cotton dust respectively. Multivariable binary logistic regression analyses was performed to identify variables associated with respiratory symptoms and adjusted odds ratio (AOR) was used to determine the strength of associations. Significance level was obtained at 95% confidence interval (CI) and p-value ≤0.05.

Results: The prevalence of self-reported respiratory symptoms was 47.8% (95% CI: 41.3, 53.7%) and 15.3% (95% CI: 9.6, 22.3%) among exposed and control groups respectively. Sex (AOR = 2.1, 95% CI: 1.29, 3.45), service year (AOR = 2.38, 95% CI: 1.19, 4.71) and ventilation (AOR = 2.4, 95% CI: 1.17, 4.91) were factors significantly associated with respiratory symptoms. Furthermore, working department such as; ginning (AOR = 5.1, 95% CI: 2.13, 12.16), spinning (AOR = 4.96, 95% CI: 2.18, 11.29), weaving (AOR = 5.9, 95% CI: 2.46, 14.27) and blowing working departments (AOR = 5.14, 95% CI: 1.4, 18.94) were significantly associated with respiratory disorders.

Conclusions: The prevalence of self-reported respiratory symptoms was higher among workers exposed to cotton dust than unexposed workers. Sex, service year, working department and work unit ventilation were predictor variables for respiratory symptoms. Thus, reducing exposure to dust, adequate ventilation and improving the hygiene of working departments are needed to reduce respiratory symptoms.

Keywords: Respiratory symptoms, Cotton dust, Textile factory workers, Northwest Ethiopia

* Correspondence: sintayehudaba2004@gmail.com
Department of Environmental and Occupational Health and Safety, Institute of Public Health, University of Gondar, Gondar, Ethiopia

Background

Occupational respiratory diseases are a major global public health problem that account for up to 30% of all registered work related diseases and 10–20% of deaths are caused by respiratory problems [1]. Owing to an exposure to occupational airborne particulates, an estimated 386, 000 deaths and nearly 6.6 million disability adjusted life years (DALYs) occurred among workers [2]. With respect to cotton dust exposure, chest tightness was the most common respiratory symptom (20.3%). About 14.2% of cotton processing workers were encountering byssinosis [3].

The ginning, spinning and weaving process of textile industry generate large amount of cotton dust. The dust consists of different size and type of particles, such as ground-up plant matter, fiber, bacteria, fungi, soil, pesticides, non-cotton matter, and other contaminants [4, 5]. Exposure to the cotton dust led to respiratory problems, such as cough, phlegm, wheezing, shortness of breath, chest tightness, chronic bronchitis, and byssinosis [6–8]. Exposure to cotton dust has also profound effect on pulmonary function [8]. Byssinosis is a chronic respiratory disease that is seen among workers exposed to cotton dust [9, 10]. The type and concentration of dust, duration of exposure and genetic factors are interplaying the diseases of the respiratory system induced by occupational dusts [11, 12]. Moreover, working in the department where there is higher exposure of cotton dust such as spinning and weaving and being aged were found to be the risk factors for respiratory problems related to cotton dust [10].

Respiratory problems related to coton dust start to decline in developed countries as a result of stringent measures taken by the employers and workers. However, the problems are quite neglected in developing countries [13, 14] and there is lack of health information.

Textile industry is one of the major manufacturing industry, which is established across the developed and developing countries including Africa [15]. In developing countries, notably in Africa, the cotton industry occupies an important place. The cotton sector is expanding considering the size of cotton production and the number of people employed in this sector [10]. In Ethiopia, textile industry or cotton sector is the main economic motor that attracts numerous work forces [16]. However, the workers are at risk of cotton dust related respiratory problems. But the degree of the problem is not well known and there is a scarcity of data showing these kinds of health issues and its risk factors in Ethiopia.

Therefore, this study was conducted to assess cotton dust exposure, self-reported respiratory symptoms and associated factors among textile factory workers.

Methods

Study design and study population

A Comparative cross-sectional study design was employed in northwest Ethiopia textile factory.

The source population of this study was all workers in northwest Ethiopia textile factories and those who were worked in ginning, spinning, weaving and blowing departments. Those workers who worked for more than 1 year were included in the study. However, workers with previous exposure to other occupational dust such as silica, coal dust and who have history of smoking were excluded. Moreover, workers who had history of asthma or chronic obstructive pulmonary disease (COPD) before joining to the work were also excluded from this study.

Regarding the activities carried out in working unit, Ginning section involves the process of separating of the cotton fibers from the seed for the conversion of the cotton into a continuous thread. Cotton ginning consists simple operations, which was done mechanically. During the ginning process, dust fibers and lint are generated which can be inhaled by workers.

Blowing section is the initial stage in spinning process. Blow department is consisting of different machines in which the supplied compressed bales are opened, cleaned, dust removed, mixing or blending performed for making uniform lap of definite length. It is sued in succession to open and clean the cotton fiber according to the required amount of degree.

The Spinning department uses machines in order to produce cotton into threads of required size from the locks of cotton.

The Weaving department comprises different activities such as winding, warping, gluing and weaving. Then, cloth is obtained from the chain threads placed vertically and the weft threads placed horizontally. Cloths are afterwards stocked in the warehouse.

The source population for unexposed group were both the general administration staff members of the textile factories and external workers in the informal sectors located in the surroundings (estimated to be 200–500 meter far from technical department of textile factory) having at least 1 year of job activities. Those who have history of smoking, asthma or COPD were excluded from unexposed group.

Sample size determination

The sample size was determined using double population proportion formula using EpiInfo software considering the following assumptions: proportion of respiratory symptoms among exposed group (36.9%) [10], proportion of respiratory symptoms among unexposed group (21.2%) [10], 95% confidence interval, 80% power, margin of error (5%), 2:1 ratio of exposed to unexposed groups. A total of 413 study participants, 276 exposed and 137 unexposed groups were included in this study.

Sampling procedures

Study subjects from the exposed groups were selected using stratified sampling technique, assuming that workers in different departments would exhibit different level of exposure to cotton dust. Study subjects were allocated to each stratum proportionally and selected by simple random sampling. Whereas, the unexposed groups were selected by simple random sampling technique using their salary payment roaster sheet, which was obtained from their respective offices.

Measurment of variables

Respiratory symptoms, the primary outcome variable of the study was determined by the presence of one or more respiratory symptoms such as, cough, phlegm, wheezing, dyspnea, chest pain and breathlessness among workers.

Ventilation condition, the ventilation condition of the working units was reported as adequate if the working unit furnished with functional mechanical ventilation system (ventilator, Local exhaust ventilation system) and natural ventilation systems (doors, windows and any other openings). Lack of obstruction of air flow in the unit also considered and if the data collector senses sufficient air circulation in the working unit; fair if there is functional mechanical ventilation system and natural systems, but obstructed air flow due to poor design of the working units; and inadequate if the unit lacks functional mechanical and natural ventilation system, and if the air flow obstructed by adjacent buildings and poor layout of the unit.

Data collection procedures

The data were collected by using a modified questionnaire of medical research council (MRC) of Great Britain and work place observation checklists. The questionnaire consisted of three parts, like socio-demographic, environmental and behavioral factors, and respiratory symptoms. Face-to-face interview and observation of the working units were performed to collect data. Prior to the data collection, training was given for data collectors and supervisors for 3 days on procedures, techniques and ways of collecting the data. Clear introduction explaining the purpose and objective of the study was provided to the respondents on the first page of the questionnaire before data collection. In addition continuous and strict supervision and on spot checking was carried out during the data collection process.

Data processing and analysis

The data were checked, coded and entered in to epidemiological information package (EPi-info) version 7. 2.0.1 and exported to statistical package for social sciences (SPSS) version 20 for further analysis. For most variables, data were presented as frequencies and percentages. Univariate logistic regression analysis was performed primarily to select variables for the final model on the basis of p-value < 0.2. Multivariable binary logistic regressions analysis was employed to control the possible effect of confounders and finally the variables which had significant association were identified on the basis of AOR with 95% CI and p-value ≤ 0.05.

Results

Demographic and socio-economic characteristics of the study participants

Of the total 413 questionnaires (276 exposed and 137 unexposed) distributed, 401 (270 exposed and 131 unexposed) completed and valid questionnaires were analyzed, which gives a response rate of 97.1%.

Two third, 169 (62.6%) of exposed and half, 66 (50.4%) of unexposed participants were males. The mean age (± SD) of the respondents among exposed and unexposed was 28.24 (± 7.58) and 29.79 years (± 7.4) respectively (Table 1).

Table 1 Demographic and socio-economic characteristics of textile factory workers, northwest Ethiopia, 2017 ($N = 413$)

Variables	Exposed frequency (%)	Unexposed frequency (%)
Sex		
Female	101 (37.4%)	65 (49.6%)
Male	169 (62.6%)	66 (50.4%)
Age(years)		
≤ 29	199 (73.7%)	74 (56.5%)
30–39	43 (15.9%)	42 (32.1%)
≥ 40	28 (10.4%)	15 (11.5%)
Mean ± SD	28.24 ± 7.58	29.79 ± 7.4
Marital status		
Single	158 (58.5%)	54 (41.2%)
Married	109 (40.4%)	76 (58%)
Divorced/Widowed	3 (1.1%)	1 (0.8%)
Years of service in current industry (years)		
1–2	56 (20.7%)	14 (10.7%)
2–5	118 (43.7%)	83 (63.4%)
≥ 6	96 (35.6%)	34 (26.0%)
Monthly salary		
≤ 1500	163 (60.4%)	37 (28.2%)
1501–2500	87 (32.2%)	46 (35.1%)
≥ 2501	20 (7.4%)	48 (36.6%)

Workplace condition

The overall conditions of employees and the working environment were observed to see workers exposure to cotton dust. Accordingly, poor indoor air quality at working environment was observed. Working environments were characterized with excessive dust and there was no a documented functioning housekeeping program. Moreover, most of the data collectors were experienced sudden sneezing upon entering the working unit in the textile industries and it was observed that worker's eye brows, hair, nostrils and cloths were covered with dust particle.

Although, natural ventilation systems (doors, windows and other opening) were present, the air flow in different working units was obstructed due to poor design and layout of the working units. The working units lacked functional mechanical ventilation system. In addition, working units were poorly illuminated. We observed that all the working units had no warning signs and safety instruction procedures. Safety procedures were not posted indicating whether employees cotton dust exposure is kept at the accepted levels. None of the plants practiced wet mopping to minimize cotton dust exposure. We also found that all of the workers did not use respirator, face shields, and other PPE to minimize cotton dust exposure.

Respiratory symptoms

This study revealed that the prevalence of self-reported cotton dust induced respiratory symptoms were 47.8% (95% CI: 41.3, 53.7%) among exposed and 15.3% (95% CI: 9.6, 22.3%) among unexposed groups. Cough (28.1%), phlegm (19.6%), chest tightness (30%) and dyspnea (21.11%) were the commonest respiratory symptoms reported by the exposed groups. Significanct differences of respiratory symptoms were observed between exposed and unexposed participants and there were more signs of respiratory tract irritations among exposed workers than the unexposed participants (*P*-value ≤0.05) (Table 2).

Association of cotton dust exposure with respiratory symptoms

High prevalence of respiratory symptoms was reported among exposed participants than unexposed to cotton dust (*P*-value ≤0.001). Twenty (15.3%) of unexposed workers and 129 (47.8%) workers exposed to cotton dust experienced one or more respiratory symptoms.

Table 2 Prevalence of respiratory symptoms among textile factory workers, northwest Ethiopia, 2017 ($N = 413$)

Respiratory symptoms	Exposed *n* (%)	Unexposed *n* (%)	*P*-value
Cough	76 (28.1%)	13 (9.9%)	≤ 0.001
Phlegm	53 (19.6%)	4 (3.1%)	≤ 0.001
Chest tightness	81 (30%)	11 (8.4%)	≤ 0.001
Dyspnea	57 (27.1%)	6 (4.6%)	≤ 0.001

Factors associated with respiratory symptoms

In the bivariate binary logistic regression sex, monthly salary, ventilation of the working unit, working departments and PPE use had *p*-value < 0.2. However, only sex, service year and ventilation of the working units had statistically significant association with respiratory symptoms in the multivariable binary logistic regression analysis (Table 3).

According to this study male respondents had 2.1 times higher odds of developing respiratory symptoms when compared to female participants (AOR = 2.1, 95% CI: 1.29, 3.45). Employees with two to 5 years of service year had 2.38 times higher odds of having respiratory symptoms than employees with less than 2 years of work experience (AOR = 2.38, 95% CI: 1.19, 4.71).

Moreover, working department was significantly associated with respiratory symptoms. The prevalence of respiratory symptoms was higher in ginning (50%), blowing (50%), weaving (48.8%) and spinning departments (44.4%). Respondents in ginning and spinning working departments had 5.1 and 4.96 times higher odds of developing respiratory symptoms respectively than workers in administrative units and other sectors (AOR = 5.1, 95% CI: 2.13, 12.16, and AOR = 4.96, 95% CI: 2.18, 11.29). Furthermore, workers in weaving and blowing working departments had 5.9 and 5.14 times higher odds of having respiratory symptoms respectively compared to workers in administrative units and other sectors (AOR = 5.9, 95% CI: 2.46, 14.27, and AOR = 5.14, 95% CI: 1.4, 18.94).

Workers in inadequatly ventilated working units had 2.4 times higher odds of developing respiratory symptoms compared to their counter parts (AOR = 2.4, 95% CI: 1.17, 4.91).

Discussion

In the current study, the prevalence of self reported respiratory symptoms was higher among participants exposed to cotton dust (47.8%) than unexposed respondents (15.3%). The result of this study is in line with the reports of other similar studies outside Africa, like India [17], Pakistan [18] and China [19]. This might be due to the fact that exposure to dust from cotton during weaving, spinning, ginning and packaging are higher among textile workers. Hence, occupational exposure to cotton dust has been linked with respiratory disorders.

According to this study, male respondents had higher odds of developing respiratory symptoms. This finding is supported by study done in Shanghai and Lancashire cotton industries indicating that male textile workers are

Table 3 Multi variable analysis of factors associated with Factors associated with respiratory symptoms among textile factory workers, northwest Ethiopia, 2017 ($N = 413$)

Variables	Respiratory symptoms		COR (95% CI)	AOR (95% CI)
	No	Yes		
Sex				
Female	123	43	1.00	1.00
Male	129	106	2.35 (1.53, 3.62)	2.1 (1.29, 3.45)*
Age(years)				
≤ 29	170	103	1.00	1.00
30–39	56	29	0.86 (0.51, 1.43)	1.6 (0.81, 3.14)
≥ 40	26	17	1.1 (0.56, 2.1)	1.63 (0.67, 3.98)
Marital status				
Single	124	88	1.00	1.00
Married	125	60	0.68 (0.45, 1.02)	0.8 (0.48, 1.39)
Divorced/Widowed	3	1	0.47 (0.05, 4.6)	0.45 (0.04, 5.18)
Educational level				
Primary school	20	12	1.00	1.00
Secondary school	43	44	1.7 (0.74, 3.91)	1.66 (0.67, 4.1)
Diploma and above	189	93	0.82 (0.38, 1.75)	1.29 (0.51, 3.27)
Monthly salary				
≤ 1500	123	77	1.00	1.00
1501–2500	77	56	1.16 (0.74, 1.82)	1.3 (0.79, 2.26)
≥ 2501	52	16	0.49 (0.26, 0.92)	0.87 (0.38, 1.98)
Years of service in current industry (years)				
1–2	49	21	1.00	1.00
2–5	121	80	1.5 (0.86, 2.77)	2.38 (1.19, 4.71)*
≥6	82	48	1.4 (0.73, 2.55)	1.51 (0.68, 3.36)
Working department				
Ginning	41	41	5.5 (2.92, 10.56)	5.1 (2.13, 12.16)**
Spinning	50	40	4.4 (2.36, 8.35)	4.96 (2.18. 11.29)**
Weaving	43	41	5.3 (2. 8, 10.04)	5.9 (2.46, 14.27)**
Blowing	7	7	5.6 (1.76, 17.5)	5.14 (1.4, 18.94)*
Administration/informal sector	111	20	1.00	1.00
Ventilation of the working unit				
Adequate	58	16	1.00	1.00
Fair	127	70	1.99 (1.07, 3.74)	2.1 (1.07, 4.19)*
Inadequate	67	63	3.41 (1.78, 6.54)	2.4 (1.17, 4.91)*
PPE use				
No	148	61	1.00	1.00
Yes	104	88	2.05 (1.36, 3.1)	099 (0.59, 1.66)

Note: * = P-value ≤0.05, ** = p-value ≤0.001

at higher risk of having respiratory symptoms than female textile workers [20, 21]. The difference in respiratory symptoms might be explained due to the fact that male workers have longer service year in this study and have higher cumulative dust exposure. Other possible reason is, female workers are usually assigned in less hazardous department in cotton industries [20, 21]. However, this finding is contrary to studies done in Greek [22], Denmark [23] and China [24].

Employees who have longer service years had higher odds of having respiratory symptoms. This finding was similar with studies done in Egypt [25] and India [24, 26]. This result shows, the longer the duration of exposure to cotton dust the higher the presence of respiratory symptoms. This can be justified as more experienced workers had prolonged exposure to cotton dust in cotton industries they are at greatest risk for developing respiratory symptoms [22, 23].

Moreover, working department was significantly associated factor with respiratory symptoms. The prevalence of respiratory symptoms was higher in ginning, weaving, spinning and blowing departments. This finding is similar with studies done in Pakistan in 2015 [27] and in 2017 [28] and in Egypt [25]. This is due to the fact that worker in higher cotton dust exposure work environment such as blowing are more likely to develop respiratory symptoms than those workers with in administrative areas where there is less cotton dust exposure [18]. Furthermore, cotton dust is high in these working units because of the work nature and poor environmental conditions [29].

Ventilation of working units was statistically associated with respiratory symptoms. Higher odds of developing respiratory symptoms were observed among workers who worked in inadequately ventilated working units. This result is not surprising because textile industries release high level of dust in working environment [30, 31] and various studies indicated that lack of ventilation in cotton industry working environment as a major factor of developing respiratory symptoms among cotton industry workers [32]. Moreover, their effects have a tendency to be more pronounced in the case of poor ventilation [33].

Lack of the Pulmonary Function Test and measurement of cotton dust concentration to strengthen the self-reported symptoms were the limitations of this study. In addition, the possibility of healthy workers effect could not be ruled out. But through observation of overall conditions of employees and working environment, excluding workers with less than 1 year of work experience and by honestly explaining the objective and significances of the study we tried to minimize the effect.

Conclusion

The prevalence of self-reported respiratory symptoms were higher among participants exposed to cotton dust than unexposed respondents and there were more signs of respiratory tract irritations among workers exposed to to cotton dust. Sex, years of service, working department and work unit ventilation are risk factors for the presence of respiratory symptoms. Thus, reducing exposure to dusts, adequate ventilation and improving hygiene of the working department are needed to reduce respiratory problems.

Abbreviations

AOR: Adjusted odd ratio; CI: Confidence interval; COPD: Chronic obstructive pulmonary disease; DALYS: Disability-adjusted life years; ILO: International Labor Organization; IRB: Institutional review board; PPE: Personal protective equipment; SPSS: Statistical package for social sciences

Acknowledgements

We would like to thank University of Gondar, College of Medicine and Health Sciences for providing ethical clearance for this study. We also like to express our gratitude to Northwest Ethiopia textile factories and our study participants.

Funding

There is no source of funding for this study.

Authors' contributions

SDW contributed to the study design, data collection, data analysis, interpretations of the results. DHC contributed in study design, data analysis and manuscript preparation. AD contributed to the study design, data analysis, and manuscript write-up and review. ZG, BD and TG contributed in study design and review of the manuscript. AG, TH and DG contributed in interpretations of the result and manuscript review. All authors read and approved the final manuscript.

informed verbal consent from the manager and workers. The purpose of the study was explained and confidentiality of the information was assured.

Competing interests

The authors declare that they have no competing interests.

References

1. International labor organization (ILO). Action towards prevention of occupational non-communicable diseases. Geneva: International labor organization; 2011. Available from:http://www.worldpsi.org/sites/default/files/attachment/news/ilo_presenation.pdf. Accessed 20 Sept 2017.
2. Driscoll T, Nelson DI, Steenland K, Leigh J, Concha-Barrientos M, Fingerhut M, et al. The global burden of non-malignant respiratory disease due to occupational airborne exposures. Am J Ind Med. 2005;48(6):432–45.
3. Altin R, Ozkurt S, Fisekci F, Cimrin A, Zencir M, Sevinc C. Prevalence of byssinosis and respiratory symptoms among cotton mill workers. Respiration. 2002;69(1):52–6.
4. Rom W. Byssinosis and other diseases of textile workers. In: Ron WN, editor. Environmental and occupational medicine. Philadelphia: Lippincott-Raven; 1998.
5. Jacobs RR. Strategies for prevention of byssinosis. Am J Ind Med. 1987; 12(6):717–28.
6. Nagoda M, Okpapi J, Babashani M. Assessment of respiratory symptoms and lung function among textile workers at Kano textile Mills, Kano, Nigeria. Niger J Clin Pract. 2012;15(4):373–9.
7. Nafees AA, Fatmi Z, Kadir MM, Sathiakumar N. Pattern and predictors for respiratory illnesses and symptoms and lung function among textile workers in Karachi, Pakistan. Occup Environ Med. 2013;70(2):99–107.
8. Wang X, Zhang H, Sun B, Dai H, Hang J, Eisen E, et al. A 20-year follow-up study on chronic respiratory effects of exposure to cotton dust. Eur Respir J. 2005;26(5):881–6.
9. Parikh J. Byssinosis in developing countries. Br J Ind Med. 1992;49(4):217.
10. Hinson A, Schlünssen V, Agodokpessi G, Sigsgaards T, Fayomi B. The prevalence of byssinosis among cotton workers in the north of Benin. Int J Occup Environ Med. 2014;5(4):194–200.
11. Subbarao P, Mandhane PJ, Sears MR. Asthma: epidemiology, etiology and risk factors. Can Med Assoc J. 2009;181(9):E181–E90.
12. Meo SA, Al-Drees AM. Lung function among non-smoking wheat flour mill workers. Int J Occup Med Environ Health. 2005;18(3):259–64.
13. Sudha B, Meenaxi T. Occupational health hazards in textiles industry. Asian J Home Sci. 2014;9(1):267–71.
14. Haglind P, Lundholm M, Rylander R. Prevalence of byssinosis in Swedish cotton mills. Occup Environ Med. 1981;38(2):138–43.
15. Kim J-O, Traore M, Warfield C. The textile and apparel industry in developing countries. Text Prog. 2006;38(3):1–64.
16. Kumie A, Amera T, Berhane K, Samet J, Hundal N, Michael FG, et al. Occupational health and safety in Ethiopia: a review of situational analysis and needs assessment. Ethiop J Health Dev. 2016;30(1):17–27.
17. Singh MB, Fotedar R, Lakshminarayana J. Occupational morbidities and their association with nutrition and environmental factors among textile Workers of Desert Areas of Rajasthan, India. J Occup Health. 2005;47:371–7.
18. Saadia SAKA. Pulmonary function studies in Pakistani cotton ginners. Pak J Physiol. 2006;2(1):1-4.
19. Christiani D, Eisen E, Wegman D, Ye T, Lu P, Gong Z, et al. Respiratory disease in cotton textile workers in the People's Republic of China. I. Respiratory symptoms. Scand J Work Environ Health. 1986;12(1):40–5.
20. Lai PS, Hang JQ, Zhang FY, Lin X, Zheng BY, Dai HL, et al. Gender differences in the effect of occupational endotoxin exposure on impaired lung function and death: the shanghai textile worker study. Occup Environ Med. 2014;71(2):118–25. https://doi.org/10.1136/oemed-2013-101676.
21. Raza S, Fletcher A, Pickering C, Niven RM, Faragher E. Respiratory symptoms in Lancashire textile weavers. Occup Environ Med. 1999;56(8):514–9.
22. Saha A, Doctor PB, Bhagia LJ, Majumdar PK, Patel BD. A study of respiratory function among the workers engaged in ginning processes. Indian J Occup Environ Med. 2014;18(3):118.
23. Mansouri F, Pili JP, Abbasi A, Soltani M, Izadi N. Respiratory problems among cotton textile workers. Lung India. 2016;33(2):163.

24. Phakthongsuk P, Sangsupawanich P, Musigsan A, Thammakumpee G. Work-related respiratory symptoms among cotton-fabric sewing workers. Int J Occup Med Environ Health. 2007;20(1):17–24.
25. Tageldin MA, Gomaa AA, Hegazy EAM. Respiratory symptoms and pulmonary function among cotton textile workers at Misr company for spinning and weaving EL-Mahalla, Egypt. Egypt J Chest Dis Tuberc. 2017;66(2):369–76.
26. Kumar RS. Cotton dust-impact on human health and environment in the textile industry. Text Mag Madras. 2008;49(3):55.
27. Tanzil S, Nafees A. Low prevalence of asthma among textile workers in Karachi, Pakistan. J Pak Med Assoc. 2015;65(8):869–74.
28. Khan A, Moshammer H, Kundi M. Industrial hygiene, occupational safety and respiratory symptoms in the Pakistani cotton industry. BMJ Open. 2015; 5(4):e007266. http://dx.doi.org/10.1136/bmjopen-2014-007266.
29. Anyfantis ID, Rachiotis G, Hadjichristodoulou C, Gourgoulianis KI. Respiratory symptoms and lung function among Greek cotton industry workers: a cross-sectional study. Int J Occup Environ Med. 2017;8(1):32–8.
30. Kennedy SM, Christiani DC, Eisen EA, Wegman DH, Greaves IA, Olenchock SA, et al. Cotton dust and endotoxin exposure-response relationships in cotton textile workers 1–4. Am Rev Respir Dis. 1987;135(1):194–200.
31. Jannet J, Jeyanthi G. Pulmonary health status of ginning factory women laborers in Tirupur, India. Indian J Occup Environ Med. 2006;10(3):116.
32. Alemu K, Kumie A, Davey G. Byssinosis and other respiratory symptoms among factory workers in Akaki textile factory, Ethiopia. Ethiop J Health Dev. 2010;24(2):133-39. http://dx.doi.org/10.4314/ejhd.v24i2.62962.
33. Bentayeb M, Norback D, Bednarek M, Bernard A, Cai G, Cerrai S, et al. Indoor air quality, ventilation and respiratory health in elderly residents living in nursing homes in Europe. Eur Respir J. 2015;45(5):1228–38.

23

Heavy metals effect on breast cancer progression

A. Romaniuk[1], M. Lyndin[1], V. Sikora[1*], Y. Lyndina[2], S. Romaniuk[3] and K. Sikora[4]

Abstract

Background: Breast cancer is the most frequent localization of malignant process in American women and women of European countries. To date it is not possible to control the morbidity growth due to lack of effective ways of primary prevention. Comparing the incidence of breast cancer in developed countries with the countries of Asia and Africa, there is the fact of population predominance lesion in more urbanized countries. This suggests that the environment along with other factors, occupies a significant place in the initiation and progression of breast neoplasia. The impressive rates of industrial development led to the pollution of soil, surface water and, as a consequence, food by heavy metal salts.
The purposes of this paper are as follows: the chemical composition determination of neoplastic breast tissue, evaluation of the DNA methylation level, study of prognostic-important receptors expression in the breast cancer cells, establishing linkages between all the derived indicators.

Methods: In our study we used the following methods: studying of the chemical composition of breast cancer tissue by atomic absorption spectrophotometry and energy-dispersion spectrometer; immunohistochemical study of ER, PR, HER2/neu, p53, Ki-67, E-cadherin and MGMT receptors; DNA extraction and investigation by oscillating infrared spectroscopy method.

Results: The total amount of heavy metals in breast cancer tissue ranged from 51.21×10^{-3} to 84.86×10^{-3} μg/kg. We have got the following results: the growth of heavy metals in neoplastic tissue is accompanied with the increase of HER2/neu, p53, Ki-67, MGMT expression and decrease of ER and PR expression. The increment of pathological DNA methylation is accompanied with the increasing amount of heavy metals in tumor tissue.

Conclusions: Heavy metals through different pathogenetic links stimulate the progression of breast cancer and reduce its sensitivity to treatment. DNA of tumor tissue has a different level of methylation which changes with the amount of heavy metals in cancer cells. This is displayed on the synthesis of prognostically important receptors in neoplastic tissue.

Keywords: Breast cancer, Heavy metals, DNA methylation, Receptors

Background

Breast cancer (BC) is the most frequent localization of malignant process in American women and women of European countries [1]. In Ukraine, this pathology is found in 16,000 women each year (the incidence is 64.5 per 100,000 women) [2]. Nowadays it isn't possible to control the growth of morbidity due to lack of effective ways of primary prevention. Comparing the incidence of BC in developed countries with the countries of Asia and Africa, unfortunately, there is the fact of predominance lesion of population in more urbanized countries [3]. Thus, this suggests that the environment along with other factors, occupies a significant place in both the initiation and progression of breast neoplasia [4]. The impressive rates of industrial development led to the pollution of soil, surface water and, as a consequence, food by heavy metal salts.

During investigation of the environment in Ukraine it was found that the amount of iron, chromium, copper, nickel, lead and zinc salts in the ground were increased [5].

* Correspondence: v.sikora@med.sumdu.edu.ua
[1]Department of pathology, Sumy State University, st. Privokzalnaya, 31, Sumy Postal code 40022, Ukraine

It is known that the carcinogenic effect of heavy metals (HM) is realized through the mechanisms of DNA structure breach and suppression of antioxidant protection [6, 7]. Furthermore, there is information about the possibility of heavy metals influence on the expression of prognostic-important receptors in BC tissue [8, 9]. Previously, it was found that breast tissue (unaltered and affected by tumor process) can accumulate heavy metals that influence on the DNA fragmentation level and tumor cells survival [10].

It is generally known that the most important receptors in BC tissue are the estrogen receptor (ER), progesterone receptor (PR), human epidermal growth factor receptor 2 (HER2/neu), Ki-67 and p53. Moreover, ER and PR status of BC is recognized as one of the most powerful prognostic markers. If the tumor belongs to steroid-positive variant, it is managed and controlled by anti-estrogen drugs [11]. Contrary to this, the expression of HER2/neu indicates the tumor resistance to chemotherapy, including tamoxifen, aggressiveness of cancer [12]. The degree of differentiation and malignancy of BC is largely determined by proliferative activity of tumor cells. Study of Ki-67 protein that is expressed in all cells that came from G_0-phase allows to determine "hidden" proliferative potential of neoplasia and to evaluate its malignancy extent [13]. Pathological p53 presents in 18%-25% of BC cases. Functional inactivation of wild type (wt) p53 and synthesis of mutant type (mt) p53 are associated with early recurrences, poorer course and resistance to chemotherapy [14].

DNA methylation, the accession of methyl groups to the nitrogenous bases, is a modification of DNA without changing its nucleotide sequence [15]. "Silence" of tumor suppressor genes by DNA methylation is a powerful molecular mechanism by which DNA methylation can initiate cancer. It also substantiates therapy that aims to inhibit DNA methylation, and reactivation of blocked tumor suppressor genes [16]. It has been described a significant correlation between DNA methylation and expression of BC key genes such as MYC, TERT, TP63 and others [17]. However, hypomethylation is no less important because the critical genes of growth and metastasis are hypomethylated in cancer tissue [18].

O6-methyguanine-DNA methyltransferase (MGMT), with its gene being located on the chromosome 10, eliminates DNA damage by alkylating agents, removing their cytotoxic effect [19]. Afferent protein sequence is combined with damaged nucleic acid and without changing DNA structure takes alkyl residue [20]. Nevertheless, inactivated MGMT may enter into relationship with receptors for steroid hormones, inhibiting their function, thereby blocking the signal transmission for cell division [21]. There is information about inhibitory effect of heavy metal salts on MGMT activity. It has been shown that the expression of MGMT in tumor cells can be increased, demonstrating BC resistance against chemotherapy [22], and can be decreased (due to methylation of MGMT promoter), providing the possibility of "cancer" cells enter into apoptosis [23]. MGMT-positive status of the tissue is correlated with the identification of luminal molecular types of BC and low cell proliferative activity [24]. Considering this, it was proposed to examine the expression of MGMT as a separate prognostic factor of breast malignancy [23].

In summary we can say that nowadays the question remains open concerning the relationship between the tumor chemical composition, DNA methylation and expression of prognostic receptors of BC tissue.

The **objectives** of this paper are as follows: the chemical composition determination of neoplastic breast tissue, evaluation of the DNA methylation level, study of prognostic-important receptors expression in the BC cells, establishing linkages between all the derived indicators.

Methods

The tissue (40 samples of BC tissue and 20 samples of intact breast tissue) received during the postoperative biopsy was kept in the refrigerator. It became the subject of the further investigation after the establishing of the histological diagnosis. The diagnosis of invasive ductal carcinoma (IDC) with varying of malignancy degree (by Scarff-Bloom-Richardson) was found after the standard hematoxylin eosin staining of prepared slices.

Studying of the chemical composition of BC tissue

Tissue samples for atomic absorption spectrophotometry were weighed with an accuracy of 0.001 g. Then they were burned in a muffle furnace at a temperature 450 °C for removing the organic matrix. The resulting ash was dissolved in a mixture of hydrochloric (2 ml) and nitric (1 ml) acids. The resulting solution was analyzed by C115 – 01 spectrophotometer with flame and electrothermal atomiser. Each microelement (increased amount of which is inherent for the Ukraine) content was measured at a specific wavelength: Zn – 213.9 nm, Cu – 324.7 nm, Pb – 283.3 nm, Cr – 357.9 nm, Fe – 248.3 nm and Ni – 240.7 nm. Measurements and calculations were performed by «AAS-SPECTR» program.

Paraffin sections (of 5 μm thickness) for energy dispersive spectrometry were subjected to dewaxing and applied on spectral pure graphite rods. Chemical composition was studied by means of the scanning electron microscope with energy-dispersion spectrometer [25]. Digital images of the specimen and the indicators of microelements content were identified by Magellanes and VCU software.

Table 1 Antibody for immunohistochemical reaction («Thermo Fisher Scientific», USA)

Antibody	Host	Clone	Dilution	Cellular localization
ERα	Rabbit	SP1	1:200	Nuclear
PR	Rabbit	YR85	1:150	Nuclear
HER2/neu	Rabbit	SP3	1:100	Membrane
p53	Mouse	SP5	1:100	Nuclear
Ki-67	Rabbit	SP6	1:100	Nuclear
MGMT	Mouse	MT3.1	1:50	Cytoplasmic and nuclear
E-cadherin	Rabbit	67A4	1:100	Membrane

Immunohistochemical study

The material for the immunohistochemical reaction was fixed in 10% neutral formalin for 24 h, after that paraffin blocks were made of it. Then sections of 3-4 µm thickness were made and they were subjected to the standard process of dehydration in xylol and alcohols of rising concentration. Immunohistochemical reaction consisted of 2 stages. During the first stage the incubation with primary rabbit antibodies («Thermo Fisher Scientific», USA) in different dilutions in tissue sections took place (Table 1). Then we conducted the receptor visualization using detection systems «UltraVision Quanto Detection System HRP DAB Chromogen» («Thermo Fisher Scientific», USA). We visualized the cell structural components using diaminobenzidine, which painted them in a brown color. We have performed immunohistochemical reaction with E-cadherin for the purpose of the differential diagnosis between high degree malignant invasive lobular carcinoma and IDC. The positive reaction took place only in IDC.

DNA extraction and investigation

DNA was extracted from the tissue using a lysis buffer which consisted of 30 mM hydroxymethylamino-methane, 10 mM ethylenediamine-tetraacetic acid, 1% sodium dodecyl sulfate and 5 mg proteinase K (pH 8.0). DNA was purified with phenol-chloroform extraction and the following precipitation in absolute ethanol.

DNA methylation level was determined at the Institute for Single Crystals, National Academy of Sciences (Ukraine) using the oscillating infrared spectroscopy method. An obligatory condition was the deprivation of samples of auxiliary substances (absolute ethanol, chloroform, phenol and others) that were used for DNA extraction, and that could overcharge DNA spectrum. Obtained DNA product was triturated with KBr and placed into tablets for infrared spectroscopy on the SpectrumOne spectrometer. Spectrum analysis was performed by OridionVersion8 program.

Statistical analysis of the results

Mathematical calculations were done using Microsoft Excel 2010 with 12.0.5 Attestat option. We have found such indicators as chi-squared Pearson's test, Pearson's correlation coefficient (with statistical significance $p < 0.05$).

Results

The invasive ductal carcinoma is characterized by the formation of nests, clusters and trabeculas, though some tumors are characterized by solid growth with a small amount of stroma. Some part of the tumor has clear tubular structures with lumen in the center. The cells are quite variable in structure. The cytoplasm is often broad and eosinophilic. The nuclei are round, monomorphic or with polymorphism and well-visible nucleoli. The mitotic activity varies greatly - from full absence to 10-20 or more in one field of view (Fig. 1).

Using atomic absorption spectrophotometry of IDC tissue it has been found that the content of iron was from 38.46×10^{-3} to 69.63×10^{-3} µg/kg (average 59.73×10^{-3} µg/kg), copper – from 2.8×10^{-3} to 9.11×10^{-3} µg/kg (average 5.66×10^{-3} µg/kg), chromium – from 0 to 6.1×10^{-3} µg/kg (average 2.41×10^{-3} µg/kg), zinc – from 1.89×10^{-3} to

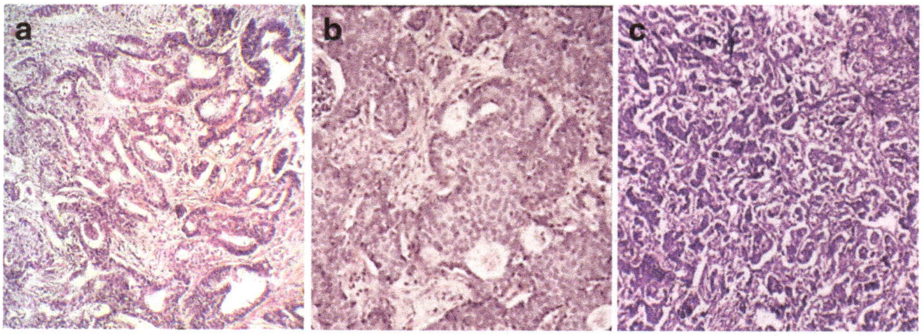

Fig. 1 Invasive ductal carcinoma of varying degrees of malignancy by Scarff-Bloom-Richardson. **a** – well-differentiated carcinoma, **b** – moderately differentiated carcinoma, **c** – poorly differentiated carcinoma. Staining with hematoxylin and eosin. Magnification ×100

6.4 × 10^{-3} μg/kg (average 4.25 × 10^{-3} μg/kg), lead – from 0 to 0.6 × 10^{-3} μg/kg (average 0.11 × 10^{-3} μg/kg) and nickel – from 0.08 × 10^{-3} to 0.52 × 10^{-3} μg/kg (average 0.3 × 10^{-3} μg/kg). The total amount of HM ranged from 51.21 × 10^{-3} to 84.86 × 10^{-3} μg/kg (average 72.44 × 10^{-3} μg/kg). In near located intact breast tissue these levels were much lower: iron on the average 34,26 × 10^{-3} μg/kg, copper – 2.73 × 10^{-3} μg/kg, chromium – 0.92 × 10^{-3} μg/kg, zinc – 1.67 × 10^{-3} μg/kg, lead – 0.04 × 10^{-3} μg/kg and nickel – 0.1 × 10^{-3} μg/kg (Table 2).

In order to determine the spatial features of HM localization in "cancer" tissue we studied the chemical composition of IDC by energy dispersion method on scanning electron microscope. This process took place in two functional modes: local scanning of the sample surface at different zoom levels and focal scanning, considering trace-element composition of parenchymal and stromal components of BC tissue (Fig. 2). Such macroelements as calcium, phosphorus, potassium, sulfur and sodium dominated in neoplastic tissue. Such heavy metals as zinc, iron, copper, chromium, nickel and lead are encountered in different proportions among other microelements. We have found that HM accumulated more in the parenchymal component of tumor tissue ($p < 0.05$). Comparing the data of two studies on the detection of the chemical composition we've got identical results – if the concentration of HM in a gram of tumor was increased then the percentage content also grew that have been obtained using energy-dispersive method of study ($p < 0.05$). The relationship ($r = 0.62$, $p < 0.01$) between the HM accumulation in the foci of neoplasia and the degree of malignancy of BC has been established.

Immunohistochemical analysis has revealed different variants of receptors expression. 63% of tumors were ER-positive that was evaluated according to D.C.Allred recommendations. In 50% of cases we have revealed the presence of PR. Investigating the presence of HER2/neu receptors we have found that 12 samples were receptor positive. Studying the expression of Ki-67 receptor we have found that IDC tissue in 87.5% of cases possessed varying degree of proliferative activity. The presence of mutated proapoptotic protein p53 (mt p53) has been found in 37.5% of samples of BC (the possibility to identify wt p53 protein was absent due to the short time of its existence and its below a threshold level – this number is impossible to detect by immunohistochemical studies). The examples of receptor-positive variants of BC tissues are shown in Fig. 3. The results of statistical data processing of immunohistochemical studies have found that in our research the correlative connections were as follows: the positive correlative connections between ER and PR ($r = 0.85$, $p < 0.01$), p53 and Ki-67 ($r = 0.55$, $p < 0.01$); the negative correlative connections between ER and HER2/neu ($r = -0.56$, $p < 0.01$), PR and

Table 2 The content of HM in cancerous and healthy breast tissue (×10^{-3} μg/kg)

	Iron	Copper	Zinc	Leac	Chromium	Nickel	Total
1.	41.36	4.23	3.74	0.16	1.46	0.26	51.21
2.	44.17	3.42	4.17	0.09	0.72	0.34	52.91
3.	38.46	4.3	4.[illegible]	0.18	5.1	0.42	53.06
4.	39.65	4.71	5.11	0.14	3.41	0.23	53.25
5.	51.27	5.57	1.89	0.14	1.32	0.28	60.47
6.	52.26	4.32	4.08	0.01	0.65	0.34	61.66
7.	49.38	6.56	3.35	0.15	2.46	0.29	62.19
8.	52.44	4.89	3.29	0	1.78	0.28	62.68
9.	47.81	6.32	3.89	0.07	4.53	0.28	62.9
10.	53.48	5.82	3.23	0.18	1.56	0.32	64.59
11.	52.4	5.61	5.09	0.14	1.78	0.29	65.31
12.	56.54	3.56	3.54	0.01	2.12	0.3	66.07
13.	55.84	6.18	3.65	0	2.11	0.25	68.03
14.	54.63	6.19	5.33	0.16	3.1	0.35	69.76
15.	61.41	5.13	2.93	0.08	0.78	0.26	70.59
16.	60.87	3.65	4.48	0.19	2.23	0.28	71.7
17.	62.62	2.8	4.1	0.09	2.47	0.34	72.42
18.	61.89	3.69	4.44	0.16	2.32	0.34	72.84
19.	60.55	6.21	3.45	0.06	2.51	0.32	73.1
20.	68.39	4.81	2.8	0.09	0	0.16	76.25
21.	64.33	7.25	3.36	0	1.52	0.29	76.75
22.	64.48	5.25	4.88	0.04	2.86	0.36	77.87
23.	65.86	4.23	3.86	0.03	3.62	0.28	77.88
24.	63.81	5.26	5.23	0.11	3.51	0.27	78.19
25.	62.57	8.11	5.69	0.03	1.85	0.35	78.6
26.	63.23	8.66	5.73	0.14	1.69	0.08	79.58
27.	65.59	6.36	4.77	0.19	2.45	0.26	79.62
28.	65.21	7.63	4.11	0	2.56	0.28	79.79
29.	69.63	5.77	2.75	0.14	1.32	0.28	79.89
30.	68.12	5.11	2.84	0.11	3.54	0.28	80
31.	67.54	2.99	5.65	0.08	3.66	0.28	80.21
32.	66.25	7.36	4.23	0.14	2.36	0.32	80.71
33.	68.33	7.68	3.65	0.11	0.92	0.33	81.02
34.	68.87	5.12	4.26	0.08	2.66	0.3	81.29
35.	68.65	5.36	3.96	0	3.15	0.29	81.41
36.	67.2	5.17	6.11	0.12	2.63	0.3	81.53
37.	67.25	6.29	4.85	0.06	3.6	0.25	82.3
38.	66.65	8.62	4.42	0.16	2.24	0.29	82.38
39.	68.11	6.59	6.38	0	1.86	0.35	83.29
40.	62.13	9.11	6.4	0.6	6.1	0.52	84.86
Minimum value	38.46	2.8	1.89	0	0	0.08	51.21
Maximum value	69.63	9.11	6.4	0.6	6.1	0.52	84.86
Average value	59.73	5.66	4.25	0.11	2.41	0.3	72.44
Average value in healthy breast tissue	34.26	2.73	1.67	0.04	0.92	0.1	39.72

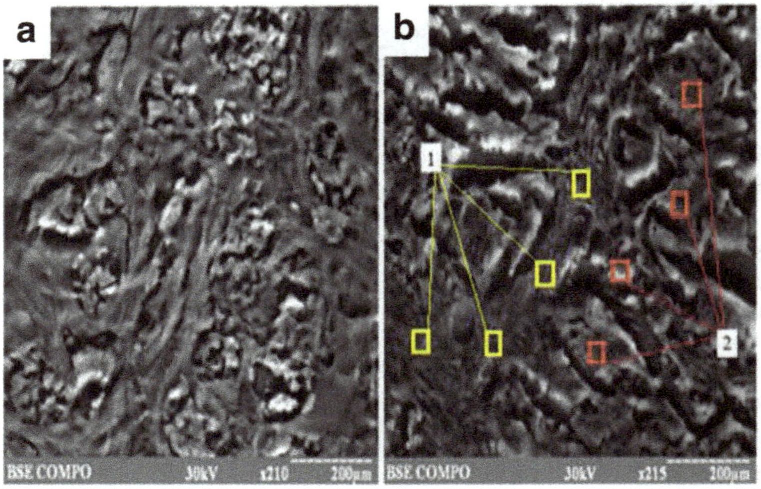

Fig. 2 The scanning images of IDC tissue. **a** – local scanning of the sample surface (x210), **b** – focal scanning (x215): 1 – stromal component of tissue, 2 – parenchymal component of tissue

HER2/neu ($r = -0.58$, $p < 0.01$), ER and Ki-67 ($r = -0.37$, $p < 0.05$), PR and Ki-67 ($r = -0.33$, $p < 0.05$).

The patterns of MGMT expression, according to the recommendations of the manufacturer of the antibodies, were cytoplasm and nucleus (Fig. 4). In our studies it has been received more pronounced nuclear localization of MGMT. This confirms the basic function of MGMT, which carries an alkyl residue (methyl-, ethyl-, n-propil- and others) from O^6 position of guanine on its 145th active site which respectively is localized in the nucleus of "cancer" cells. We have not established the cases in which pattern of expression was only cytoplasm. During research we have revealed the following results: 17 cases (42.5%) of IDC were MGMT-positive and 23 samples (57.5%) – MGMT-negative. Cytoplasmic expression of MGMT has been found in almost 30% of BC cases. Investigating the combination of MGMT and ER expression we have revealed an interesting pattern – during the increase of MGMT expression the level of steroid hormone receptors decreased ($r = -0.5$, $p < 0.01$).

According to the results of spectroscopy, the range of DNA fluctuations is located within 400–4000cm^{-1}. We conventionally divided obtained infrared DNA spectra into three areas: the first area corresponded to the spectrum of nitrogenous bases fluctuations (4000-2000 cm^{-1}), the second – the fluctuations of deoxyribose CH_2-groups (1700-1500 cm^{-1}) and the third – the fluctuations of the deoxyribose and phosphate groups in the skeleton of DNA molecules (1300-1000 cm^{-1}). The spectra were divided into weak ≤5%, average – 5-20% and

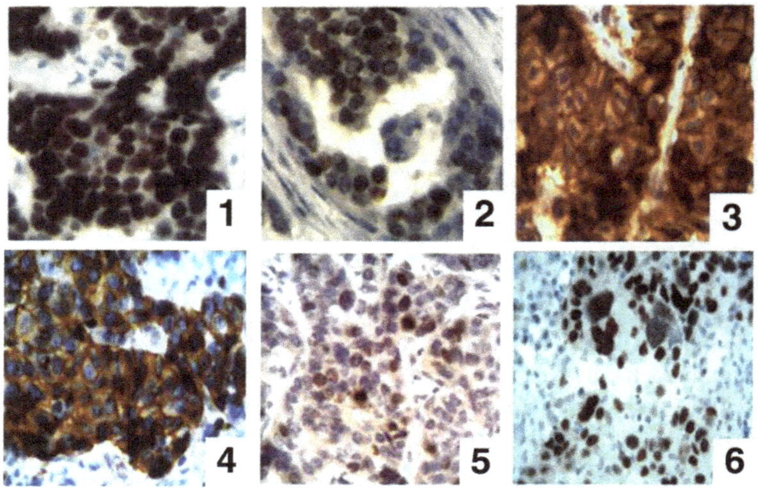

Fig. 3 The immunohistochemical study of BC tissue. **1** – ER, **2** – PR, **3** – HER2/neu, **4** – E-cadherin, **5** – Ki-67, **6** – p53. Magnification ×400

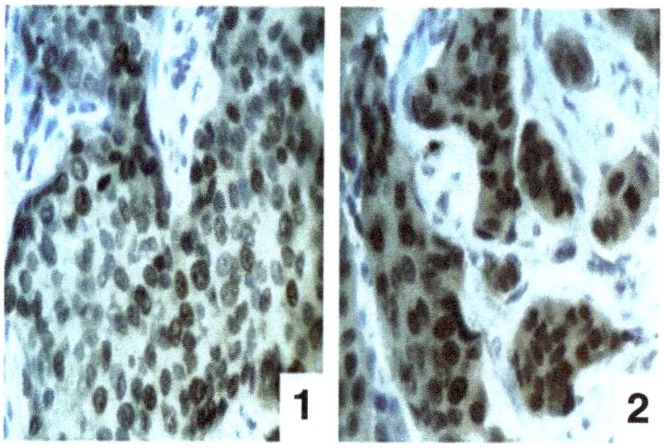

Fig. 4 The immunohistochemical study of MGMT. **1** – IDC tissue with nuclear localization of the enzyme, **2** – IDC tissue with nuclear and cytoplasmic localization of the enzyme. Magnification ×400

strong – ≥20%, depending on the intensity of infrared absorption. The attention was also paid to the level of manifestation of vibrational spectrum and its length. The main purpose of the study was to identify the DNA methylation level by the indicators of the deviation of absorptive waves in 2850 cm^{-1}-3050 cm^{-1} range, corresponding to methyl (-CH_3) group fluctuations.

The results have shown that the spectrum of methyl group fluctuation was in the range from 2893 cm^{-1} to 3048 cm^{-1} and it presented in 92.5% (37 cases) as one peak, and in 7.5% (3 cases) there was the splitting of infrared fluctuations of -CH_3 groups (Fig. 5). The peak of -CH_3 fluctuations was in the range from 2920 cm^{-1} to 2991 cm^{-1}. Its intensity was in the range from 76.15% to 98.72% (average 89.71%), it being a strong peak. Therefore as -CH_3 fluctuations is in the range of fluctuations of nitrogenous bases (4000-2000 cm^{-1}), we can assume that the process of pathological methylation takes place in the adenine, guanine and cytosine or thymine additionally adds a methyl group. We found moderate positive correlative relationship between the level of MGMT expression and DNA methylation levels ($r = 0.53$, $p < 0.01$), between the level of infrared spectrum absorption and level of p53 expression ($r = 0.32$, $p < 0.01$). We observed the tendency of decreasing the expression of ER and PR with the growth of abnormal DNA methylation.

Comparing the results of the chemical composition of IDC tissue with results of immunohistochemical investigations we have got the following results: the growth of HM in neoplastic tissue is accompanied with the increase of HER2/neu ($r = 0.36$, $p < 0.05$), p53 (r = 0.53, p < 0.01), Ki-67 ($r = 0.47$, $p < 0.01$), MGMT ($r = 0.34$, p < 0.05) expression and decrease of ER ($r = -0.71$, p < 0.01) and PR ($r = -0.66$, p < 0.01) expression. The growth of pathological DNA methylation is also accompanied with the increasing amount of HM in tumor tissue ($r = 0.41$, p < 0.01).

General information concerning the presence of correlation connections between different BC indicators are presented in Table 3.

It should be noted that all the molecular-genetic indicators of IDC progression authentically increased while reducing of tumor differentiation degree.

Discussion

Our present is characterized by the growing influence of environmental factors upon human health. Without a

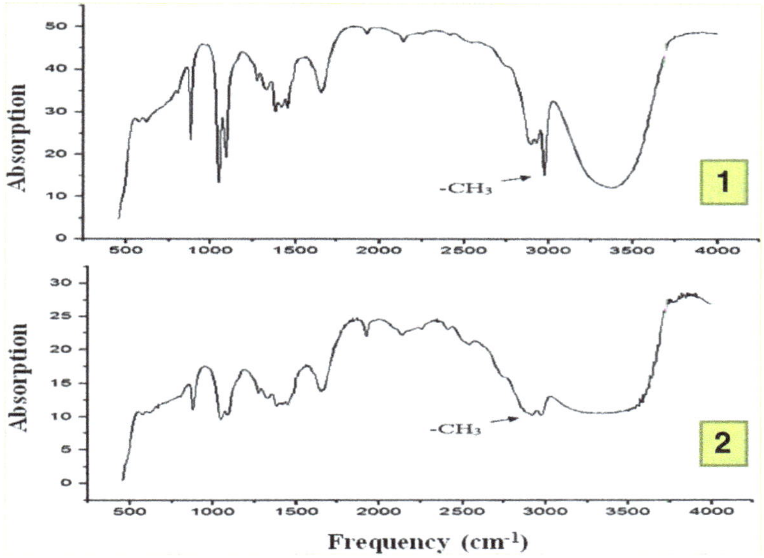

Fig. 5 Infrared spectrum of DNA. **1** – spectrum with one peak of methyl group fluctuation, **2** – spectrum with the splitting of infrared fluctuations of -CH3 groups

Table 3 Factor analysis of IDC indicators

	HM	ER	PR	HER2/neu	Ki-67	P53	MGMT	IRS
HM	1	-0,71083	-0,65867	0,35888	0,46852	0,53194	0,33878	0,41066
ER	-0,71083	1	0,85496	-0,56184	-0,3719	-0,28936	-0,50235	-0,30911
PR	-0,65867	0,85496	1	-0,58187	-0,3285	-0,27685	-0,50022	-0,289655
HER2/neu	0,35889	-0,56184	-0,58187	1	0,22818	0.22583	0,20967	0,03736839
Ki-67	0,468522	-0,3719	-0,3285	0,22818	1	0,54678	0,24542	0,17198477
P53	0,531949	-0,28936	-0,27685	0.22583	0,54678	1	0,20152	0,31904601
MGMT	0,33878	-0,50235	-0,50022	0,20967	0,24542	0,20152	1	0,5265685
IRS	0,41066	-0,30911	-0,28966	0,03736	0,17198	0,31904	0,52656	1

IRS infra red spectrum. **Orange color** – a negative correlation between HM and ER, HM and PR, ER and HER2/neu, ER and Ki-67, ER and MGMT, PR and HER2/neu, PR and Ki-67, PR and MGMT. **Green color** - a positive correlation between HM and HER2/neu, HM and Ki-67, HM and P53, HM and MGMT, HM and IRS, P53 and Ki-67, IRS and P53, IRS and MGMT. **Blue color** - intersection of the same indicators

doubt, HM are vital micro elements which are included in the vital functions of all body cells. But their function is changing when they arrive in excessive quantities to the intracellular environment, showing their toxic functions. According to the results of spectrophotometry IDC tissue contains in its composition different amount of HM. The reason is that the cancer cells at the expense of disorders of endo-exocytosis of chemicals accumulate HM, in accordance with the growth of their number in the blood vessels (due to the increased receipts of HM to the body). We can explain the increase of heavy elements concentration in the neoplastic tissue with the progression of carcinogenesis at the expense of violation of regulatory mechanisms of HM assimilation and utilization by tumor cells. Increasing level of cell anaplasia leads to blocking the synthesis of enzymes involved in maintaining of intracellular homeostasis. On the other hand, these microelements stimulate this imbalance by supporting of HM ominous impact on the course of malignancy.

HM accumulation impacts on cell phenotype. This process is realized through a block of steroid receptors that reduces the sensitivity of cancer cells to antihormone therapy. This is due to DNA methylation and increases the amount of MGMT (see below), the initiation of inflammation and inhibition of ESR genes transcription [26], depletion of ER and progression of phenotypic simplification [27].

On the other hand, heavy microelements activate antiapoptotic function and proliferative potential of cells by the synthesis of mt p53 [10]. As shown by our study MGMT protein is no exception. Its quantity grows with increasing HM intracellular content. We explain the protein growth level through different effects of heavy metals on MGMT synthesis. In our opinion one of the possible points in this chain is their impact on cell DNA. In this case HM might lead to the increment of methyl group accession to the DNA molecule. This fact is not accidental, because the HM are involved in many intracellular processes, including the transfer of electrons and active groups (-CH_3, -O, -S) [28]. We have found a positive correlative relationship between DNA methylation level and the amount of HM in the tumor tissue during our study.

The general scheme of pathological DNA methylation and MGMT synthesis is as follows (Scheme 1). An exogenous revenue of heavy metal salts into the body leads to their deposition in tumor tissue [29]. On the one hand they block the reparative systems [7], on the other hand they can stimulate the transfer of -CH_3 groups [28]. As a result methyl groups are joined to thymine (only thymine ($C_5H_6N_2O_2$) has in its composition in norm -CH_3 group) and -CH3 groups to other nitrogen bases. The excessive abnormal DNA methylation can stimulate the reparative system activation, which is represented by MGMT protein, which permanently removes attached -CH_3 group from nitrogenous bases [20].

Inactivated MGMT enters into relationship with receptors for steroid hormones inhibiting their function [21]. This fact is confirmed by the presence of a negative correlative connection between the MGMT expression and steroid receptors. The lack of relationship between the MGMT, p53 and Ki-67 expression indicates separate enzyme impact on the course of the malignant process that does not depend on the presence of other disorders in the pathogenesis [23]. Instead, the level of p53 protein

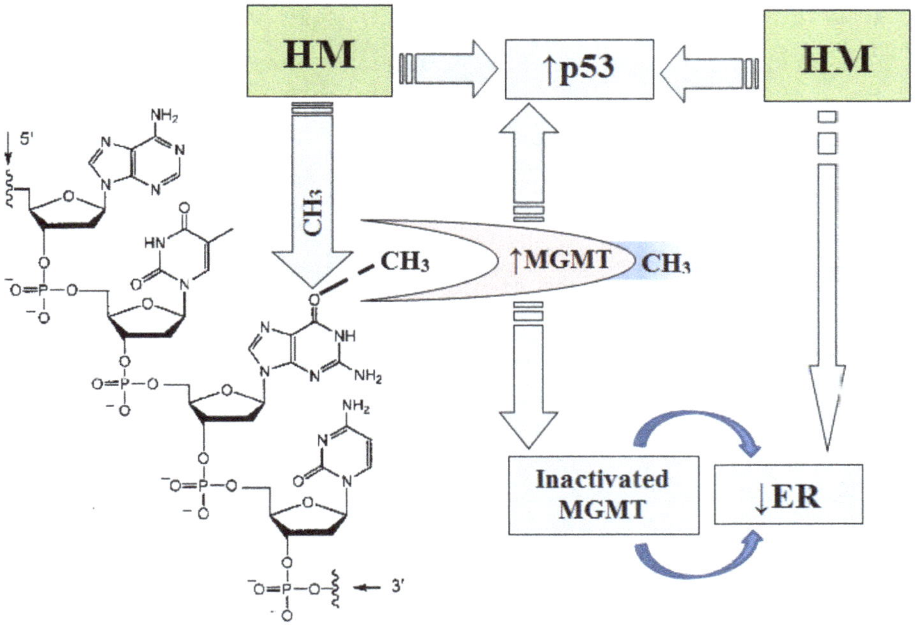

Scheme 1 The pathological DNA methylation and its effect on the receptor profile of tumor tissue

expression increased together with increasing of the level of DNA methylation. This indicates the impact of the methylation on cancer cells pro-apoptotic function [17].

The relationship between the expression of ER and PR, ER and HER2/neu, PR and HER2/neu, p53 and Ki-67, ER and Ki-67, PR and Ki-67 indicate the presence of close cooperation between the various links of IDC progression [10, 30].

Conclusions

Heavy metals are accumulated in breast cancer tissue. The total amount of them range from 51.21×10^{-3} to 84.86×10^{-3} μg/kg (average 72.44×10^{-3} μg/kg) in this tumor. They are accumulated more in the parenchymal component of tumor tissue. We have established the relationship between the heavy metals accumulation in the foci of neoplasia and degree of breast cancer malignancy.

DNA of tumor tissue has a different level of methylation which changes with the amount of heavy metals in cancer cells (a positive correlation between the amount of heavy metals in the neoplastic tissue and DNA methylation level has been established – $r = 0.41$, $p < 0.05$). This is displayed on the synthesis of prognostically important receptors (MGMT, p53) in neoplastic tissue. Inactivated MGMT can enter into relationship with receptors for steroid hormones inhibiting their function.

The growth of heavy metals in neoplastic tissue is accompanied with the increase of HER2/neu, p53, Ki-67, MGMT expression and decrease of ER and PR expression. The relationship between the expression of ER and PR, ER and HER2/neu, PR and HER2/neu, p53 and Ki-67, ER and Ki-67, PR and Ki-67 indicate the presence of close cooperation between various links of invasive ductal carcinoma progression.

Heavy metals through different pathogenetic links stimulate the progression of breast cancer and reduce its sensitivity to treatment.

Abbreviations

BC: Breast cancer; ER: Estrogen receptor; HER2/neu: Human epidermal growth factor receptor 2; HM: Heavy metals; IDC: Invasive ductal carcinoma; MGMT: O6-methyguanine-DNA methyltransferase; mt p53: Mutant type p53; PR: Progesterone receptor; wt p53: Wild type p53

Acknowledgements

We thank Zolotarova Vera who helped in the conduction of immunohistochemical reactions.

Funding

The work was carried out with the support of the research theme "Development of the diagnosis method of the reproductive systemorgans tumors using cellular adhesion molecules of cancer-embryonic antigen"(state registration number 62.12.01 - 01.17/20.3П) and an internal grant from the Sumy State University "Protein of heat shock as prognostic markers for malignant tumors development in the reproductive system".

Authors' contributions

All authors agreed to be accountable for all aspects of the work and ensuring accuracy and integrity and approved the final version of this manuscript. ML, AR and VS were responsible for final approval of the article, analysis and interpretation of the data. SR, YL and KS were involved in the writing of the manuscript, participated in writing and editing the manuscript.

Competing interests

The authors declare that they have no competing interests.

Author details

[1]Department of pathology, Sumy State University, st. Privokzalnaya, 31, Sumy Postal code 40022, Ukraine. [2]Department of normal anatomy, Sumy State University, Sumy, Ukraine. [3]Cardiology department of Sumy regional hospital, Sumy, Ukraine. [4]Sumy Regional Clinical Perinatal Center, Sumy, Ukraine.

References

1. Lakhani SR, Ellis IO, Schnitt SJ, Tan PH, van de Vijver MJ. WHO classification of tumours of the breast. IARC/world health organization classification of tumours. Lyon, France: WHO Press; 2012.
2. Zotov AS, Belik EO. Mastopathy and breast cancer. Moscow: MEDpress-inform; 2005. p. 112.
3. Verkooijen HM, Fioretta G, Vlastos G, Morabia A, Schubert H, Sappino AP, Pelte MF, Schäfer P, Kurtz J, Bouchardy C. Important increase of invasive lobular breast cancer incidence in Geneva, Switzerland. Int J Cancer. 2003; 104(6):778–81.
4. Parkin DM, Bray F, Ferlay J, Pisani P. Global cancer statistics, 2002. CA Cancer J Clin. 2005;55(2):74–108.
5. Vashkulat NP. Establish levels of heavy metals in soils in Ukraine. Environ Health. 2002;2:44–6.
6. Bont DR, Larebeke NV. Endogenous DNA damage in humans: a review of quantitative data. Mutagenesis. 2004;19(3):169–85.
7. Xi H. Does iron have a role in breast cancer? Lancet Oncol. 2008;9(8):803–7.
8. Taylor KM, Vichova P, Jordan N, Hiscox S, Hendley R, Nicholson RI. ZIP7-mediated intracellular zinc transport contributes to aberrant growth factor signaling in antihormone-resistant breast cancer cells. Endocrinology. 2008; 149:4912–20.
9. Lowndes SA, Sheldon HV, Cai S, Taylor JM, Harris AL. Copper chelator ATN-224 inhibits endothelial function by multiple mechanisms. Microvasc Res. 2009;77(3):314–26.
10. Romaniuk A, Lyndin M, Moskalenko R, Kuzenko Y, Gladchenko O, Lyndina Y. Pathogenetic mechanisms of heavy metals effect on proapoptotic and proliferative potential of breast cancer. Intervent Med Appl Sci. 2015;7(2):63–7.
11. Geyer FC, Rodrigues DN, Weigelt B, Reis-Filho JS. Molecular classification of estrogen receptor-positive/luminal breast cancers. Adv Anat Pathol. 2012;19: 39–53.
12. Nair BC, Vallabhaneni S, Tekmal RR, Vadlamudi RK. Roscovitine confers tumor suppressive effect on therapy-resistant breast tumor cells. Breast Cancer Res. 2011;13:80–9.
13. Weigel MT, Dowsett M. Current and emerging biomarkers in breast cancer: prognosis and prediction. Endocr Relat Cancer. 2010;17:245–62.
14. Eldar A, Rozenberg H, Diskin-Posner Y, Rohs R, Shakked Z. Structural studies of p53 inactivation by DNA-contact mutations and its rescue by suppressor mutations via alternative protein – DNA interactions. Nucl Acids Res. 2013; 41:1–12.
15. Buck-Koehntop BA, Defossez PA. On how mammalian transcription factors recognize methylated DNA. Epigenetics. 2013;8(2):131–7.
16. Hansen KD, Timp W, Bravo HC, Sabunciyan S, Langmead B, McDonald OG, Wen B, Wu H, Liu Y, Diep D, Briem E, Zhang K, Irizarry RA, Feinberg AP. Increased methylation variation in epigenetic domains across cancer types. Nat Genet. 2011;43(8):768–75.
17. Heyn H, Sayols S, Moutinho C, Vidal E, Sanchez-Mut JV, Stefansson OA, Nadal E, Moran S, Eyfjord JE, Gonzalez-Suarez E, Pujana MA, Esteller M. Linkage of DNA Methylation quantitative trait loci to human cancer risk. Cell Rep. 2014;7(2):331–8.
18. Stefanska B, Huang J, Bhattacharyya B, Suderman M, Hallett M, Han ZG, Szyf M. Definition of the landscape of promoter DNA hypomethylation in liver cancer. Cancer Res. 2011;71(17):5891–903.
19. Jacinto FV, Esteller M. MGMT hypermethylation: a prognostic foe, a predictive friend. DNA Rpair. 2007;6(8):1155–60.
20. Munot K, Bell SM, Lane S, Horgan K, Hanby AM, Speirs V. Pattern of expression of genes linked to epigenetic silencing in human breast cancer. Hum Pathol. 2006;37(8):989–99.
21. Teo AK, Oh HK, Ali RB, Li BF. The modified human DNA repair enzyme O6-Methylguanine-DNA Methyltransferase is a negative regulator of Estrogen receptor-mediated transcription upon alkylation DNA damage. Mol Cell Biol. 2001;21(20):7105–14.
22. Sharma S, Salehi F, Scheithauer BW, Rotondo F, Syro LV, Kovacs K. Role of MGMT in tumor development, progression, diagnosis, treatment and prognosis. Anticancer Res. 2009;29(10):3759–68.
23. Fumagalli C, Pruneri G, Possanzini P, Manzotti M, Barile M, Feroce I, Colleoni M, Bonanni B, Maisonneuve P, Radice P, Viale G, Barberis M. Methylation of O6-methylguanine-DNA methyltransferase (MGMT) promoter gene in triple-negative breast cancer patients. Breast Cancer Res Treat. 2012;134(1):131–7.
24. Neto JC, Ikoma MM, Carvalho KC, Vassallo J, De Brot M, Gobbi H, Soares FA, Rocha RM. MGMT and PTEN as potential prognostic markers in breast cancer. Exp Mol Pathol. 2012;92(1):20–6.
25. Kuzenko YV. Method: chemical and morphological studying of paraffin sections. Morphologia. 2014;8(2):89–92.
26. Romaniuk A, Lyndin M. Immune microenvironment as a factor of breast cancer progression. Diagn Pathol. 2015;10:79.
27. Romaniuk AM, Lyndin MS, Moskalenko RA, Zolotarova AV. Evaluation of the receptors estrogen, progesterone and her2/neu expression in the breast cancer tissue under the influence of trace elements on the body. J Clin Exp Med Res. 2014;2(2):168–75.
28. Arita A, Costa M. Epigenetics in metal carcinogenesis: nickel, arsenic, chromium and cadmium. Metallomics. 2009;1(3):222–8.
29. Silva MP, Soave DF, Ribeiro-Silva A, Poletti ME. Trace elements as tumor biomarkers and prognostic factors in breast cancer: a study through energy dispersive x-ray fluorescence. BMC Res Notes. 2012;5:194.
30. Davion S, Sullivan M, Rohan S, Siziopikou KP. p53 expression in triple negative breast carcinomas: evidence of age-related and racial differences. Journal of Cancer Therapy. 2012;3:649–54.

Is it useful to combine sputum cytology and low-dose spiral computed tomography for early detection of lung cancer in formerly asbestos-exposed power industry workers?

Michael K Felten[1*], Lars Knoll[1], Christian Schikowsky[1], Marco Das[2,7], Christian Feldhaus[3], Kurt G Hering[4], Alfred Böcking[5,6] and Thomas Kraus[1]

Abstract

Background: Low-dose spiral computed tomography (LDSCT) in comparison to conventional chest X-ray proved to be a highly sensitive method of diagnosing early stage lung cancer. However, centrally located early stage lung tumours remain a diagnostic challenge. We determined the practicability and efficacy of early detection of lung cancer when combining LDSCT and sputum cytology.

Methods: Of a cohort of 4446 formerly asbestos exposed power industry workers, we examined a subgroup of 187 (4.2%) high risk participants for lung cancer at least once with both LDSCT and sputum cytology. After the examination period the participants were followed-up for more than three years.

Results: The examinations resulted in the diagnosis of lung cancer in 12 participants (6.4%). Six were in clinical stage I. We found 10 non-small cell lung carcinomas and one small cell lung carcinoma. Sputum specimens showed suspicious pathological findings in seven cases and in 11 cases the results of LDSCT indicated malignancies. The overall sensitivity and specificity of sputum cytology was 58.0% and 98% with positive (PPV) and negative (NPV) predictive values of 70% and 97%. For LDSCT we calculated the sensitivity and specificity of 92% and 97%. The PPV and NPV were 65% and 99% respectively.

Conclusions: Our results confirmed that in surveillance programmes a combination of sputum cytology and LDSCT is well feasible and accepted by the participants. Sputum examination alone is not effective enough for the detection of lung cancer, especially at early stage. Even in well- defined risk groups highly exposed to asbestos, we cannot recommend the use of combined LDSCT and sputum cytology examinations as long as no survival benefit has been proved for the combination of both methods. For ensuring low rates of false-positive and false-negative results, programme planners must closely cooperate with experienced medical practitioners and pathologists in a well-functioning interdisciplinary network.

Keywords: Lung cancer, Sputum cytology, Computed tomography, Asbestos

* Correspondence: mfelten@ukaachen.de
[1]Institute of Occupational and Social Medicine, Medical Faculty, RWTH Aachen University, Aachen, Germany
Full list of author information is available at the end of the article

Background

Lung cancer remains one of the leading types of cancer in the world. In 2008 1.61 million new cases of lung cancer occurred and 1.38 million people died [1]. According to the American Cancer Society, the total number of deaths from all types of lung cancer in the United States for the year 2010 still exceeded that from colon-, breast- and prostate cancers combined [2]. The huge and worldwide public health importance of lung cancer urgently calls for effective and affordable health interventions. The primary objectives should be early detection and treatment in addition to smoking cessation programmes. In the 1970s, the National Cancer Institute of America sponsored three mass-screening programmes using chest X-rays and sputum cytology [3-5]. No differences in mortality were observed between the intervention and control groups [6]. As a result of these and other studies, mass screening for lung cancer was not recommended [7]. In recent studies, where the highly sensitive method of low-dose spiral computed tomography (LDSCT) was used instead of conventional chest X-rays, a higher detection rate of early-stage lung cancers could be demonstrated. But the design of these uncontrolled and non-randomised studies was unsuitable to demonstrate that screening with LDSCT decreases mortality [8]. Consequently, medical guidelines did not recommend lung cancer screening in individuals, when they do not have specific symptoms or an increased disease risk [9,10]. Recent results from the National Lung Screening Trial confirmed a decreasing effect of LDSCT screening on mortality, particularly in those with a high risk of lung cancer [11].

Smoking is the predominant risk factor for lung cancer with a 23 times higher risk in male smokers compared to non-smokers [2,12]. Additional environmental and occupational risk factors are also relevant for the development of lung cancer. Exposure to asbestos dust, especially in combination with cigarette smoke, is a main occupational cause of lung malignancies [13-16]. The health effects of asbestos dust are difficult to measure and control. Some reasons for that are the long latency periods (12–37 years) between exposure and the occurrence of lung cancer and the widespread, unprotected use in the past [17].

In this study, we tested the hypothesis that non-automated sputum cytology may be particularly useful for the diagnosis of centrally located tumours [18,19], whereas LDSCT is more capable of detecting tumours in the peripheral parts of the lung. Following that notion, the best detection rates of early stage lung cancer would be in theory expected by applying both methods. We examined the practicability and efficacy of lung cancer screening in a group of power industry workers, who were heavily exposed to asbestos dust in the past.

Methods

Our study cohort included 5632 formerly asbestos exposed employees of a major provider of electrical power in Germany. They had been enrolled after confirming by signature some contact with asbestos fibres in the past and giving written consent to participate. Most participants had been involved in general maintenance and repair work in various installations of power generation, including lignite fuelled power plants. Routine occupational tasks involved the handling of asbestos and asbestos containing materials such as the removal of asbestos lagging around the turbines and the spraying of asbestos pulp. The work was carried out without effective personal protective measures or technical ventilation [20].

All medical examinations were done in the framework of a health surveillance programme, which had been set up for the formerly exposed employees with the primary objective to detect newly developing lung cancers in an early stage. Before starting the examinations, we recorded age, tobacco consumption and duration of asbestos exposure for all 5632 participants, assuming that these were the major risk factors for lung cancer development. The required data were collected via self-administered questionnaires. Based on this information, all study participants were allocated to one of three risk groups with an assumed low, medium and high risk of developing lung cancer. For risk stratification, we combined the factors duration of asbestos exposure in years, age and smoking status as follows: duration × $[\text{age}/50]^3$ × smoking (0.1 = non-smoker, 0.3 = ex-smoker, 1.0 = smoker) [21]. Between March 2002 and December 2006 a total of 4446 (78.9%) participants were examined at least once for asbestos related diseases. Routine examinations included occupational history, medical history, standard interview on current respiratory symptoms, physical examination of the thorax and lung function testing. In contrast to the standard chest X-ray in the other participants, the high risk group was examined annually with LDSCT of the thorax and sputum cytology. Automated sputum-cytometry with certified instruments was not available in Germany at the time sputum samples were obtained for this study. Out of those examined, 3182 participants belonged to the low, 1001 to the medium and 263 to the high risk group. For the analysis presented here, we focused on high risk participants who were not older than 75 years on the reference date of 1 September 2002. This was based on the assumption that all other participants, particularly those in the low risk group and those older than 75 years, would have benefitted significantly less from a combined examination with sputum cytology and LDSCT. That way we ensured for most of our study group an acceptable balance between the likelihood of lung cancer and the possible harms from false-positive sputum findings. Participants, who did not submit a sputum sample to the study laboratory, refused to participate in one of the two screening methods or had no usable results because of other reasons, were excluded from the analysis (n = 76). Our evaluation included 187 high risk participants who fulfilled all admission criteria [21]. They represented 4.2% of those examined (n = 4446) and 3.3% of the total cohort (n = 5632). The research was performed according to the principles of the World Medical Association's Declaration of Helsinki and obtained approval by the Institutional Review Board of the Medical Faculty of RWTH Aachen University (registration number EK2205).

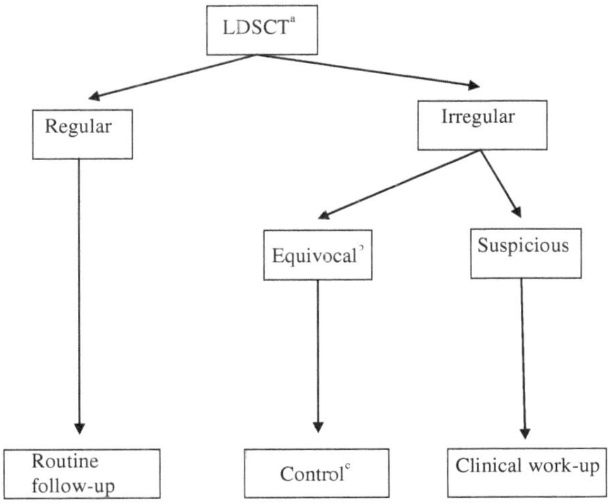

Figure 1 Flow chart for processing the findings of the low-dose spiral computed tomography of the thorax. [a]LDSCT = low-dose spiral computed tomography, [b]Non calcified nodules 6 - ≤10 mm, [c]3, 6 or 12 month follow-up with LDSCT, depending on size of nodule.

Computed tomography scans

Computed tomography examinations were carried out in a low-dose spiral technique applying 10 $mAs_{eff.}$ for persons weighing less than 80 kg, and 20 $mAs_{eff.}$ for persons weighing more than 80 kg. No contrast material was administered. All CT-scans were performed with a 16-slice MDCT scanner (SOMATOM Sensation 16, Siemens Medical Solutions, Forchheim, Germany) using the following parameters: 16 × 0.75 mm collimation, rotation time 0.5 sec, table feed/rotation 18 mm. For lung nodule detection a stack of images was reconstructed with 1 mm slice thickness and 0.5 mm increment using a sharp reconstruction kernel (Siemens B50 kernel) and a window centre of –400 HU and a width of 2000 HU. The initial reading was done by an experienced clinical radiologist (MD) at a standard PACS reading workstation (Barco, Philips/Sectra, Stockholm, Sweden). Data were then transferred to a workstation for further evaluation using dedicated lung analysis software (LungCare™, Siemens Medical Solutions, Forchheim, Germany). All CT-scans were routinely re-read by an occupational physician with special experience in the diagnosis of asbestos related diseases (TK). The follow-up algorithm applied for lung nodules has been described elsewhere [21]. In cases with suspicious lung nodules and other pathological findings we recommended a clinical work-up in cooperation with the clinical departments of Internal Medicine, Diagnostic Radiology, Heart and Thorax Surgery, and Radiotherapy (Figure 1).

Sputum cytology

During medical examination, all participants were instructed in detail on how to generate good sputum samples, how to deposit them in the prepared containers and how to send them to the study laboratory in prepaid envelopes. For sputum collection we used plastic tubes with a screw cap, one for each specimen, containing ca. 50 ml of a fixing solution with 50% ethanol, 2% carbowax 1540 and 0.006% rifampicin [22].

The cytological results were categorized in "regular" for normal or inflammatory sputa and "irregular" or "equivocal" for sputa with squamous cell metaplasia in combination with mild or moderate dysplasia (Figure 2). Further categories were "suspicious" for sputa with squamous cell metaplasia and severe dysplasia or very few abnormal cells, and "pathological" for sputa containing malignant cells. In cases of "insufficient" sputum specimens, we requested the participants to send in a new sputum sample as soon as possible. If the assessment was "equivocal" we asked the participants to collect a second set of samples after about three months. In cases of "suspicious" or "pathological" results, we recommended immediate clinical work-up. Appointments with clinicians could be arranged at any time in the framework of the surveillance programme.

A pathological sputum result was considered truly positive if it was confirmed by tissue biopsy or the LDSCT finding clearly indicated lung cancer. Diagnosed lung tumours were classified according to the TNM staging system and their radiological localisation [23]. Tumours located distal to the segmental bronchus were classified as peripheral, all others were considered as centrally located.

Re-examination

In July 2006 when this study was terminated, 187 participants had been examined at least once with a combination of LDSCT and sputum cytology. Re-examinations after one year and later were possible only in those participants who had their initial examination in or before July 2005. Other reasons for missing re-examination data were refusal to participate again, lack of consent to one of the two investigations and inability to attend because of various reasons such as disease, death or moving

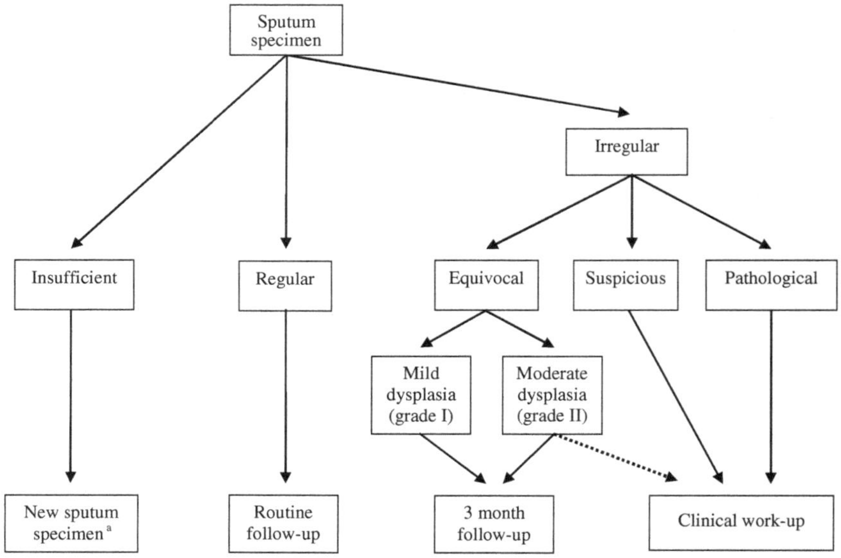

Figure 2 Flow chart for processing the sputum findings. [a]Participants were requested to send in a new sputum sample as soon as possible.

away. Of the group of 187 participants, 117 (62%) were re-examined with both methods one year, 66 (35%) two years and 12 (6%) three years after the initial contact. Thus our data pool included the results of 382 parallel examinations with sputum cytology and CT-scan of the thorax.

Follow-up period

Between August 2006 and the end of 2009 we recorded all new cases of lung cancer in the cohort and analysed their pre diagnosis results during the active study period. That provided us with some indication on the predictive value of LDSCT and sputum cytology. As the study design precluded retrospective analysis of the clinical records backwards from 2009, we evaluated the occupational disease register of the BGETEM as the main secondary source. As an additional source of information, we used death certificates filed before the end of 2009 and indicating the diagnosis of lung cancer.

Statistical analysis

The sensitivity and specificity of the cytological and radiological investigations was tested against the final diagnosis of lung cancer after three years of follow-up. Furthermore, we calculated the positive (PPV) and negative predictive values (NPV) of sputum cytology and computed tomography. As gold standard for diagnosis, we used the biopsy results obtained in the process of clinical work-up. Calculations of statistical parameters such as sensitivity and specificity were based on the combined results of LDSCT and cytology obtained in the active study period (baseline and re-examination).

Results

The burden of asbestos exposure and the results for the risk factors age, latency period and cigarette smoke are shown in Table 1. Latency is defined here as the time period between first exposure to asbestos and the date of the initial examination, covering periods of up to 60 years. As some participants were exposed from the beginning of their apprenticeship until retirement age there was a wide range of exposure duration of approximately 35 years. When comparing mean age and latency period, it seems that asbestos exposure started for many participants in their mid-twenties. The mean pack year value was calculated including the results of the active smokers and participants with smoking periods of less than one year.

New cases of lung cancer during the examination period

In the active study period 12 participants were newly diagnosed with lung cancer (6.4%), 11 of them confirmed with lung tissue biopsy (Table 2). One of the 12 patients (case number four) died suddenly before the diagnosis could be confirmed with lung biopsy. As the patient had clear clinical signs with weight loss of 28 kg within six months together with a fast growing lung nodule

Table 1 Asbestos exposure and other risk factors in the study group (n =187)

	Mean	SD	Range
Age (years)	65.8	5.8	46 – 78
Time since first exposure (years)	40.4	7.8	26 – 60
Duration of asbestos exposure (years)	29.5	7.7	15 – 49
Pack years	44.7	47.9	0 – 118

Table 2 Cases of lung cancer among 187 high risk participants with CT scan and sputum examination

No.	Examination[a]	Location[b]	Diagnosis[c]	Histology[d]	Stage	Survival[e]
1	b	per	CT + spu	SQC	IIIa	
2	r	per	CT + spu	SQC	Ia	29
3	b	per	CT	ADO	Ia	
4[g]	b	per	CT			7
5	r	per	CT	LAC	IIIb	23
6	b	per	CT	ADO	Ia	64
7	b	cen	CT + spu	SQC	IV	21
8	b	cen	CT + spu	SQC	Ia	
9	r	cen	CT + spu	SQC	IIb	33
10	b	cen	CT + spu	SQC	Ib	18
11	b	cen	CT	SMC	Ia	28
12	r	cen	spu	SQC	IIIb	72
13	i	cen		SMC	IIb	14
14	i					35
15[h]	f					
16	f			SMC	IIIb	k
17	f			SMC	IIb	k
18	f				IIIb	k

[a]Examination with significant result: b = baseline, r = re-examination, i = interval, f = follow-up.
[b]Location of tumour: per = peripheral, cen = central.
[c]Result indicating diagnosis: CT = low-dose spiral computed tomography, spu = sputum cytology.
[d]Histology of lung carcinoma: SQC = squamous cell, ADO = adeno, LAC = large cell, SMC = small cell.
[e]Survival time after beginning of initial clinical symptoms indicating the disease (months).
[g]Died suddenly 2004 before biopsy could be taken, diagnosis unequivocal clinically and on CT.
[h]Died 2008 with lung cancer after refusing further examinations.
[k]Alive by the end of follow-up.
In patients with missing data the documented histories were incomplete or could not be retrieved in time.

reaching 4.7 cm in diameter on CT scan, we considered him also as a confirmed case of progressive lung cancer. Eight lung cancers were diagnosed at the first combined examination (baseline), four at the first re-examination and two in the interval between the baseline examination and the first re-examination. One of the two (case number 13) was diagnosed in an external hospital after symptoms developed. We found ten cases of non-small cell lung carcinoma (NSCLC) and one small cell lung carcinoma (SCLC). Of the 11 participants with biopsy confirmation, six were in clinical stage I, one in stage II, three in stage III and one in stage IV. In half of the 12 confirmed cases the tumours were located in the periphery of the lung.

Sputum cytology

In seven cases with newly diagnosed primary lung cancer, sputum specimens showed suspicious or pathological findings (Table 3). In three other cases with suspicious or pathological sputum specimens, no malignant lung tumours were detected and therefore considered as false positive (false positive rate 1.7%). In the remaining five

Table 3 Participants with newly diagnosed lung cancer during the examination period: comparison of sputum cytology with the results of low-dose spiral computed tomography (LDSCT) of the thorax for the whole cohort (n = 187)

	Lung cancer	No lung cancer[a]	Total[b]
Sputum cytology			
Suspicious or pathological[c]	7	3	10
Regular or equivocal[d]	5	172	177
LDSCT			
Suspicious	11	6	17
Regular	1	169	170
Cytology and LDSCT			
At least one positive	12	8[e]	20
Both negative	0	167	167

[a]Including six lung cancer patients falling ill outside the examination period.
[b]The totals of test results in each group add up to n = 187.
[c]In at least one sputum sample.
[d]In all samples tested.
[e]In one participant, both results were positive.

cases with confirmed lung cancer, the sputum results showed no signs of malignancy and were considered as false negative (false-negative rate 42%). Four of these were peripheral tumours. When comparing the results of sputum cytology with the total number of confirmed lung cancer cases mostly diagnosed with biopsy, we calculated the sensitivity and specificity of cytology with 58% and 98%. The positive (PPV) and negative (NPV) predictive values were 70% and 97%.

Computed tomography

In 11 cases the results of computed tomography indicated malignant lung disease (Table 3). One lung cancer that could not be detected on LDSCT was a patient with a central nodule later diagnosed as squamous cell carcinoma. As the simultaneously done sputum cytology showed a pathological result, that case was counted as a false negative CT result (false negative rate 8.3%). In another six cases with radiological signs of pulmonary or pleural malignant disease the results of clinical work-up did not confirm the radiological diagnosis. Three patients suffered from tuberculoma, an atypical pneumonia and one was diagnosed with dystelectasis of unknown origin. Another two patients showed radiological signs of progressive pleural thickening, consistent with early stage malignant pleural mesothelioma. After explorative surgery including pleural and pulmonary biopsies the final diagnosis of chronic proliferative pleurisy with signs of early lung fibrosis was made. The remaining patient had a large pulmonary nodule, which showed no signs of growth over a period of 46 months and was therefore no longer seen as suspicious (false positive rate 3.4%). For the CT results, we calculated a sensitivity and specificity of 92% and 97%. The PPV and NPV were 65% and 99% respectively. When combining the results of both methods (Table 3), we obtained an overall sensitivity and specificity of 100% and 95%, with a PPV of 60% and a NPV of 100%.

New cases during follow-up

Of the remaining six patients with lung cancer indicated in Table 2 (cases 13 to 18), two developed their disease in the period between routine examinations (interval) and four after the examination period in August 2006 and the conclusion of follow-up by the end of 2009 (follow-up). None of these patients had pathological or equivocal findings on LDSCT or with sputum cytology in the baseline or re-examinations. The time period between last examination and recorded date of diagnosis lay between 17 and 19 months. In three of the patients we could secure a histological confirmation of the diagnosis lung cancer, one patient died in the year 2008 after refusing further examinations.

Discussion

The various forms of lung cancer are increasingly common and remain difficult to treat. As long as occupational and environmental causes of lung cancer, such as exposure to asbestos dust and tobacco smoking, cannot be abolished and the chance of recovery mainly depends on the stage of the disease, the early detection of lung cancer is the primary objective of focused health interventions. As the search for an effective biomarker indicating early disease was not successful so far, a combination of sensitive radiological imaging and a filter for detecting high risk individuals seems the most promising approach at present. Our study was based on the simultaneous use of sensitive, state-of-the-art radiological imaging and elaborate sputum cytology applied to a highly selected group of individuals. In theory, the combined use of imaging and cytology should help to further reduce the "blind spot" of radiological imaging regarding the early detection of central lung tumours. Other complementary screening strategies for lung cancer are under investigation, but they are either too invasive as a first-step screening method, such as fluorescence bronchoscopy, or their practical value has not been proven yet, such as exhaled breath analysis [24,25]. Our hypothesis was that parallel cytology could detect invisible, early stage central tumours or quickly confirm the malignant nature of tumours with a difficult location for taking biopsies. However, our highly selected but small study group together with the limited follow-up period were serious limitations for testing that hypothesis. It was possible that we might have missed some patients with newly diagnosed lung cancer, who were alive and were not reported to the BGETEM as suspect cases of occupational lung cancer. We would also have missed deceased lung cancer patients with a false or misleading diagnosis on their death certificates. From a practical point of view, the secondary objective of establishing a novel approach under routine working conditions appeared almost as important. While sputum cytology in combination with other screening methods has been tested before, there are no recent reports on larger scale use together with LDSCT in asbestos exposed individuals [25-27]. Our evaluation should therefore also be seen as a contribution to the debate, whether or not a formerly asbestos exposed participant of an early detection programme for lung cancer is willing to undergo additional, often inconvenient sputum testing. Large scale health programmes, even in individuals with an increased risk of disease, would be open for criticism when launched without convincing evidence of both, increased survival and reduced all-cause mortality. Due to scope and design of the study, we could not assess the overall effectiveness of lung cancer screening in asbestos exposed individuals. However, our results provide good indication of the value of a combined approach using CT-scans and sputum cytology.

When focussing on the occupational risk of lung cancer caused by the exposure to airborne asbestos, the identification of high-risk individuals is complicated by the formerly widespread, unprotected use of asbestos and the extremely long latency periods between exposure and disease. In our effort to form a high-risk group, who would benefit most from lung cancer screening, we linked the data on asbestos exposure with age and smoking habits, which resulted in a highly selected group of 4.2% of the total [21]. We could therefore assume with some certainty that the participants most at risk of developing lung cancer were included in the study group. However, it was also clear that the exposure data based on self-administered questionnaires might have been affected by a potential recall bias, especially in those who had started work several decades before. The data on cumulative exposure to asbestos and tobacco smoke (Table 1) should therefore be seen in the light of the long time periods since first exposure, stretching in some over an entire working life, and interpreted with caution.

Examination methods

In large-scale surveillance programmes, examination methods must be easy to handle and fit into tight working schedules. The methods should be standardized, not invasive and easily tolerated by the participants. The values for sensitivity and specificity should be well over 90%. In the light of these requirements, LDSCT seems to be an examination method, which is well suited for health surveillance. CT-scans can be performed within a few seconds, not causing any physical inconvenience or requiring a specific activity by the patient. The method of sputum collection at home is not invasive and is also a well-accepted procedure. Nevertheless, this technique is little standardized and the collection of sputum samples at home precludes technical guidance by an experienced person. It was therefore impractical to use induced sputum samples which would have required some technical support for the saline aerosol inhalation as usually only available at hospital. It was however clear that sputum induction would have allowed better quality samples and more valid results. In the context of our study, the approach of routine sputum sampling still proved to be a well feasible and acceptable surveillance method.

False-positive results

For participants with false positive results, the examination with LDSCT or sputum cytology had significant consequences. They usually underwent invasive and actually unnecessary examinations such as lung biopsy or thoracotomy with the risk of adverse effects and potentially even affecting the survival time of the individual. Health surveillance programmes for the early detection of lung cancer with high rates of false positive findings would be ineffective and difficult to justify. Humphrey et al. described recent LDSCT studies in which the false positive rates ranged from 5% to 50% of prevalence and 3% to 12% of incidence [8]. While in our study the false positive rates were minimal in comparison (1.7% with 3 of 175 sputum examinations and 3.4% with 6 of 175 LDSCT examinations), the positive predictive values of 70% and 65% respectively, and the resulting precision of sputum cytology and LDSCT were unsatisfactory. When combining the results of both methods, the resulting PPV of 60% was still lower. This was accompanied by a corresponding increase of sensitivity to 100%. Eight participants had to undergo actually unnecessary further investigations, which were however limited to sputum and CT controls after three months in the three participants with irregular sputum results. When defining as "false-positive" only those results leading to invasive clinical work up with negative outcome, we had no false positive sputum results.

Another important aspect when considering the consequences of false positive screening results was the fact that individuals informed on the results will usually experience an extended period of anxiety and concern before the results were confirmed false. That was also the case with one of our participants, who was admitted to a psychiatric institution for treatment of depression after being informed that a lung nodule suspicious of lung cancer had been found. It seems therefore essential that large scale early detection programmes for life threatening diseases such as lung cancer are carried out with the support of a network of specialists also including psychologists and psychiatrists, who can attend to individual patients.

Sputum findings

In a review of 16 representative studies to assess the sensitivity of sputum cytology, values ranging from 42% to 97% were calculated, depending on the location of the lesions [19]. However, the variety of methods made it difficult to assess the validity of these data. In our study, the calculated sensitivity of sputum cytology was with 58% low in comparison with the value for LDSCT of 92%. We considered the finding that one centrally located lung tumour invisible on LDSCT was detected by sputum cytology (in stage IIIb) as at least demonstrating the potential benefit of the method in a surveillance effort.

One of the false negative cases was equivocal for sputa with squamous cell metaplasia with moderate dysplasia (grade II). For such cases, we recommended a control sputum examination after three months (Figure 2). If immediate clinical work-up (Figure 2, dotted line) would be done, the rate of false-negative findings could be reduced and sensitivity improved. However, the positive predictive value would also have decreased from 70% to 53.8%, resulting in a reduced precision of sputum cytology and more false-positive results. To identify malignant cells by means of sputum cytology requires experienced personnel with a high degree of expertise. Sputum analysis using DNA image cytometry as an automated computer-assisted method to detect malignant cells may be an alternative, which is more suitable for widespread routine use. Sputum cytometry alone or better in combination with sputum cytology might increase the sensitivity of sputum examinations by 70 to 90% [28-30].

Location of lung tumours

The importance of tumour location on the sensitivity of sputum cytology has been described in previous studies [19,31]. Most of them showed decreased sensitivity for peripherally located masses, others could not find any difference. Our results seemed to indicate that centrally located tumours were diagnosed more often by sputum cytology (83%) than peripheral tumours (33%). One plausible explanation might be the closer contact of central tumours to the bronchogenic system. It may well be that in cases with a centrally located tumour the closer contact to the bronchogenic system could compensate for the higher risk of a false negative result of the CT scan. That risk is further increased by the standard technique of CT without contrast material.

Follow-up

Participants with normal examination results, who were diagnosed with lung cancer during follow-up, might be seen as "false negative" cases. However, the delay between examination and diagnosis let it appear unlikely that any signs of a developing carcinoma could have been picked up by CT scan or sputum cytology. The fact that four cases among a group of about 200 over a period of more than three years corresponded roughly with the expected true incidence may also indicate that specific symptoms and detectable signs of disease developed only after the examinations. As none of the participants with false positive results developed disease during follow-up, we can assume that they were truly false positive cases and the applied algorithm was effective in ruling out early stage lung disease.

Conclusions

Our results confirmed that (1) in surveillance programmes a combination of sputum cytology and LDSCT is well feasible and accepted by the participants. (2) Sputum examination alone is not effective for the detection of early stage lung cancer. (3) In high risk individuals, the combination of LDSCT scans and sputum cytology is probably more effective in detecting early lung cancer than LDSCT alone. However, the combination of both methods cannot be generally recommended as long as there is no evidence of a significant reduction of mortality and an improvement in overall survival. (4) For keeping false-positive and false-negative findings low, it is essential to ensure close cooperation with experienced clinicians and pathologists in a well-established interdisciplinary network.

Competing interests

The authors declare that they have no competing interests. This survey was supported financially by the Institution for Statutory Accident Insurance and Prevention in the Energy, Textile, Electrical and Media Industry (BGETEM, grant number 360057) and RWE Power AG (grant number 370221) with unrestricted grants to the Medical Faculty, RWTH Aachen University.

Authors' contributions

MKF and LK organized the cohort, examined most of the participants, managed the survey data and drafted the manuscript. TK, KGH and CF conceived the survey and planned the building of the cohort. TK and AB managed the collection of the sputum samples, AB organised and supervised their examination and interpreted the results. MD and TK read the CT-scans and interpreted the results. LK and CS did the statistical analysis of the survey data. All authors read and approved the final manuscript.

Acknowledgements

The authors wish to thank the doctors and staff of the investigation centres involved for sharing their knowledge and experience. Dr. J. Hüdepohl and PD Dr. W. Zschiesche of the Institution for Statutory Accident Insurance and Prevention in the Energy, Textile, Electrical and Media Industry (BGETEM) supported the building of the cohort and helped to design the framework of the survey. We also thank Dr. C.H. Winter, Stuttgart for his critical reading of the manuscript and his numerous other contributions. The various contributions and good will of many others, who supported our work, is gratefully acknowledged. We are also grateful to Kathy Bischof for reviewing the manuscript.

Author details

[1]Institute of Occupational and Social Medicine, Medical Faculty, RWTH Aachen University, Aachen, Germany. [2]Department of Diagnostic Radiology, Medical Faculty, RWTH Aachen University, Aachen, Germany. [3]RWE Power AG, Essen, Germany. [4]Department of Diagnostic Radiology, Knappschaftskrankenhaus, Dortmund, Germany. [5]Institute of Cytopathology, Heinrich Heine University, Düsseldorf, Germany. [6]Institute of Pathology, Düren Hospital, Düren, Germany. [7]Department of Radiology, Maastricht University Medical Centre, Maastricht, Netherlands.

References

1. **GLOBOCAN 2008, cancer incidence and mortality worldwide: IARC cancer base No. 10 [Internet].** http://globocan.iarc.fr.
2. American Cancer Society: *Cancer Facts and Figures 2010.* Atlanta: American Cancer Society; 2010.
3. Fontana RS, Sanderson DR, Taylor WF, Woolner LB, Miller WE, Muhm JR, Uhlenhopp MA: **Early lung cancer detection: results of the initial (prevalence) radiologic and cytologic screening in the Mayo Clinic study.** *Am Rev Respir Dis* 1984, **130:**561–565.
4. Frost JK, Ball WC Jr, Levin ML, Tockman MS, Baker RR, Carter D, Eggleston JC, Erozan YS, Gupta PK, Khouri NF, Marsh BR, Stitik FP: **Early lung cancer detection: results of the initial (prevalence) radiologic and cytologic screening in the Johns Hopkins study.** *Am Rev Respir Dis* 1984, **130:**549–554.
5. Flehinger BJ, Melamed MR, Zaman MB, Heelan RT, Perchick WB, Martini N: **Early lung cancer detection: results of the initial (prevalence) radiologic and cytologic screening in the Memorial Sloan-Kettering study.** *Am Rev Respir Dis* 1984, **130:**555–560.

6. Fontana RS, Sanderson DR, Woolner LB, Taylor WF, Miller WE, Muhm JR: **Lung cancer screening: the Mayo program.** *J Occup Med* 1986, **28:**746–750.
7. Eddy DM: **Screening for lung cancer.** *Ann Intern Med* 1989, **111:**232–237.
8. Humphrey LL, Teutsch S, Johnson M: **Lung cancer screening with sputum cytologic examination, chest radiography, and computed tomography: an update for the U.S. Preventive Services Task Force.** *Ann Intern Med* 2004, **140:**740–753.
9. Aberle DR, Adams AM, Berg CD, Black WC, Clapp JD, Fagerstrom RM, Gareen IF, Gatsonis C, Marcus PM, Sicks JD: **Reduced lung-cancer mortality with low-dose computed tomographic screening.** *N Engl J Med* 2011, **365:**395–409.
10. Raji OY, Duffy SW, Agbaje OF, Baker SG, Christiani DC, Cassidy A, Field JK: **Predictive accuracy of the Liverpool Lung Project risk model for stratifying patients for computed tomography screening for lung cancer: a case–control and cohort validation study.** *Ann Intern Med* 2012, **157:**242–250.
11. Kovalchik SA, Tammemagi M, Berg CD, Caporaso NE, Riley TL, Korch M, Silvestri GA, Chaturvedi AK, Katki HA: **Targeting of low-dose CT screening according to the risk of lung-cancer death.** *N Engl J Med* 2013, **369:**245–254.
12. **The 2004 United States Surgeon General's Report: the health consequences of smoking.** *N S W Public Health Bull* 2004, **15:**107.
13. Hammond EC, Selikoff IJ, Seidman H: **Asbestos exposure, cigarette smoking and death rates.** *Ann N Y Acad Sci* 1979, **330:**473–490.
14. Woitowitz HJ, Rodelsperger K: **Chrysotile asbestos and mesothelioma.** *Am J Ind Med* 1991, **19:**551–553.
15. Rösler JA, Woitowitz HJ, Lange HJ, Ulm K, Woitowitz RH, Rödelsberger K: **Forschungsbericht Asbest IV. Asbesteinwirkung am Arbeitsplatz und Sterblichkeit an bösartigen Tumoren in der Bundesrepublik Deutschland.** *Schriftenreihe des Hauptverbandes der Gewerblichen Berufsgenossenschaften, Sankt Augustin* 1993, **4:**1–160.
16. Henderson DW, Jones ML, De Klerk N, Leigh J, Musk AW, Shilkin KB, Williams VM: **The diagnosis and attribution of asbestos-related diseases in an Australian context: report of the Adelaide Workshop on Asbestos-Related Diseases. October 6–7, 2000.** *Int J Occup Environ Health* 2004, **10:**40–46.
17. Selikoff IJ, Hammond EC, Seidman H: **Latency of asbestos disease among insulation workers in the United States and Canada.** *Cancer* 1980, **46:**2736–2740.
18. Rivera MP, Detterbeck F, Mehta AC: **Diagnosis of lung cancer: the guidelines.** *Chest* 2003, **123:**129S–136S.
19. Schreiber G, McCrory DC: **Performance characteristics of different modalities for diagnosis of suspected lung cancer: summary of published evidence.** *Chest* 2003, **123:**115S–128S.
20. Felten MK, Knoll L, Eisenhawer C, Ackermann D, Khatab K, Hudepohl J, Zschiesche W, Kraus T: **Retrospective exposure assessment to airborne asbestos among power industry workers.** *J Occup Med Toxicol* 2010, **5:**15.
21. Das M, Muhlenbruch G, Mahnken AH, Hering KG, Sirbu H, Zschiesche W, Knoll L, Felten MK, Kraus T, Gunther RW, Wildberger JE: **Asbestos Surveillance Program Aachen (ASPA): initial results from baseline screening for lung cancer in asbestos-exposed high-risk individuals using low-dose multidetector-row CT.** *Eur Radiol* 2007, **17:**1193–1199.
22. Saccomanno G, Saunders RP, Archer VE, Auerbach O, Kuschner M, Beckler PA: **Cancer of the lung: the cytology of sputum prior to the development of carcinoma.** *Acta Cytol* 1965, **9:**413–423.
23. Mountain CF: **Revisions in the International System for Staging Lung Cancer.** *Chest* 1997, **111:**1710–1717.
24. Lam S, MacAulay C, LeRiche JC, Palcic B: **Detection and localization of early lung cancer by fluorescence bronchoscopy.** *Cancer* 2000, **89:**2468–2473.
25. Mascaux C, Peled N, Garg K, Kato Y, Wynes MW, Hirsch FR: **Early detection and screening of lung cancer.** *Expert Rev Mol Diagn* 2010, **10:**799–815.
26. Lam B, Lam SY, Wong MP, Ooi CG, Fong DY, Lam DC, Lai AY, Tam CM, Pang CB, Ip MS, Lam WK: **Sputum cytology examination followed by autofluorescence bronchoscopy: a practical way of identifying early stage lung cancer in central airway.** *Lung Cancer* 2009, **64:**289–294.
27. Swensen SJ, Jett JR, Hartman TE, Midthun DE, Sloan JA, Sykes AM, Aughenbaugh GL, Clemens MA: **Lung cancer screening with CT: Mayo Clinic experience.** *Radiology* 2003, **226:**756–761.
28. Marek W, Kotschy-Lang N, Muti A, Kohler CH, Nielsen L, Topalidis TH, Atay Z, Nakhosteen JA: **Can semi-automated image cytometry on induced sputum become a screening tool for lung cancer? Evaluation of quantitative semi-automated sputum cytometry on radon- and uranium-exposed workers.** *Eur Respir J* 2001, **18:**942–950.
29. Marek W, Richartz G, Philippou S, Marek L, Kotschy-Lang N: **Sputum screening for lung cancer in radon exposed uranium miners: a comparison of semi-automated sputum cytometry and conventional cytology.** *J Physiol Pharmacol* 2007, **58**(Suppl 5):349–361.
30. Palcic B, Garner DM, Beveridge J, Sun XR, Doudkine A, MacAulay C, Lam S, Payne PW: **Increase of sensitivity of sputum cytology using high-resolution image cytometry: field study results.** *Cytometry* 2002, **50:**168–176.
31. Boecking A, Biesterfeld S, Chatelain R, Gien-Gerlach G, Esser E: **Diagnosis of bronchial carcinoma on sections of paraffin-embedded sputum: sensitivity and specificity of an alternative to routine cytology.** *Acta Cytol* 1992, **36:**37–47.

Diisocyanate-induced asthma in Switzerland: long-term course and patients' self-assessment after a 12-year follow-up

Martin Rüegger, Doreen Droste, Markus Hofmann, Marcel Jost and David Miedinger*

Abstract

Background: Isocyanates are among the most common causes of occupational asthma (OA) in Switzerland. Patients with OA have been shown to have unfavourable medical, socioeconomic and psychological outcomes. We investigated long-term asthma and the socio-economic outcomes of diisocyanate-induced asthma (DIA) in Switzerland.

Patients and methods: We conducted an observational study on 49 patients with DIA and followed 35 of these patients over a mean exposure-free interval of 12 ± 0.5 (range 11.0-13.0) years. At the initial and follow-up examinations, we recorded data on respiratory symptoms and asthma medication; measured the lung function; and tested for bronchial hyperreactivity. We allowed the patients to assess their state of health and overall satisfaction using a visual analogue scale (VAS) at these visits.

Results: The 35 patients whom we could follow had a median symptomatic exposure time of 12 months, interquartile range (IQR) 26 months and a median overall exposure time of 51 (IQR 104) months. Their subjective symptoms ($p < 0.001$) and the use of asthma medication ($p = 0.002$), particularly the use of inhaled corticosteroids ($p < 0.001$), decreased by nearly 50%. At the same time, the self-assessment of the patients' state of health and overall satisfaction increased considerably according to both symptomatology and income. In contrast, slight reductions in terms of FVC% predicted from 102% to 96% ($p = 0.04$), of FEV1% predicted from 91% to 87% ($p = 0.06$) and of the FEV1/FVC ratio of 3%; ($p = 0.01$) were observed while NSBHR positivity did not change significantly. In univariate as well as multivariate logistic analyses we showed significant associations between age, duration of exposure and FEV1/FVC ratio with persistent asthma symptoms and NSBHR.

Conclusions: We found that the patients' symptoms, the extent of their therapy and the decrease in their lung volumes during the follow-up period were similar to the findings in the literature. The same hold true for some prognostic factors, whereas the patients' self-assessment of their state of health and overall satisfaction improved considerably.

Keywords: Occupational asthma, Diisocyanate asthma, Long-term follow-up, Self-assessment

Background

For more than two decades diisocyanates, a group of highly reactive and widely used chemicals, were one of the most common causes of occupational asthma in industrialised countries [1] though the incidence of diisocyanate induced occupational asthma (DIA) seems to have decreased over recent years [2-4].

* Correspondence: david.miedinger@suva.ch
Department of Occupational Medicine, Swiss National Insurance Fund Suva, Fluhmattstr. 1, CH 6002 Lucerne, Switzerland

Follow-up studies published during the last 20 years have shown a poor outcome for DIA even in the absence of additional exposure to the offending agent. Approximately 50-82% of persons who suffer from DIA do not recover completely and need continuous anti-asthmatic therapy [5-8]. According to the literature, recovery depends on a series of prognostic factors, such as the lung volume at the beginning of exposure [9], the time of diagnosis [10,11], the degree of bronchial hyperreactivity [9], the length of exposure time [12,13], the duration of symptomatic exposure [11,14,15] and possibly the duration of follow-up [16,17].

Until the early 1990s, there were only clinical follow-up studies on DIA that explored short time periods [7,8,12,13,18]. Therefore, we decided to do a long-term study with our own DIA patients beginning in 1993 and covering a time period of at least 10 years. Subsequently, in 2000 and in 2003, two carefully conducted studies on the outcome of patients with DIA over a 12-year follow-up were published [19,20].

The aim of our study was to investigate the long-term outcome of DIA in a non-preselected group of patients; we focussed on asthma symptoms, the need for treatment, changes in lung function and on nonspecific bronchial hyperreactivity (NSBHR). Further we wanted to evaluate the factors that were associated with persistent asthma symptoms and NSBHR [16] as well as the individual state of health and overall satisfaction at follow-up.

Materials and methods

All patients with suspected DIA reported to Suva (Swiss Accident Insurance Fund) between 1993 and 1995 were eligible for the study. Patients were included if the combination of their history and their spirometric findings, peak expiratory flow (PEF) recordings or inhalation challenge test results confirmed the diagnosis [21]. All of the patients gave their informed consent to participate in the study.

The patients who were admitted to our study had been exposed to one or more of the following diisocyanates: toluene diisocyanate (TDI), diphenylmethane diisocyanate (MDI), hexamethylene diisocyanate (HDI), naphthylene diisocyanate (NDI) or isophorone diisocyanate (IPDI) or one of their reactive prepolymers either continuously or intermittently.

We performed an uncontrolled observational study over 12 years. For each subject, a detailed clinical and occupational history was recorded and lung function and bronchoprovocation tests were performed between 1993 and 1995, i.e., at the time of diagnosis (T0), and again in 2006, at the time of re-evaluation (T1). The participants' longitudinal results are presented with data available at T0 and T1.

The data were recorded by one of Suva's occupational physicians at three different locations (Lausanne, Lucerne and Winterthur) during 1993–1995 (T0) and again in 2006 (T1) by DD as part of her doctoral thesis except two patients who were interviewed and examined by MH, and two others by their family doctors because of the patients' limited mobility. To ensure uniformity of questioning a checklist was used that had been established before. Most of the data have been collected routinely when evaluating notified cases in order to determine causality of occupational asthma (OA).

The subject's history included upper airway symptoms, such as nasal flow and itching, and lower airway symptoms, such as irritation, cough, wheezing, dyspnoea, chest tightness, and their temporal relationship to work. Additionally, information on the use of asthma medications, smoking habits, isocyanate exposure and current workplace as well as socioeconomic aspects were gathered.

In 2006, the subjects were asked to report their state of health as well as their overall satisfaction using two identical 10 cm neutral VASs. These measures reflect subjective factors in a global manner but correlate highly with several standard questionnaires and are accurate and useful for assessing symptoms, such as pain, anxiety and psychological distress [22]. Patients had to enter one mark retrospectively for the time T0 and another mark for the current time, T1. The second VAS mark could not be set until the first one was covered. The left end of the scale (0 cm) signified the worst rating conceivable, whereas the right end (10 cm) indicated the optimal rating.

Between 1993 and 1995, all patients had a walk-through visit by an occupational physician to confirm exposure to isocyanates and to exclude relevant co-exposure to other sensitizers or irritants that might have caused the reported symptoms (results not reported).

All of the patients underwent routine clinical examinations as well as standard lung function tests at one of Suva's three occupational medical centres. The tests conducted at time T0 and T1 included forced vital capacity (FVC), forced expiratory volume in 1 second (FEV1) and the FEV1/FVC ratio, which in most cases were measured by whole-body plethysmography (Jaeger MasterLab Germany, Vmax Autobox, VIASYS Healthcare Inc., SensorMedics, California, USA). The values published by the European Respiratory Society were used as reference values [23]. A significant obstructive ventilatory impairment was assumed to be present when the FEV1/FVC ratio was <0.7 [24].

To test NSBHR with acetyl-β-methylcholine chloride inhalation, Mefar dosimeters (Mefar MB3, Brescia, Italy) were used. The results were expressed as the cumulative doses required to provoke an FEV1 reduction of 20% (PD_{20}) graded according to the ATS scheme which was slightly modified [25]. If the FEV1 was <70% of the predicted value, the test was not performed, and the reversibility was checked by inhaling two puffs of salbutamol (200 µg DA). Generally we defined NSBHR in the participants as having a fall in FEV1 of >20% by inhaling ≤2 mg methacholine or having an increase in FEV1 of >10% after inhalation of salbutamol.

To confirm respiratory tract sensitisation to diisocyanates at T0, 31 of the 49 patients underwent a specific-inhalation challenge in the Thurgau-Schaffhausen Alpine Clinic in Davos according to a standardised protocol with the relevant diisocyanates or isocyanate-containing products.

Tests were positive if an FEV1 decrease of at least 20% could be demonstrated and if the dose response curve showed a typically shaped immediate, late or dual reaction [26].

To compare the results between the beginning and the end of the follow-up examinations, only complete data sets were accounted for; i.e., those of dropouts were discarded. In order to check for prognostic factors we also stratified participants according to their FEV1% predicted, FEV1/FVC ratio at T0 and a change in FEV1% predicted between T0 and T1.

Continuous variables are reported as a mean ± standard deviation (SD) or median plus interquartile range (IQR) when non-normally distributed. Statistical tests applied were the Kolmogorov-Smirnov, the McNemar's-, paired t-, Sign-, Wilcoxons-Mann–Whitney- and the chi-squared test. After performing univariate analyses, a logistic regression analysis with staggered inclusion of co-variates was performed to evaluate the effects of different variables on dependent variables such as "persistent asthma symptoms" and "persistent bronchial hyperresponsiveness at follow-up". In the "a priori" models we selected some variables (age at diagnosis, total exposure time, exposure time with symptoms) that were already shown to be associated with asthma outcome [16]. In the "a posteriori" models we included co-variates in whom univariate analyses showed significant or borderline associations with the dependent variables. Statistical analyses were performed by applying the PSPP software package [27]. To calculate mean values ± SD, median values and IQRs, Microsoft Excel for Mac Version 14.3.9 software was used. A $p < 0.05$ was considered to be statistically significant.

Results

Forty-nine patients (47 males, 2 females; mean age, 38 ± 13 years) were considered for inclusion into the study. These patients represented all individuals who claimed compensation between 1993 and 1995 and for whom the diagnosis of DIA could be established. Most of the study participants were car spray painters, industrial spray painters, furniture spray painters, carpenters and cabinet makers (49%), followed by polyurethane foam casters and moulders (37%) and other craftsmen (14%).

We observed that 86% of the subjects were no longer being exposed to isocyanates when the diagnosis of OA was made (T0). They had ended their exposure on average one month before the investigation (range, 30 months before to 7 months thereafter) because Suva declared 44 of them unsuitable for further isocyanate-related occupational activities (declaration of "unsuitability" [DOU]) [28]. Five patients could not be declared unsuitable because three of them were self-employed persons, one received an invalidity pension for a non-occupational disease and one was affected from DIA very early during his apprenticeship so that a DOU was not indicated. In practice, the DOU resulted in nearly all of the patients changing their workplace or their employer. The median overall isocyanate exposure time of the whole cohort was 57 months (IQR 108 months), and the median symptomatic exposure time was 16 months (IQR 30 months).

After a mean interval of 12 years (range, 11.0–13.0 years), 35 of the 49 patients could be contacted and agreed to be re-examined, corresponding to a re-examination rate of 71.4%. Figure 1 summarizes the flow of patients and the reasons for non-follow up. Twenty-two subjects (63%) were still working. One of them remained at the original workplace as a car spray painter but had switched to non-isocyanate-containing varnishes, 4 (11%) had relocated to completely isocyanate-free workplaces within the same company, and 17 (49%) had changed their job as well as their employer to avoid further isocyanate exposure. Thirteen subjects were no longer occupationally active, 7 due to premature or regular retirement; 3 were on social welfare, 2 were unemployed and one was on long-term sick leave unrelated to DIA.

The characteristics of the 35 participating subjects and the 14 dropouts are shown in Table 1. Except for the lower PD_{20} at T0 for those that were not re-examined later, the other variables did not significantly differ from those of the individuals that were re-investigated for this study.

Table 2 represents the changes in symptoms, asthma therapy, health status and overall satisfaction for those participants for whom follow-up data was available. It shows a significant decline in the frequency of symptoms, use of asthma medication - especially inhaled corticosteroids - and an increase in subjective health status and overall satisfaction.

Table 3 summarizes the results of pulmonary function tests for the 35 subjects who were re-examined for this study. Lung function values were slightly lower at T1 compared to T0 reaching the level of significance only for FEV% predicted and for the FEV1/FVC ratio. 34 of 35 participants were tested for NSBHR either by methacholine challenge or by bronchodilatation with salbutamol. While 23 subjects (68%) were positive at the time of diagnosis their number decreased to 17 (50%) at T1, a result that did not reach statistical significance ($p = 0.22$). When focussing on the 26 participants whose tests were done by the same method on both occasions (22 by methacholine and 4 by bronchodilatation) the number of positive results again dropped from 18 to 15 (14 methacholine and 4 bronchodilatation tests at T0; 14 methacholine and 1 bronchodilatation test at T1) a decline that again did not reach statistical significance. The same was true for those 22 patients who underwent methacholine challenge tests (median of PD_{20} 0.95 mg (IQR 1.68 mg) at T0 versus 0.70 mg (IQR 1.66 mg; $p = 0.81$) at T1.

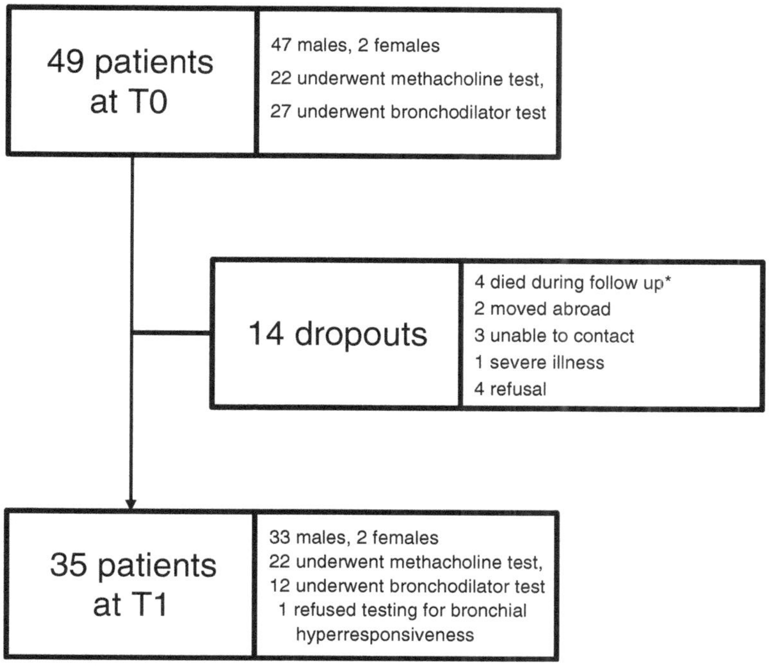

Figure 1 Flow-chart of recruited patients. Legend: T0 = time of diagnosis, T1 = time of re-evaluation. *Reasons for death (coronary heart disease (n = 1), aspiration pneumonia (n = 1), unknown (n = 2)).

Table 1 Baseline characteristics of participants and dropouts at T0 (n = 49)

	Participants (n = 35)	Dropouts (n = 14)	p-value
Age at diagnosis	39 ± 13	36 ± 13	0.53
Sex (males)	33 (94%)	14 (100%)	1.0
FVC% predicted	102 ± 17	97 ± 13	0.37
FEV1% predicted	91 ± 16	90 ± 16	0.89
FEV1/FVC	75 ± 9	74 ± 10	0.50
PD_{20} (mg)	0.95 (1.7)	0.30 (0.5)	0.03
NSBHR positivity	23 (68%)	11 (92%)	0.13
Total exposure time (months)	51 (104)	74 (89)	0.77
Time with symptoms (months)	12 (26)	24 (31)	0.38
Smokers	10 (29%)	6 (43%)	0.5
Pack-years*	25 (24)	13 (14)	0.16
Upper airway symptoms	28 (80%)	11 (79)	1.0
Asthma symptoms	34 (97%)	14 (100)	1.0
Asthma medication	31 (91%)	8 (89)	1.0

Legend: FVC = forced expiratory vital capacity. FEV1 = forced expiratory volume in 1 second. NSBHR = nonspecific bronchial hyperreactivity. PD20 = provocative dose of methacholine producing a fall in FEV1 of 20%. *Pack-years for smokers and ex-smokers added. Data is presented as mean ± SD, median and interquartile range (IQR) or number (%).

Tables 4, 5 and 6 show baseline characteristics according to lung function at T0 and lung function loss during follow-up. Age, FEV1/FVC, smoking variables and exposure data in those individuals with FEV1 < 80% predicted at T0 were not different from those with better lung function. The same was true for those with ≥15% loss of FEV1% predicted between T0 and T1. Individuals with a FEV1/FVC ratio <0.7 at T0 had a lower FEV1% predicted and a higher tobacco consumption than those with higher FEV1/FVC ratio.

Table 2 Change in symptoms, therapy and visual analogue scale (VAS) ratings between T0 and T1 (n = 35)

	T0	T1	p-value
Upper airway symptoms	28 (80%)	9 (26%)	<0.001
Asthma symptoms	34 (97%)	20 (57%)	<0.001
Use of asthma medication*	31 (91%)	19 (56%)	0.002
Short acting beta2 agonists	19 (56%)	13 (38%)	0.18
Long acting beta2 agonists	10 (29%)	10 (29%)	1.0
Inhalable corticosteroids	26 (76%)	10 (29%)	<0.001
Smokers	10 (29 %)	14 (40%)	0.05
VAS (cm) health status	1.2 (2.9)	8.0 (4.0)	<0.001
VAS (cm) overall satisfaction	2.1 (6.1)	8.3 (3.4)	<0.001

Legend: Upper airway symptoms (conjunctivitis, rhinitis, hoarseness, pharyngeal irritant sensations); asthma symptoms (irritation, wheezing, chronic cough, chest tightness and dyspnoea); VAS = visual analogue scale. Data is presented as mean ± SD, median and interquartile range (IQR) or number (%). *n = 34.

Table 3 Results of lung function and hyperreactivity testing at T0 and T1

	T0	T1	p-value
FVC% predicted	102 ± 17	96 ± 17	0.04
FEV1% predicted	91 ± 16	87 ± 18	0.06
FEV1/FVC	76 ± 9	73 ± 8	0.01
PD_{20} (mg)	0.95 (1.7)	0.70 (1.7)	0.81

Legend: FVC = forced vital capacity. FEV1 = forced expiratory volume in one second. PD20 = provocative dose of methacholine causing a 20% fall in FEV1. NSBHR = nonspecific bronchial hyperreactivity.
Data is presented as mean ± SD or median and interquartile range (IQR).

The results of the multivariate logistic regression analysis can be seen in Table 7. In the "a priori" models age was associated with persistent asthma symptoms at follow-up (p = 0.02) and persistent NSBHR was associated with total exposure time (p = 0.04). In the predictive "a posteriori" model the degree of airflow limitation at diagnosis was associated with persistent asthma symptoms at T1 (p = 0.05). Asthma medication (p < 0.001) and age (p = 0.06) at T1 were associated with asthma symptoms both at follow up.

Discussion

The aim of our 12-year follow-up study was to investigate the long-term outcome of patients with DIA, to check for possible prognostic factors and to compare these results obtained in Switzerland with those reported in the literature, primarily of the two previously cited larger cohorts of patients with DIA [19,20]. We found that at a mean of 12 years after removal from exposure to the offending diisocyanates, the majority of the patients reported fewer respiratory symptoms, decreased asthma medication use and a better self-reported overall health status while lung function values at follow up were slightly lower compared to normal.

At T1, 14 of the initially evaluated 49 patients at T0 could not be retraced (dropout rate 28.6%). The 35 patients who could be followed until T1 represent a small sample size, a fact that weakened the informative value of our results. Piirilä (8% non-responders in their first phase questionnaire survey) and, particularly, Padoan and co-workers (no non-responders) did clearly better in this regard. Nevertheless, the 71.4% who re-participated in our study were within the range of other but shorter follow-up studies [15,29-32]. When analysing our data retrospectively, dropouts were having a more pronounced bronchial hyperreactivity (p = 0.03) at diagnosis compared to participants. With respect to all the other variables such as smoking status, job groups (data not shown), age, the presence of airway symptoms, the level of FVC and FEV1% predicted as well as the FEV1/FVC ratio or the overall exposure time period, we could not find any significant differences between study participants and dropouts. Thus we believe that the participants represent fairly well the whole study group, a fact that might outweigh to some extent its small sample size.

Based on the average number of the Swiss working population of 4 millions during 1993 – 1995 (Swiss

Table 4 Baseline characteristics of patients according to their FEV1 at T0

	FEV1 ≥ 80% pred. (n = 28)	FEV1 < 80% pred. (n = 7)	p-value
Age	38 ± 13	42 ± 10	0.44
FEV1/FVC	77 ± 8	72 ± 11	0.20
Current smoking	8 (29%)	2 (29%)	1.0
Pack years*	7 (15)	20 (13)	0.37
Total exposure time (months)	51 (99)	53 (129)	0.68
Symptomatic exposure time (months)	13 (34)	8 (14)	0.22

Legend: FVC = forced expiratory vital capacity. FEV1 = forced expiratory volume in 1 second. *Pack-years for smokers and ex-smokers added.
Data is presented as mean ± SD, median and interquartile range (IQR) or number (%).

Table 5 Baseline characteristics of patients according to their FEV1/FVC ratio at T0

	FEV1/FVC ≥ 0.7 (n = 25)	FEV1/FVC < 0.7 (n = 10)	p-value
Age (years)	37 ± 14	42 ± 9	0.34
FEV1% predicted	95 ± 13	83 ± 20	<0.001
Current smoking	7 (28%)	3 (30%)	1.00
Pack years*	5 (12)	20 (20)	<0.001
Total exposure time (months)	44 (80)	145 (143)	0.16
Symptomatic exposure time (months)	11 (15)	19 (33)	0.31

Legend: FVC = forced expiratory vital capacity. FEV1 = forced expiratory volume in 1 second. *Pack-years for smokers and ex-smokers added.
Data is presented as mean ± SD, median and interquartile range (IQR) or number (%).

Table 6 Baseline characteristics of patients according to their FEV1 loss between T0 and T1

	FEV1 loss < 15% (n = 28)	FEV1 loss ≥15% (n = 7)	p-value
Age	37 ± 13	45 ± 10	0.11
FEV1% pred.at T0	90 ± 17	98 ± 13	0.25
FEV1/FVC at T0	77 ± 9	72 ± 7	0.25
Current smoking	8 (29%)	2 (29%)	1.0
Pack years*	11 (17)	11 (17)	0.42
Total exposure time (months)	46 (91)	62 (169)	0.32
Symptomatic exposure time (months)	11 (19)	19 (49)	0.40

Legend: FVC = forced expiratory vital capacity. FEV1 = forced expiratory volume in 1 second. *Pack-years for smokers and ex-smokers added.
Data is presented as mean ± SD, median and interquartile range (IQR) or number (%).

Table 7 Multivariate logistic regression analysis of predictors for persistent asthma at follow-up

	"A priori"		"A posteriori"	
			Predictive	Descriptive
	Model 1	Model 2	Model 3	Model 4
Dependent variables	Persistent asthma symptoms at follow-up	Persistent NSBHR at follow-up	Persistent asthma symptoms at follow-up	Persistent asthma symptoms at follow-up
Co-variates				
Age at T0	0.08 (p = 0.02)	0.03 (p = 0.35)	0.04 (p = 0.27)	
Age at T1				0.09 (p = 0.06)
Total exposure time		−0.02 (p = 0.04)		
Symptomatic exposure time	0.01 (p = 0.37)	0.03 (p = 0.10)		
Upper airway symptoms at T0			−1.91 (p = 0.12)	
Upper airway symptoms at T1				1.36 (p = 0.29)
FEV1/FVC at T0			−0.11 (p = 0.05)	
Asthma medication at T1				2.85 (p < 0.001)
Intercept	−2.90	−0.32	9.01	−5.98
R^2	0.22	0.28	0.39	0.55

Legend: FVC = forced expiratory vital capacity, FEV1 = forced expiratory volume in 1 second. NSBHBR = non specific bronchial hyperreactivity. R^2 = Nagelkerke R Square. Data are presented as B-coefficient (p-value).

Federal Statistical Office) the 49 DIA cases correspond to a yearly incidence rate of 4.1 cases/million which is somewhat higher than in France by ONAP indicating 3.5 cases/million [33] but considerably lower than the 10.8 cases/million reported by the PROPULSE program in Québec, Canada [34]. To note that both these sentinel programs became active during the 1990ies i.e. during the same time period when we were following-up our patients and – more important - that we report on legally compensated cases only unlike those published from Québec and from France.

Removing an asthmatic worker from the offending agent leads to an improvement in asthma severity, a fact that was confirmed by Rachiotis and co-workers [16] when doing a systematic literature review and meta-analysis on the outcome of occupational asthma after cessation of exposure. The authors found a pooled rate of symptomatic recovery of 32% (95% CI 26%–38%). This finding is in agreement with the results of a recent review issued by Baur and co-workers [21], who found that, on average, 33.7% of patients (95% CI 23.6%–45.6%) no longer exhibited symptoms after complete cessation of exposure to the offending agent. These results indicate that usually more than 50% of the subjects remain symptomatic, which is in line with our figures showing that 57% of the patients continued to complain of asthma symptoms at follow up, a finding that is slightly better than that observed in the studies by Piirilä and Padoan [19,20], in which more than two thirds of the patients remained asthmatic.

In our study most of the patients were still on anti-asthmatic medication at follow-up; more than half of them were taking it on a regular basis, whereas 10 were still inhaling corticosteroids. These results are comparable to those of both the Piirilä and the Padoan studies, in which 66% and 60%, respectively, of the patients required some form of anti-asthmatic treatment at the end of their follow-up, approximately half of them again on a regular basis in the Piirilä study [19]. According to an extended literature survey that was conducted by the Agency for Healthcare Research and Quality (AHRQ), the proportion of OA patients who require medication after cessation of exposure ranges from 17% to 100%, depending to a great extent on the characteristics of the cohort and on exposure. Furthermore, the AHRQ data suggest that 4 years after removal of the offending low-molecular-weight agent, approximately half of the patients are still under treatment [35], which is in line with what we have observed.

In contrast to the Piirilä and the Padoan studies, we asked the patients to assess their individual state of health as well as their overall satisfaction using a VAS. To the best of our knowledge, these factors have not been addressed in another comparable long-term DIA study. On a group basis, we observed a statistically significant increase in self-reported health status and overall satisfaction between T0 and T1, results that were comparable to those of the Karvala study, in which the overall quality of life parameter in patients with occupational asthma to moulds was reported to be between 6.5 and 7.4 [36]. When we stratified our VAS ratings according to the presence or the absence of symptoms, we observed that those without asthma symptoms at follow-up were reporting even better satisfaction than those with persistent symptoms (data not shown). Assuming that by far the majority of "normal persons" would not set their VAS mark precisely on 10 but rather somewhat lower, our results for the group without symptoms at follow-up do not likely differ from what could be expected from healthy people.

We admit that VAS results have to be interpreted with caution. First of all one can argue that patients who could not be followed up – dropouts - would have been more seriously diseased judging their quality of life significantly lower than the participants thus biasing the observed results in a too optimistic direction. However we think that this hypothesis is not very probable, as – with the exception of PD_{20} – there were no significantly different baseline characteristics between participants and dropouts (Table 1). Secondly there is no doubt that any self-assessment, especially if done retrospectively, is subjective and can thus be biased. However we had no indication for subjects to under or over report their state of health at T0 or T1 except that – in theory - some over-reporting could have been expected because the interviewers were physicians who were employed by Suva the compensating body. Such a tendency could have biased the VAS markings towards a lower level at T0 as well as at T1 thus not decisively change the absolute amount of improvement we observed.

Complete cessation of exposure to the offending agent improves symptoms as well as lung function [37] but is associated with worse socioeconomic outcomes [15,35,38], thereby increasing anxiety and depressive symptoms [31,39-41] that, in turn, have a negative impact on asthma outcome. When examining the data on socioeconomic factors at T1, we found that those 13 patients who were not working lost on average 19.2% of their income, 7 of them after retiring regularly or prematurely, incurring an income reduction either way. Those who were still economically active (22 of 35) had a salary increase of 13.7% (after retraining) or a slight loss of 6% (without retraining) [42]. To look at the impact of both symptoms and income on overall satisfaction at the end of the follow-up, we found that persisting asthmatic symptoms entailed a clearly lower VAS ranking than the loss of income. It is obvious that the latter does not reflect all aspects of possible socioeconomic problems. Nevertheless, we think that once financial problems have been managed and an alternative job is found, to the patients' satisfaction, psychological distress will be alleviated, resulting in better tolerability of the remaining symptoms, as observed by Piirilä and Keskinen [19,43].

Lung function in the participants was lower than those reported in the Piirilä and the Padoan studies (99.6% and 98.8% predicted respectively) [19,20]. According to the literature, the lungs are not completely developed by late adolescence, with lung function values not plateauing until early in the third decade of life [44]. Two of our 35 subjects were only 17 and 18 years old at diagnosis, a fact that could explain the slight reduction in the average lung volumes at the beginning of the study but not an isolated decrease in FEV1.

The decreases in FVC% predicted as well as in the FEV1/FVC ratio between T0 and T1 were small but significant, whereas the FEV1% predicted changed only insignificantly even though the number of patients with overt airflow limitation remained numerically constant ($n = 10$). These results are again consistent with those of Piirilä, Padoan and others, indicating slight but overt lung function deterioration during follow-up.

When specifically looking at the observed small FEV1/FVC decrease, which is based on a fixed lower limit of 0.7 instead of using calculated limits of normal, as has been recommended earlier [45,46], we believe that this decrease might be attributed, at least in part, to the physiological loss of elastic recoil by ageing. This argument holds true only if one assumes that any substantial recovery of the lung volume of our subjects occurred during the approximately one-month time period between the cessation of exposure and the examination at T0, outweighing the observed volume decrease. In any case it is questionable whether the observed small lung function decreases are clinically relevant. Another possible explanation for the decrease in lung volumes might be persisting diisocyanate exposure. However, this can be largely ruled out because 86% of the subjects had been removed from any further contact by the time of T0, although 9 persons reported having had sporadic and unintended diisocyanate exposures during the follow-up period.

Overall there was a trend for a decrease in the number of individuals with NSBHR having either a positive challenge test to methacholine or a significant reversibility after inhalation of a short acting bronchodilatator. However when considering PD_{20} in individuals who underwent methacholine testing at the beginning and at the end of the follow up period, no significant change could be observed. It is well known that the duration of symptomatic exposure and the level of NSBHR are risk factors for persistent NSBHR and that some individuals keep their NSBHR despite complete removal from the exposing allergen in the workplace [16,21,47]. We believe that two factors might explain our result: Firstly our NSBHR test pairs are incomplete, potentially biasing the result in favour of those subjects doing worse; and secondly we observed an overall increase of active smokers during follow-up (Table 2), which by itself might be a risk factor for NSBHR [48].

When analysing our participants according to their lung function at T0 or its change during follow up (Tables 4, 5 and 6) we did not find any significant differences concerning age and exposure parameters between affected and non affected individuals, FEV1 and tobacco consumption for the patients with a FEV1/FVC ratio <0.7 (Table 5) excluded, though some of the criteria we looked at are known prognostic factors of OA [9,16,21].

The presence of airflow limitation is a known prognostic factor for asthma, COPD and other (respiratory) diseases. When we compared the patients having an FEV1/FVC ratio <0.7 with those who were non-obstructive at T0 (Table 5) we found the former to have started with a significantly lower FEV1% predicted and to have had a significantly higher tobacco consumption while the other parameters did not differ between the two groups (Table 5) [16,21]. Again these results are very well comparable with what has been published in the literature except for tobacco consumption that is not an accepted risk factor for DIA [6,9]. Nevertheless we assume that in some of our patients airflow limitation at T0 was due to both isocyanate as well as tobacco exposure, the latter playing an explicit role as aggravating factor as it is known that smoking adversely affects asthma outcome due to altered airway inflammation and corticosteroid insensitivity contributing therefore to a high rate of symptom persistence and lung function loss at follow-up [49]. Further it is possible that some of our subjects started their isocyanate exposure with a pre-existing airflow limitation, a hypothesis we cannot prove because we do not dispose of any medical data for the time when they started their isocyanate exposure.

When we further stratified our cohort according to the FEV1 loss that was observed between T0 and T1 (Table 6) we largely obtained the same results: The "marked decliners" (FEV1 loss ≥15% predicted) tended to be older, to have a lower FEV1% predicted at T0 and a longer total diisocyanate as well as a symptomatic exposure time.

Finally we tried to identify factors that were associated with the long-term outcome such as persistent asthmatic symptoms and NSBHR by performing a multivariate logistic regression analysis. Several studies did report that duration of (symptomatic) exposure and age at diagnosis are associated with adverse outcomes of occupational and non-occupational asthma [9,16,21]. This is what we could confirm in the "a priori model" as age and exposure time were associated with DIA outcomes. In the "a posteriori model" the FEV1/FVC ratio was the factor that best predicted persistent asthma symptoms at follow-up. Finally age and asthma medication at follow-up were the co-variates that were associated with persistent asthma symptoms at follow-up. To note that age might be linked to the length of exposure, two variables that have not been clearly disentangled until now [9]. However in our sample age and total exposure time did not correlate at all (Pearson Correlation Coefficient = 0.11, $p = 0.47$) while total exposure time showed only a moderate correlation with symptomatic exposure time (Pearson Correlation Coefficient = 0.53, $p < 0.001$). Rachiotis and co-workers found - based on 2 studies only – older patients to be more likely to completely recover from NSBHR while 5 out of 6 other cited studies reported shorter durations of exposure to be associated with a better outcome in terms of physiological recovery respectively NSBHR. Rachiotis' result is supported – at least in tendency - by Baur and colleagues [21] who pointed to the fact that the data from the literature they based their report upon were mostly not significant. To conclude there is no firmly established association between NSBHR and independent variables such as age and duration of exposure while NSBHR positivity at the time of diagnosis is a negative prognostic factor [9,21].

The finding of an association between the FEV1/FVC ratio at T0 and the persistence of asthma symptoms at T1 is supported by the review of Maestrelli and co-workers who stated that impaired lung function at diagnosis had a negative role on the outcome of OA though they report only isolated data on FEV1 and FVC but not on their ratio.

In retrospect, we recognised that medical examinations dating back to the start of exposure would have been very helpful enabling us to look for individuals at risk when further exposed to noxious substances at their workplaces. As part of preventive measures, we would recommend reasonable medical pre-employment or at least surveillance programs to be introduced not only for all isocyanate-exposed workers but for all persons at risk to develop occupational asthma [1,21,50,51].

Conclusion

In conclusion, we found that more than 50% of our 35 subjects suffering from DIA reported to remain symptomatic, had worse lung function and were in need of therapy for asthma after an exposure-free follow-up period of 12 years. In contrast, the patients' self-assessment of their health and overall satisfaction increased considerably during the observation period, which is primarily a consequence of becoming symptom free and having satisfactorily resolved their socioeconomic problems. Persistence of asthma symptoms and NSBHR was associated with age, exposure time and lung function at the time of diagnosis (T0). Our results suggest that surveillance programs as well as information on occupational risks for asthma and early symptoms recognition should be offered to the workforce thereby not excluding older and experienced workers as they are still at risk for DIA the latter being characterized by worse outcomes. Finally workers and especially patients with diagnosed occupational asthma should receive counselling on smoking cessation as continuous smoking may adversely affect asthma outcomes.

Abbreviations
DIA: Diisocyanate asthma; NSBHR: Non-specific bronchial hyperreactivity; DOU: Declaration of unfitness; OA: Occupational asthma; PEF: Peak expiratory flow; VAS: Visual analogue scale.

Competing interests
The authors declare that they have no competing interests.

Authors' contributions
MR was involved in the initial planning of the study. He also drafted and revised the manuscript. DD performed all but four of the follow-up examinations. She also wrote a doctoral thesis evaluating additional data that were not included in the present paper. MH conducted two of the remaining follow-up examinations. MJ was the initiator of the study and the former chief occupational physician and head of Suvas' occupational medical department. DM critically revised the study results and contributed substantial medical as well as statistical input. All of the co-authors read and approved the final manuscript.

Acknowledgements
First, all the authors would like to thank all of the patients for their participation and their former and active colleagues of the occupational medical department of Suva who performed the initial medical examinations at T0 as well as the on-site visits at the different work places. We extend our special appreciation to the laboratory staff from Lucerne, Lausanne and Winterthur, who performed all of the lung function tests, and finally, to B. Villiger and F. Schwarz from the former Thurgau Schaffhausen Alpine Clinic in Davos for conducting the specific bronchoprovocation tests.

Funding
The costs of the examinations as well as other expenses, such as for travelling, were covered by Suva. There was no additional third party funding.

References
1. Baur X, Aasen TB, Sherwood Burge P, Heederik D, Henneberger PK, Maestrelli P, Schlünssen V, Vandenplas O, Wilken D: **The management of work-related asthma guidelines: a broader perspective.** *Respir Rev* 2012, **21**:125–139.
2. Paris C, Ngatchou-Wandji J, Luc A, McNamee R, Bensefa-Colas L, Larabi L, Telle-Lamberton M, Herin F, Bergeret A, Bonneterre V, Brochard P, Choudat D, Dupas D, Garnier R, Pairon JC, Agius RM, Ameille J: **Work-related asthma in France: recent trends for the period 2001–2009.** *Occup Environ Med* 2012, **69**:391–397.
3. Buyantseva LV, Liss GM, Ribeiro M, Manno M, Luce CE, Tarlo SM: **Reduction in diisocyanate and non-diisocyanate sensitizer-induced occupational asthma in Ontario.** *J Occup Environ Med* 2011, **53**:420–426.
4. Vandenplas O, Lantin AC, D'Alpaos V, Larbanois A, Hoet P, Vandeweerdt M, Thimpont J, Speybroeck N: **Time trends in occupational asthma in Belgium.** *Respir Med* 2011, **105**:1364–1372.
5. Piirilä PL, Meuronen A, Majuri M-L, Luukkonen R, Mäntylä T, Wolff HJ, Nordman H, Alenius H, Laitinen A: **Inflammation and functional outcome in diisocyanate-induced asthma after cessation of exposure.** *Allergy* 2008, **63**:583–591.
6. Mapp CE, Boschetto P, Maestrelli P, Fabbri LM: **Occupational asthma, state of the art.** *Am J Respir Crit Care Med* 2005, **172**:280–305.
7. Mapp CE, Corona PC, De Marzo N, Fabbri LM: **Persistent asthma due to isocyanates: a follow-up study of subjects with occupational asthma due to toluene diisocyanate (TDI).** *Am Rev Respir Dis* 1988, **137**:1326–1329.
8. Lozewicz S, Assoufi BK, Hawkins R, Taylor AJ: **Outcome of asthma induced by isocyanates.** *Br J Dis Chest* 1987, **81**:14–22.
9. Maestrelli P, Schlünssen V, Mason P, Sigsgaard T: **Contribution of host factors and workplace exposure to the outcome of occupational asthma.** *Eur Respir Rev* 2012, **21**:88–96.
10. Tarlo SM, Balmes J, Balkissoon R, Beach J, Beckett W, Bernstein D, Blanc PD, Brooks SM, Cowl CT, Daroowalla F, Harber P, Lemiere C, Liss GM, Pacheco KA, Redlich CA, Rowe B, Heitzer J: **Diagnosis and management of work-related asthma: American College Of Chest Physicians Consensus Statement.** *Chest* 2008, **134**(Suppl 3):1S–41S.
11. Park HS, Nahm DH: **Prognostic factors for toluene diisocyanate-induced occupational asthma after removal from exposure.** *Clin Exp Allergy* 1997, **27**:145–150.
12. Pisati G, Baruffini A, Zedda S: **Toluene diisocyanate induced asthma: outcome according to persistence or cessation of exposure.** *Br J Ind Med* 1993, **50**:60–64.
13. Rosenberg N, Garnier R, Rousselin X, Mertz R, Gervais P: **Clinical and socio-professional fate of isocyanate-induced asthma.** *Clin Allergy* 1987, **17**:55–61.
14. Pisati G, Baruffini A, Bernabeo F, Cerri S, Mangili A: **Rechallenging subjects with occupational asthma due to toluene diisocyanate (TDI), after long-term removal from exposure.** *Arch Occup Environ Health* 2007, **80**:298–305.
15. Gannon PFG, Weir DC, Robertson AS, Sherwood Burge P: **Health., employment, and financial outcomes in workers with occupational asthma.** *Br J Ind Med* 1993, **50**:491–496.
16. Rachiotis G, Savani R, Brant A, MacNeill St J, Newman Taylor A, Cullinan P: **Outcome of occupational asthma after cessation of exposure: a systematic review.** *Thorax* 2007, **62**:147–152.
17. Perfetti L, Cartier A, Ghezzo H, Gautrin D, Malo JL: **Follow-up of occupational asthma after removal from or diminution of exposure to the responsible agent: relevance of the length of the interval from cessation of exposure.** *Chest* 1988, **114**:298–403.
18. Paggiaro PL, Vagaggini B, Dente FL, Bacci E, Bancalari L, Carrara M, Di Franco A, Giannini D, Giuntini C: **Bronchial hyperresponsiveness and toluene diisocyanate. Long-term change in sensitized asthmatic subjects.** *Chest* 1993, **103**:1123–1128.
19. Piirilä PL, Nordman H, Keskinen HM, Luukkonen R, Salo S-P, Tuomi TO, Tuppurainen M: **Long-term follow-up of hexamethylene diisocyanate-, diphenylmethane diisocyanate-, and toluenediisocyanate-induced asthma.** *Am J Respir Crit Care Med* 2000, **162**:516–522.
20. Padoan M, Pozzato V, Simoni M, Zedda L, Milan G, Bononi I, Piola C, Maestrelli P, Boschetto P, Mapp CE: **Long-term follow-up of toluene diisocyanate-induced asthma.** *Eur Respir J* 2003, **21**:637–640.
21. Baur X, Sigsgaard T, Aasen TB, Burge PS, Heederik D, Henneberger P, Maestrelli P, Rooyackers J, Schlünssen V, Vandenplas O, Wilken D: **Guidelines for the management of work-related asthma. ERS Task Force Report.** *Eur Respir J* 2012, **39**:529–545.
22. de Boer AGEM, van Lanschot JJB, Stalmeier PFM, van Sandick JW, Hulscher JBF, de Haes JCJM, Sprangers MAG: **Is a single-item visual analogue scale as valid, reliable and responsive as multi-item scales in measuring quality of life?** *Qual Life Res* 2004, **13**:311–320.
23. Quanjer PH, Tammeling GJ, Cotes JE, Pedersen OF, Peslin R, Yernault JC: **Lung volumes and forced ventilatory flows: Report working party standardization of lung function tests, European Community for steel and coal. Official statement of the European Respiratory Society.** *Eur Respir J* 1993, **16**(suppl):5–40.
24. Celli BR, MacNee W: **Standards for the diagnosis and treatment of patients with COPD: a summary of the ATS/ERS position paper.** *Eur Respir J* 2004, **23**:932–946.
25. American Thoracic Society: **Guidelines for methacholine and exercise challenge testing – 1999.** *Am J Respir Crit Care Med* 2000, **161**:309–329.
26. Vandenplas O, Malo JL: **Inhalation challenges with agents causing occupational asthma.** *Eur Respir J* 1997, **10**:2612–2629.
27. Pfaff B, Darrington J, Stover J, Satman MH, Williams J, Kiefte M, Kobly P, van Son R: *GNU PSPP. Version 0.8.2.* Boston: Free Software Foundation; 2014:2014.
28. Jost M, Rast H: **Assessment of the suitability of workers based on the Swiss Law on Accident Insurance–declaration of unsuitability/declaration of conditional suitability. [Article in German].** *Ther Umsch* 2007, **64**:437–442.
29. Lemière C, Chaboillez S, Welman M, Maghni K: **Outcome of occupational asthma after removal from exposure: A follow-up study.** *Can Respir J* 2010, **17**:61–66.
30. Gautrin D, Ghezzo H, Infante-Rivard C, Magnan M, L'Archevêque J, Suarthana E, Malo JL: **Long-term outcomes in a prospective cohort of apprentices exposed to high-molecular-weight agents.** *Am J Respir Crit Care Med* 2008, **177**:871–879.
31. Labrecque M, Khemici E, Cartier A, Malo JL, Turcot J: **Impairment in workers with isocyanate-induced occupational asthma and removed from exposure in the province of Québec between 1985 and 2002.** *J Occup Environ Med* 2006, **48**:1093–1098.

32. Maghni K, Lemière C, Ghezzo H, Yuquan W, Malo JL: **Airway inflammation after cessation of exposure to agents causing occupational asthma.** *Am J Respir Crit Care Med* 2004, **169:**367–372.
33. Ameille J, Pauli G, Calastreng-Crinquand A, Vervloët D, Iwatsubo Y, Popin E, Bayeux-Dunglas MC, Kopferschmitt-Kubler MC, and the corresponding members ofthe ONAP: **Reported incidence of occupational asthma in France, 1996–99: the ONAP programme.** *Occup Environ Med* 2003, **60:**136–141.
34. Provencher S, Labrèche FP, De Guire L: **Physician based surveillance system for occupational respiratory diseases: the experience of PROPULSE, Quebec, Canada.** *Occup Environ Med* 1997, **54:**272–276.
35. Beach J, Rowe BH, Blitz S, Crumley E, Hooton N, Russell K, Spooner C, Klassen T: **Diagnosis and management of work-related asthma.** In *Evidence Report/Technology Assessment Number 129.* Prepared for Agency for Healthcare Research and Quality, U.S. Department of Health and Human Services, 540 Gaither Road, Rockville, MD 20850: AHRQ Publication; 2005. www.ahrq.gov.
36. Karvala K, Uitti J, Luukkonen R, Nordman H: **Quality of life of patients with asthma related to damp and moldy work environments.** *Scand J Work Environ Health* 2013, **39:**96–105.
37. Vandenplas O, Dressel H, Nowak D, Jamart J: **What is the optimal management option for occupational asthma?** *Eur Respir Rev* 2012, **21:**97–104.
38. Vandenplas O, Dressel H, Wilken D, Jamart J, Heederik D, Maestrelli P, Sigsgaard T, Henneberger P, Baur X: **Management of occupational asthma: cessation or reduction of exposure? A systematic review of available evidence.** *Eur Respir J* 2011, **38:**804–811.
39. Miedinger D, Lavoie KL, L'Archeveque J, Ghezzo H, Malo JL: **Identification of clinically significant psychological distress and psychiatric morbidity by examining quality of life in subjects with occupational asthma.** *Health Qual Life Outcomes* 2011, **9:**76.
40. Miedinger D, Lavoie KL, L'Archevêque J, Ghezzo H, Zunzunuegui MV, Malo JL: **Quality-of-life, psychological, and cost outcomes 2 years after diagnosis of occupational asthma.** *J Occup Environ Med* 2011, **53:**231–238.
41. Lavoie KL, Joseph M, Bacon SL: **Psychological distress and occupational asthma.** *Curr Opin Allergy Clin Immunol* 2009, **9:**103–109.
42. Rüegger M, Droste D, Hofmann M, Jost M: **Socioeconomic consequences of isocyanate-induced occupational asthma: results of a 12-year follow-up study [abstract].** *Swiss Med Wkly* 2009, **139**(suppl 171):6S.
43. Piirilä PL, Keskinen HK, Luukonen R, Salo S-P, Tuppurainen M, Nordmann H: **Work, Unemployment and Life Satisfaction among patients with diisocyanate induced asthma-a prospective study.** *J Occup Health* 2005, **47:**112–118.
44. Stanojevic S, Wade A, Stocks J: **Reference values for lung function: past, present and future.** *Eur Respir J* 2010, **36:**12–19.
45. Swanney MP, Ruppel G, Enricht PL, Pedersen OF, Crapo RO, Miller MR, Jensen RL, Falaschetti E, Schouten JP, Hankinson JL, Stocks J, Quanjer PH: **Using the lower limit of normal for the FEV1 /FVC ratio reduces the misclassification of airway obstruction.** *Thorax* 2008, **63:**1046–1051.
46. Pellegrino R, Viegi G, Brusasco V, Crapo RO, Burgos F, Casaburi R, Coates A, van der Grinten CPM, Gustafsson P, Hankinson J, Jensen R, Johnson DC, MacIntyre N, McKay R, Miller MR, Navajas D, Pedersen OF, Wanger J: **Interpretative strategies for lung function tests.** *Eur Respir J* 2005, **26:**948–968.
47. Malo JL, Cartier A, Ghezzo H, Lafrance M, McCants M, Lehrer SB: **Patterns of improvement in spirometry, bronchial hyperresponsiveness, and specific IgE antibody levels after cessation of exposure in occupational asthma caused by snow-crab processing.** *Am Rev Respir Dis* 1988, **138:**807–812.
48. Pride NB: **Bronchial hyperreactivity in smokers.** *Eur Respir J* 1988, **5:**485–487.
49. Polosa R, Thomson NC: **Smoking and asthma: dangerous liaisons.** *Eur Respir J* 2013, **41:**716–726.
50. Labrècque M, Malo JL, Alaoui KM, Rabhi K: **Medical surveillance programme for diisocyanate exposure.** *Occup Environ Med* 2011, **68:**302–307.
51. Wilken D, Baur X, Barbinova L, Preisser A, Meyer E, Rooyackers J, Heederik D: **What are the benefits of medical screening and surveillance?** *Eur Respir Rev* 2012, **21:**105–111.

26

Occupational accident and disease claims, work-related stress and job satisfaction of physiotherapists

Birte Brattig[1], Anja Schablon[1], Albert Nienhaus[1,2,3*] and Claudia Peters[1]

Abstract

Introduction: Physiotherapists are exposed to diverse occupational demands. Until now, little has been known about the interaction between occupational stress and the job satisfaction of physiotherapists. This paper aims to examine their work-related stress and job satisfaction. It will analyse accidents at work and occupational diseases of physiotherapists along with work-related physical and psychosocial stress and job satisfaction.

Method: We analysed routine data of the German Institute for Statutory Accident Insurance and Prevention in the Health and Welfare Services (BGW) on accidents at work and occurring en route to/from work as well as occupational diseases of physiotherapists. Work-related stress and job satisfaction were examined in a cross-sectional survey using a standard questionnaire to be completed by subjects themselves.

Results: Between 2007 and 2011, 1,229 cases of occupational disease were reported to the BGW. The majority of reports involved skin diseases (73%). Stumbles and falls were the most frequent causes of accidents at work (42.9%). Eighty-five physiotherapists all over Germany took part in the survey. They experience high quantitative demands at work. The main physical demands consist of a torso posture between 45° and 90° and high hand activity. Of the 85 subjects, 51% suffer from complaints of the musculoskeletal system in the neck and thoracic spine area and 24% have skin diseases. Most physiotherapists (88%) are satisfied with their work overall. This is aided by a high degree of influence on their work and breaks, by practical application of skills and expert knowledge, high regard for their profession, varied work and a good atmosphere at work. Reservations tend to be about statutory regulations and the social benefits provided by the German healthcare system.

Conclusion: Overall, despite high demands and stress relating to the adequacy of resources, the majority of physiotherapists surveyed seem to be satisfied with their job. The main focus of action to promote the health of physiotherapists should be on preventing skin disease, problems of the musculoskeletal system and accidents caused by stumbles and falls.

Keywords: Working conditions, Physiotherapist, Job satisfaction, Accidents, Occupational disease

Introduction

Physiotherapists are exposed to diverse demands at work. Awkward postures, when administering treatments such as massages or when transferring immobile patients, can lead to musculoskeletal complaints [1-6]. This impacts on job satisfaction and the willingness to continue in the profession [7]. Until now, few studies in Germany have explored physical stress on physiotherapists. Psychosocial demands can also influence physiotherapists' job satisfaction. A study by Gröbel [8] examined psychosocial stress factors affecting salaried physiotherapists in the state of Hesse, Germany, and their consequences. It found that the quantitative and emotional demands of work tended to be viewed as moderate and that job satisfaction was rated as high. Until now, no studies have been conducted in Germany on the interaction between physical and psychosocial stress and the job satisfaction of physiotherapists.

* Correspondence: a.nienhaus@uke.de
[1]University Medical Center Hamburg-Eppendorf (UKE), Institute for Health Services Research in Dermatology and Nursing (CVcare), Hamburg, Germany
[2]Institute for Statutory Accident Insurance and Prevention in the Health and Welfare Services (BGW), Department of Occupational Health Research, Hamburg, Germany
Full list of author information is available at the end of the article

This paper analyses routine data on accidents at work and occupational diseases of physiotherapists who work in physiotherapy practices and are insured with the Institute for Statutory Accident Insurance and Prevention in the Health and Welfare Services (BGW). A survey of work-related physical and psychosocial stress and the job satisfaction of physiotherapists was also conducted.

Material and methods

The Institute for Statutory Accident Insurance and Prevention in the Health and Welfare Services (BGW) routinely records reports of accidents at work and occupational diseases [9,10]. Along with information about the accident and resulting injury, or the type of occupational disease and confirmed cause of illness, the BGW documents the affected person's activity. It distinguishes between accidents at the workplace or during working hours and accidents on the way to and from work. Accidents that lead to more than three days' incapacity for work are notifiable. The circumstances that lead to the injury are documented in more detail in a 7% random sample of all notifiable accidents. It is obligatory to report a disease if there are reasonable grounds for suspecting that the disease was caused by exposure at the workplace. For instance, contact with an infectious agent is not notifiable, but an occupationally acquired infection is notifiable [10,11]. Some occupational diseases are subject to a proviso. They can only be recognised if the disease led to relinquishment of the stressful work. This applies mainly to skin diseases and disc-related complaints of the lumbar spine.

In 2011, 136,998 full-time members of the occupational group of physiotherapists were insured with the BGW. The number of full-time workers is calculated on the basis of the number of monthly hours worked by an insured person. A part-time worker who works 80 hours per month is equivalent to 0.5 full-time workers. We analysed accidents at work and en route to/from work, along with occupational diseases, for the years 2007–2011.

In 2012, we also conducted a cross-sectional survey to examine work-related stress and job satisfaction among physiotherapists. In order to obtain a random sample of subjects for this survey, we randomly selected from the BGW dataset of all insured physiotherapists the addresses of 210 salaried, freelance or self-employed physiotherapists working in outpatient practices. After matching the address data, inter alia via the Deutscher Verband für Physiotherapie (ZVK) [12], subjects were sent an anonymous questionnaire plus a separate declaration of consent and a stamped addressed return envelope.

For the survey, we developed a standard questionnaire containing 84 items to be completed by the subjects themselves. In addition to socio-demographic information, there were questions on occupation-specific aspects. In order to quantify physical stress and demands at the workplace, frequent postures, average hand activity and exhaustion at the end of a working day were recorded. In addition, subjects were asked about contact with persons with infectious diseases.

Several questions were taken from the Copenhagen Psychosocial Questionnaire (COPSOQ) and adjusted for the physiotherapists' field of work. The COPSOQ on psychosocial stress at work was developed at the National Institute for Occupational Health in Copenhagen [13,14] and tested, shortened and standardised for Germany [15,16]. This instrument casts light on demands and satisfaction at the workplace, the working climate and the work-privacy conflict. It has previously been used for several studies of employees in the healthcare sector [17,18].

Another section of the questionnaire is based on the Work Ability Index (WAI) [19]. This instrument is used to ascertain subjects' ability to work and state of health by recording both their assessment of their own mental and physical fitness for work and currently diagnosed diseases. For the survey of physiotherapists, the range of diseases was reduced and confined to accidental injuries, diseases of the musculoskeletal system, skin diseases, diseases of the vascular system, and mental illnesses.

The *IBM SPSS Statistics 21* program was used to carry out a univariate and bivariate analysis of the data. The study was conducted in accordance with the Federal Data Protection Act. Since it involved the analysis of routine data and an anonymous questionnaire, no ethics committee approval was obtained. The BGW's data protection officer approved the data protection concept for the study.

Results

Occupational diseases and accidents at work

In 2011, the number of insured physiotherapists in outpatient practices was equivalent to 136,998 full-time posts, an increase of 21.5% on the previous year's 112,718. In the years from 2007 to 2011, physiotherapists reported a total of 25,891 insured events to the BGW. The number of reports in 2011 (n = 6.193) increased by 44.9% compared with 2007 (n = 4.275). The report ratio rose from 17.9 to 22.6 insured events per 1,000 full-time equivalents during this period. Of the insured events reported, 47.8% were notifiable. The most frequent reports concerned accidents at work (n = 14,332, of which 44.3% were notifiable), followed by accidents en route to/from work (n = 8,681, 55.2% notifiable) and occupational diseases (n = 2,878, 42.7% notifiable). The report ratio per 1,000 full-time equivalents increased for all three types of insured event (Table 1).

The majority of insured events involved women (76.0%). Men were slightly over-represented in accidents at work,

Table 1 Insurance cases among physiotherapists in the years 2007 to 2011, BGW data

Reporting year	2007	2008	2009	2010	2011	Total
Number of full-time staff	112,718	120,451	126,679	133,134	136,998	–
Total insured events (IE)	4,275	4,673	5,090	5,660	6,193	25,891
IEs per 1,000 full-time staff	17.9	18.1	18.6	20.4	22.6	–
Notifiable IEs	2,017	2,179	2,360	2,717	3,090	12,363
Reported occupational diseases (OD)	458	510	542	600	768	2,878
ODs per 1,000 IEs	4.1	4.2	4.3	4.5	5.6	
Notifiable ODs	189	208	216	263	353	1,229
Proportion of total ODs	41	41	40	44	46	43
Occupational accidents (OA)	2,429	2,645	2,826	3,096	3,336	14,332
OAs per 1,000 IEs	21.5	22.0	22.3	23.3	24.4	
Notifiable OAs	1,058	1,188	1,197	1,369	1,534	6,346
Accidents en route to/from work (AER)	1,388	1,518	1,722	1,964	2,089	8,681
AERs per 1,000 IEs	12.3	12.6	13.6	14.8	15.2	
Notifiable AERs	770	783	947	1,085	1,203	4,788

IE insured event.
OD occupational disease.
OA occupational accident.
AER accident en route to/from work.

accounting for 26.1% of cases – as opposed to 19.4% for occupational diseases and 21.5% for accidents en route to/from work (Table 2).

Of the 1,229 cases of notifiable occupational disease, an occupational cause was confirmed in 910 cases (74.0%) and an occupational disease was recognised in 57 cases (4.6%) (Table 3). Skin diseases accounted for both the majority of cases reported (n = 897, 73.0%) and for the majority of cases where an occupational cause was confirmed (876, n = 97.7%). Disc-related diseases of the lumbar spine were the second most frequently reported (n = 85, 6.9%) and occupationally caused (n = 16, 1.8%) disease.

Of the 11 infections recognised as occupational diseases or irregular health conditions in the period under review, six involved active tuberculosis and one a latent tuberculosis infection (LTBI). There was one case each of hepatitis B and C, and one of an unspecified bacteriological infection (no table).

Around one in five occupational accidents happened en route to or from work and about half of those were road accidents. Of the accidents en route to or from work, 60.8% were road accidents (Table 4). In 68.4% of cases, the type of injury cannot be identified from the accident report. Closed fractures were the most frequent consequence of injury (14.2%). They are somewhat more frequent in accidents en route to or from work than in accidents at work (16.2% and 12.7%) (Table 5). Hands are more often affected by accidents at work than by accidents on the way to or from work (2.8% and 1.3%) (Table 6). However, in both categories of accident, the feet are more frequently affected (4.8% and 3.2%). Polytrauma or head injuries are the consequence of 2.6% of occupational accidents and 3.4% of accidents en route to or from work.

In the 7% random sample in the years from 2007 to 2011, a total of 303 notifiable occupational accidents and 195 accidents en route to or from work were recorded (Table 7). This is equivalent to 4.8% and 4.1% respectively of all notifiable events and thus somewhat lower than the 7% aimed for.

As expected, the majority of occupational accidents occurred in physiotherapy practices. However, in line with the high proportion of accidents en route to or from work, 25.1% of accidents took place on paths and roads. In the case of accidents en route to or from work,

Table 2 Gender distribution by type of insured event among physiotherapists, BGW data

	Occupational disease	Occupational accident	Accident en route to/from work	All
	N (%)	N (%)	N (%)	N (%)
Male	558 (19.4)	3,747 (26.1)	1,869 (21.5)	6,174 (23.8)
Female	2,316 (80.1)	10,563 (73.7)	6,788 (78.2)	19,667 (76.0)
Unknown	4 (0.5)	22 (0.2)	24 (0.3)	50 (0.2)
Total	2,878 (11.1)	14,332 (55.4)	8,681 (33.5)	25,891

Table 3 Type and frequency of notifiable occupational diseases (OD) among physiotherapists for the years 2007 to 2011, BGW data

OD number	N (%)	Occupational cause confirmed (and OD recognised)
5101 Severe or recurrent skin diseases	897 (73.0)	876 (28)
2108 Vertebral disc-related diseases of the lumbar spine due to many years' lifting/carrying heavy loads/extreme bending of the torso	85 (6.9)	16 (11)
2101 Tendovaginal conditions or conditions of the tendinous tissue or of the tendonor muscular attachments	49 (4.0)	2 (2)
3101 Infectious diseases	38 (3.1)	11 (11)
2109 Vertebral disc-related diseases of the cervical spine due to many years' carrying heavy loads on the shoulder	31 (2.5)	0
4301 4302 Obstructive respiratory diseases due to allergenic substances, chemical irritants or substances with a toxic effect	11 (0.9)	5 (5)
Other ODs	118 (9.6)	0
Total	1,229 (100.0)	910 (57)

paths and roads were the predominant site of the accident (95.4%). Running, walking or moving were the most frequent activities engaged in immediately before the accident, both in the case of occupational accidents (53.8%) and in the case of accidents en route to or from work (37.2%) (Table 7). Driving cars or other motor vehicles (38.8%) and the use of a bicycle or similar means of transport (22.4%) were further frequent activities in the run-up to an accident en route to or from work. These activities played a subordinate role in the case of occupational accidents, at 12.2% and 2% respectively.

In occupational accidents, slipping, stumbling or falling (42.9%) and uncoordinated, awkward movements (25.1%) were the most frequent events leading to an accident. With accidents en route to or from work, loss of control over a vehicle or means of transport (56.6%), along with slipping, stumbling or falling (34.1%) were the most frequent events leading to an accident. In keeping with these accident-triggering events, colliding with or running up against an object (37.3% and 53.1%) and being hit by a moving object (17.8% and 35.7%) were the most frequent types of contact leading to an accident. Contact with sharp, pointed objects was rarely a reason for injury (5% and 0.5%). Blows, kicks, pushes or bites were rare occurrences both in occupational accidents (2.3%) and in the case of accidents on the way to or from work (1.5%). Tools and machinery were involved in only 5.3% of occupational accidents. In the case of accidents en route to or from work, as expected, vehicles played a predominant role (52.6%). Human beings or other living things played a role in 13.2% of occupational accidents and 3.2% of accidents en route to or from work. However, only a small proportion of these accidents (7 out of 40 occupational accidents and 3 out of 7 accidents on the way to or from work) were

Table 4 Distribution of reported accidents by individual type of accident for the years 2007 to 2011 among physiotherapists, BGW data

Type of accident	Notifiable		Total
	Yes	No	
	N (col%)	N (col%)	N (col%)
Occupational accidents*	**6,346 (57.0)**	**7,986 (67.2)**	**14,332 (62.3)**
of which:			
Occupational accidents at work, no road traffic	4,796 (75.6)	6,758 (84.6)	11,554 (80.6)
Occupational accidents on business, not a road traffic accident	703 (11.1)	685 (8.6)	1,388 (9.7)
Workplace accidents on business, in road traffic*	847 (13.3)	543 (6.8)	1,390 (9.7)
Accidents en route to/from work	4,788 (43.0)	3,893 (32.8)	8,681 (37.7)
of which:			
Accidents en route to/from work, not a road traffic accident	1,781 (37.2)	1,618 (41.6)	3,399 (39.2)
Accidents en route to/from work that happened in road traffic	3,007 (62.8)	2,275 (58.4)	5,282 (60.8)
Total*	11,134 (48.4)	11,879 (51.6)	23,013 (100)

*row%.

Table 5 Type of injury for notifiable occupational accidents and accidents en route to/from work among physiotherapists, summarised for the years 2007 to 2011, BGW data

Type of injury		Type of accident		Total
		Occupational accident	Accident en route to/from work	
Not specified	Number	4,414	3,200	7,614
	%	69.6%	66.8%	68.4%
Closed, fully reversible injury	Number	178	134	312
	%	2.8%	2.8%	2.8%
Closed, bloody injuries with lasting damage to substance	Number	41	44	85
	%	0.6%	0.9%	0.8%
Torsion, sprain	Number	289	329	618
	%	4.6%	6.9%	5.6%
Dislocation	Number	41	30	71
	%	0.6%	0.6%	0.6%
Laceration, cuts	Number	461	176	637
	%	7.3%	3.7%	5.7%
Closed fracture	Number	807	778	1,585
	%	12.7%	16.2%	14.2%
Open fracture	Number	55	50	105
	%	0.9%	1.0%	0.9%
Burning, scalding, chemical burn, radioactive contamination, hypothermia, frostbite, electrical effects	Number	24	0	24
	%	0.4%	0.0%	0.2%
Other injuries	Number	34	41	75
	%	0.5%	0.9%	0.7%
Type of injury unknown or unclassifiable	Number	2	6	8
	%	0.0%	0.1%	0.1%
Total	Number	6,346	4,788	11,134
	%	100.0%	100.0%	100.0%

triggered by violence (blow, kick, push, bite) (Table 7). In three out of a total of ten such cases, animals rather than human beings were the cause of the accident (no table).

Survey of physiotherapists

Eighty-five physiotherapists took part in the survey, representing a response rate of 41%. Twice as many women as men participated in the survey. The majority were in the 40 to 49 and 50 to 59 age groups, while there were only a few representatives of the under-30 age group. Sixty-seven per cent of the subjects had been working in physiotherapy for more than 20 years and 84% were freelance or self-employed proprietors of their own practice. In response to the question about their main activities, as expected 95% of respondents stated that they frequently administered physical therapy, while 87% engaged in mobilisation and manual therapy and 46% performed lymphatic drainage. Less frequently, they mentioned electrotherapy, patient transfer or hydrotherapy. Additional activities stated primarily included massages. Table 8 contains further information about the study population.

Work demands and stress

In connection with quantitative demands at work, one in four physiotherapists said they often had to work very fast and more than half said their work mounted up. In addition, over 50% of respondents were subject to emotional stress (Table 9). One in three physiotherapists found the time spent at work to be a hindrance to their own private responsibilities. However, only 15.3% of respondents said that their work as a physiotherapist interfered with their private and family life.

As regards physical demands at work, the physiotherapists were asked to state the postures they frequently adopted while working. It seems that they often had to adopt a torso posture between 45° and 90° when working with patients. However, they rarely bent their torso to an angle of more than 90°. Only 6% treated patients in a squatting position. Physiotherapists work a lot with their

Table 6 Site of injury for notifiable occupational accidents and accidents en route to/from work among physiotherapists, summarised for the years 2007 to 2011, BGW data

Site of injury		Type of accident		Total
		Occupational accident	Accident en route to/from work	
Not specified	Number	4,414	3,200	7,614
	%	69.6%	66.8%	68.4%
Polytrauma, head	Number	167	164	331
	%	2.6%	3.4%	3.0%
Neck, spinal column, arm and leg nerve plexus	Number	206	323	529
	%	3.2%	6.7%	4.8%
Chest, shoulder girdle, back, flank, chest organs	Number	93	107	200
	%	1.5%	2.2%	1.8%
Abdomen, abdominal organs, pelvis	Number	21	32	53
	%	0.3%	0.7%	0.5%
Shoulder, upper arm, elbow	Number	260	179	439
	%	4.1%	3.7%	3.9%
Lower arm, wrist, carpus	Number	286	225	511
	%	4.5%	4.7%	4.6%
Hand	Number	175	64	239
	%	2.8%	1.3%	2.1%
Hip, thigh, patella	Number	75	96	171
	%	1.2%	2.0%	1.5%
Knee joint (excluding patella) calf	Number	345	244	589
	%	5.4%	5.1%	5.3%
Ankle, foot	Number	304	154	458
	%	4.8%	3.2%	4.1%
Total	Number	6,346	4,788	11,134
	%	100.0%	100.0%	100.0%

hands, but even though the estimated effort required for average hand activity is high, at 84% (Table 10), 79% of respondents stated that they made regular hand movements without a break.

In the case of treatment of patients with infectious diseases, the highest proportion (33%) mentioned contact with patients with multi-resistant pathogens. The next highest rate of contact was with patients with hepatitis (27%) and HIV (15%). Only a few physiotherapists came into contact with childhood diseases (6%) such as whooping cough or measles or tuberculosis (2%), while 41% of respondents stated that they had no contact with patients with infectious diseases (no table).

Job satisfaction

With regard to their mental power reserves, 81% of the physiotherapists questioned stated that they had enjoyed their work of late. Nearly all participants in this study (92.9%) had a major influence on their own work, saw it as important and meaningful (97.6%) and could decide for themselves when to take a break (76.5%). They described their work as varied and felt motivated and engaged (90.6%). Moreover, they were able to apply their learned skills and expert knowledge. In addition, 80% said that the working atmosphere among colleagues was good and nearly half of respondents said they exchanged views and information at a professional level. In contrast, there was hardly any professional interchange with medical practitioners (8%) (Table 11).

An open question was used to record which factors would further enhance the physiotherapists' job satisfaction. Around one third mentioned better pay. Some also wanted more time for patients and less bureaucracy, especially when working with health insurers and in respect of the current government directive on prescriptions for therapeutic remedies (Heilmittelrichtlinie). Also mentioned were better cooperation with doctors and a generally higher level of recognition of their profession (no table). Overall, 80% of respondents were satisfied with their work (Table 11).

Table 7 Description of occupational accidents among physiotherapists according to '7% statistics', BGW data

Circumstances of accident	Occupational accident		Accident en route to/from work	
Environment where the accident victim was located prior to the accident	N	%	N	%
Physiotherapy practice or healthcare institution	191	63.0	6	3.1
Paths, roads, public domain	76	25.1	187	95.4
Other	36	11.9	3	1.5
The activity the victim was engaged in immediately before the accident				
Handling tools	15	5.0	–	
Handling machinery	2	0.7	–	
Driving/handling power-driven conveyances (car etc.)	37	12.2	76	38.8
Driving/handling non-power-driven conveyances (bicycle etc.)	6	2.0	44	22.4
Handling objects	58	19.1	–	
Running, walking, moving	163	53.8	73	37.2
Other	12	4.0	3	1.5
Event leading to the accident				
Loss of control of tool, machinery	18	5.9	1	0.5
Loss of control of vehicle or conveyance	36	11.9	111	56.6
Slipping, stumbling, falling	130	42.9	67	34.1
Uncoordinated, inappropriate, unsuitable movements	76	25.1	5	2.6
Lifting and carrying objects	10	3.3	–	
Surprise, fright, violence	7	2.3	5	2.6
Other	26	8.6	7	3.6
Contact via which the victim was injured				
Contact with electrical current, temperatures, hazardous substances	7	2.3	1	0.5
Colliding with or running into a stationary object (the victim moves)	113	37.3	104	53.1
Contact with a sharp, pointed object	15	5.0	1	0.5
Hit by collision with a moving object	54	17.8	70	35.7
Contact with a hard or rough object	10	3.3	1	0.5
Jammed, squashed	11	3.6	2	1.0
Acute excessive physical strain	79	26.1	14	7.1
Acute excessive mental strain	1	0.3	–	
Blow, kick, push, bite	7	2.3	3	1.5
Other	5	1.7	–	
Most important object connected with the accident				
Building, building installations	139	45.9	80	40.8
Tools, machinery	16	5.3	–	
Vehicles	43	14.2	103	52.6
Office furnishings, personal equipment, kitchen appliances	50	16.5	–	
Humans and other living beings	40	13.2	7	3.6
Other	15	5.0	6	3.1
Total	303	100.0	196	100.0

Complaints and diseases

Half of the respondents mentioned a disease of the cervical and thoracic spine, 36.5% a disease of the lumbar spine and 30.6% a disease of the iliosacral joint (Table 6). Around half the physiotherapists (47%) diagnosed these diseases themselves (no table). Twenty-seven per cent of the physiotherapists said they had wrist problems (carpal tunnel syndrome, rhizarthrosis), of which 60% were self-diagnosed. Knee joint complaints (20%) were somewhat less frequent (Table 12).

Table 8 Description of study population as regards job satisfaction of and stress on physiotherapists, 2012

Study population	N	%
Total	85	100.0
Gender distribution		
Male	28	32.9
Female	57	67.1
Age		
Under 30 years	4	4.7
30–49 years	15	17.6
40–49 years	28	32.9
50–59 years	27	31.8
Over 59 years	11	12.9
Professional experience in physiotherapy		
0–10 years	12	14.1
11–20 years	16	18.8
Longer than 20 years	57	67.1
Working hours		
Full-time (≥35 hours per week)	68	80.0
Part-time (<35 hours per week)	17	20.0
Overtime in the last twelve months		
Every day	11	12.9
Several times a week	29	34.1
Several times a month	14	16.5
Several times a year	20	23.5
Never	11	12.9
Professional status		
Self-employed	71	83.5
Employee	14	16.5
Home visits		
Frequent	70	82.4
Seldom or never	15	17.6
Tasks mainly performed		
Physical therapy	81	95.3
Mobilisation/manual therapy	74	87.1
Manual lymphatic drainage	39	45.9
Electrotherapy	16	18.8
Patient transfers	14	16.5
Hydrotherapy	4	4.7

Skin diseases (skin irritation, allergic skin rash/eczema, fungal infections) had been diagnosed in one quarter of respondents. Likewise, 25% of the physiotherapists surveyed suffered slight mental problems such as mild depression, anxiety, tenseness, insomnia and burnout (Table 6).

The majority (80%) of physiotherapists assessed their current physical (74%) and mental (73%) work capacity as good compared with when they were at their best. At the time of the survey, 46% had neither a disease nor an injury that impeded their work. However, 39% said they had problems in doing their work and 27% said that as a result they were sometimes forced to work more slowly or to change their working methods.

Table 9 Work stress among physiotherapists (N = 85)

Stressor	N	%
Working fast		
Frequently	22	25.9
Seldom	63	24.1
Work is unevenly distributed and mounts up		
Frequently	53	62.4
Seldom	32	37.6
Not enough time for all tasks		
Frequently	50	58.8
Seldom	35	41.2
Work involves emotionally stressful situations		
Frequently	50	58.8
Seldom	35	41.2
Work–privacy conflict		
Work interferes with private and family life		
Yes	13	15.3
No or undecided	72	84.7
Time spent working hinders private responsibilities		
Yes	27	31.8
No or undecided	57	68.2

Table 10 Physical demands of the typical physical work performed by physiotherapists surveyed 2012

Physical demands of typical daily work	N	%
Torso inclination of 45° to 90°	47	55.3
Squatting posture	16	18.8
Torso inclination >90°	15	17.6
Kneeling posture	15	17.6
Hands above shoulder level	13	15.3
Squatting	5	5.9
Hand activity		
No regular hand activities	1	1.2
Slow movements with breaks	12	14.1
Regular movements without breaks	67	78.8
Fast movements without breaks	5	5.9
Effort required, hands		
Moderate	14	16.5
High	71	83.5

Table 11 Description of resources that positively reinforced the work of physiotherapists in 2012

Resources	N	%
High job satisfaction	68	80.0
Daily tasks performed with pleasure	69	81.2
Influence on own work activity	79	92.9
Self-determined break times	65	76.5
Views own work as important and meaningful	83	97.6
Work is varied	74	87.1
Motivated and engaged in work	77	90.6
Application of acquired skills and expert knowledge at work	79	92.9
Good working atmosphere with colleagues	68	80.0
Frequent professional interchange with colleagues	34	40.0
Frequent professional interchange with doctors	7	8.2

Of the respondents, 61% said they often felt exhausted at the end of a working day. Approximately one third had often considered leaving their profession during the previous twelve months, with 55% citing physical problems as the main reason for leaving. This was followed by poor pay (32%) and mental stress (24%). However, 59% had never considered leaving the profession. Only 4% of the physiotherapists said they were unfit for work at the time of the survey (no table). When asked about sickness in the past year, 53 (62.4%) said they had not been ill, while 34.1% had been unfit for work for up to one month and 3.5% for longer than one month (Table 12). Eighty percent of respondents said they were fairly certain that they would be able to do their work without problems in two years' time (no table).

Discussion

According to our survey, work in a forward-bending posture and repetitive hand movements involving physical

Table 12 Information on diseases that may be attributable to the profession of physiotherapist 2012

Diseases of the musculoskeletal system	N	%
Lumbar spine and thoracic spine	43	50.6
Lumbar spine	31	36.5
Iliosacral joint	26	30.6
Wrist	23	27.1
Thumb-saddle joint	23	27.1
Knee joint	17	20.0
Skin diseases	20	23.5
Minor mental illnesses	21	24.7
Unfit for work in the last twelve months		
No	53	62.4
Up to one month	29	34.1
Longer than one month	3	3.5

effort represent typical strains on physiotherapists. Back problems and hand and finger problems are correspondingly frequent. However, the design of the study as a cross-sectional study and the relatively small sample size make it impossible to analyse causal interrelations. Despite the high quantitative work demands, physiotherapists were satisfied with their job.

Complaints and diseases

The data provided by the Institute for Statutory Accident Insurance and Prevention in the Health and Welfare Services (BGW) on occupational diseases showed skin diseases (73%) to be the most frequently reported occupational disease. However, in the context of our cross-sectional study, skin diseases played a subordinate role in contrast to diseases of the musculoskeletal system. A study by Cromie [20] reported that physiotherapists who often performed hydrotherapy with their patients had a higher probability of suffering skin problems. In this case, 37% of the total suffered from skin infections. In the random sample in our study, only a few therapists treated patients with hydrotherapy. Even so, a total of 24% suffered from irritated skin, allergic rashes or eczemas and fungal infections. From this, one can deduce that along with hydrotherapy, other factors such as increased use of disinfectants in hand hygiene might be responsible.

One of the professional risks run by physiotherapists is that of contact with patients with infectious diseases. In Cromie's study [20], 13% of respondents said they had caught an infectious disease through their work as a physiotherapist. According to our analysis of the BGW data, infectious diseases played only a subordinate role as an occupational disease (3% of all reports). In the five-year survey period, 38 infections were reported and 11 were recognised as an occupational disease. Tuberculosis accounted for the highest proportion (7 out of 11). Physiotherapists who practise breathing therapies run a special risk of TB infection [11,21,22]. One case each of hepatitis B and hepatitis C virus infections were recognised as occupational diseases. Thus, blood-borne virus infections seem to be rare among physiotherapists. This is in line with the generally positive trend in blood-borne virus infections among healthcare professionals in general in Germany form whom the number of claims concerning blood-burne virus infections decreased from above 500 in the year 1999 to below 200 in the year 2009 [10]. In the cross-sectional study described here, it appears that frequent contact with patients with multi-resistant pathogens (33%) and hepatitis in physiotherapy calls for efficient hygiene measures. Matching against the infectious diseases reported indicates that hygiene measures are effective.

Physiotherapists are exposed to physical strains in their profession. The BGW data shows that 7% of the notifiable occupational diseases involved 'vertebral disc-related diseases of the lumbar spine due to many years' lifting or carrying heavy loads or extreme bending of the torso', while 2.5% reported a 'vertebral disc-related disease of the cervical spine due to many years' carrying heavy loads on the shoulder'. Admittedly, none of the cervical spine diseases reported was recognised as an occupational disease because the physiotherapists did not fulfil the work-related prerequisites for recognition. Studies by Bork, 1996 [2], Cromie, 2000 [23], Campo, 2008 [3] and Grooten, 2011 [5], also ascertained that musculoskeletal diseases in physiotherapists occurred most frequently in the lower back (lumbar spine, iliosacral). Our study, too, showed that along with a higher occurrence in the area of the cervical and thoracic spine (51%), the physiotherapists also suffered musculoskeletal diseases of the lumbar spine and iliosacral complaints, each at a frequency of around 30%. As confirmed by other studies [5,6], these appear to have been provoked by awkward body postures: 55% of the physiotherapists surveyed stated that they often had to work in a forward-bending position with their torso at an angle of 45° to 90°, which can lead to musculoskeletal problems in the spinal column area. In an occupational health study to assess strain on the lumbar spine, it was found that vertebral disc L5/S1 is subject to the most strain when lifting heavy objects and when the torso is bent at an angle of 50°. In addition, strong compressive forces impact on the disc when the torso is in a static forward-bending position at an angle of 90° [24].

As regards patient transfers, 17% of respondents in our study said that they mainly did this work themselves. Along with awkward work postures, this factor is seen as one of the most problematic as far as the development of disc-related complaints and diseases is concerned [2,6]. This problem primarily affects physiotherapists (more than 80% of those in our investigation) who make frequent home visits where they find conditions that impede optimal patient care [25].

Frequent home visits involving journeys in road traffic may also be a reason for the high number (2,778) of accidents en route to/from work reported to the BGW.

Physiotherapists often work with their hands (massages, mobilising, manual therapy), which places a great strain on the hand and thumb joints [2,5,23]. This can be a risk factor for 'tendovaginal conditions or conditions of the tendinous tissue or of the tendonor muscular attachments' that affected 4% of the physiotherapists with notifiable occupational diseases (Table 3). Almost half the therapists who worked only with their hands suffered from carpal tunnel syndrome and had to take protective and corrective measures (changing their work posture, wearing wrist braces, taking painkillers, undergoing surgery) in order to continue working in their profession [1]. Physiotherapists who suffered from diseases of the thumb-saddle joint also had to adapt their way of working to cope with the complaint [26]. A major Australian study found that mainly therapists who administered massages and manual therapy suffered from thumb-saddle joint problems. It also found increased instability in the thumb joints [27].

The majority of respondents made regular hand movements involving a great deal of hand activity without a break. As a result, more than a quarter of respondents suffered from musculoskeletal complaints of the hand or thumb-saddle joints such as carpal tunnel syndrome or rhizarthrosis. However, this study found no significant connection between frequent manual treatment (mobilisation, manual therapy) and diseases of the hand joint (no table). Nonetheless, it seems reasonable to analyse the causes of musculoskeletal complaints in physiotherapists in a more differentiated way, as is already happening in an ongoing study [28].

Some physiotherapists seemed to think that the fact that they know how work-related musculoskeletal diseases could be prevented protected them against such diseases and that they as role models ought not to suffer from any such diseases [4,29]. Others preferred to diagnose and treat themselves and had not consulted a doctor. This is attributable to the skills in this profession. Campo's 2008 study [3] showed that only 13% of all physiotherapists had consulted their doctor in a one-year period, but that more than 50% suffered from work-related musculoskeletal complaints. Our survey, too, found that roughly half of all diseases of the musculoskeletal system were self-diagnosed. Nonetheless, a visit to a doctor and further diagnosis could potentially further isolate the cause of existing symptoms and more systematic treatment might bring results more quickly or prevent illness. It might also encourage the individual's admission of illness and increase social support [4].

Work stress

Almost 40% of the physiotherapists in this study said they could do their work, but suffered from complaints, while others were forced to work more slowly or to change their working methods. Almost two thirds felt exhausted at the end of a working day. Cromie found that 17% of physiotherapists changed their specialism or even their profession on account of musculoskeletal diseases [23]. In our study, 55% said that they were most likely to leave their profession because of physical problems.

Despite this stress, 46% of the physiotherapists surveyed did not feel that their work was impaired. Nearly two thirds had not been ill in the previous year. Three quarters assessed their current fitness for work and its physical demands as good and were fairly certain that they would still be able to practise their profession in two years' time without any problems. This cannot be confirmed on the basis of the literature. In Campo's phenomenological study, most physiotherapists were worried about the future [29]. Among the physiotherapists we surveyed, work-related physical stress appeared to lead to diseases and dissatisfaction only to a limited extent.

Stress at the workplace can impact heavily on working people's psyches and satisfaction with life [30] and can lead to work-related musculoskeletal diseases or to a change of workplace [3,7]. In a 2010 study by Santos, 36% of subjects said they felt stressed. Our study found that 24% cited mental stress as the crucial reason for a possible change of profession. Stressors include insufficient independence and a lack of recognition by society in general and in the healthcare sector in particular [31]. The physiotherapists in this study would appreciate greater recognition from doctors, health insurers and society at large.

Stress can also impact on the psyche. The majority of physiotherapists assessed their current fitness for work as regards mental demands as good, one quarter as mediocre and only two subjects as poor. A quarter of those surveyed suffered from minor mental complaints. A study of healthcare workers in Cyprus [32] showed that 46% found their profession stressful and 21% were suffering from burnout.

For the physiotherapists in our study, mental stress seemed to play a subordinate role. It did not seem to impact negatively on their job satisfaction. The conflict between work and family can lead to social stress. Burtchen found in 2006 that more than 35% of the physiotherapists she surveyed cited stress in their private lives as a stress factor at work, but also that stress at the workplace was often relieved in private life [33]. Our study findings tally with those of Gröbel [8], namely that professional demands on physiotherapists tend to have only a minor effect on their private and family lives.

Job satisfaction

The results of this study show that nearly 90% of the physiotherapists surveyed were satisfied with their jobs on the whole. This is a very high percentage, but tallies with the findings of other studies that also found a high level of job satisfaction among physiotherapists [34-37]. Karasek's job-demand control model [38] says that high demands with low control may lead to health and mental deficits. At the same time, high demands accompanied by high influencing possibilities and control over the work performed minimise health stress and can improve regenerative capacities (active workers). Although high demands ensure a certain stress level, they also increase motivation [39,40]. Earlier studies [7] had already shown that physiotherapists tend to belong to the group of active workers. This is an important factor for a high level of job satisfaction.

The demands on physiotherapists are having to work quickly, unevenly distributed work that mounts up because they sometimes have less than 15 minutes per patient and too little time to complete all their tasks, which include documentation. Roughly a quarter said that having more time for patients, documentation and home visits, along with a reduction in bureaucracy, would lead to increased job satisfaction. In addition, there are emotionally stressful situations such as patients' sad stories or the working atmosphere. The physiotherapists in this study exerted a high level of control primarily because the majority of those surveyed worked independently. So in an ideal case, the therapists could decide for themselves how a treatment should proceed or when to plan breaks. Unfortunately, this is not always easy in practice because statutory regulations in particular place constraints on the welfare system. According to the duty to check, as laid down in the current 1 July 2011 directive on prescriptions for therapeutic remedies (Heilmittelrichtlinie), physiotherapists may only provide and charge for their services if there are no formal errors in the prescriptions issued by doctors [41,16]. As a result, these prescriptions must be checked for accuracy each time before treating a patient, which further reduces the little time available to therapists. Given the difficulties of working with some health insurers, a quarter of the therapists surveyed cited this as a negative factor impacting on job satisfaction. Moreover, collaboration with some medical practitioners did not always work. Only 8% of the physiotherapists surveyed said that there was sufficient communication and professional interchange with doctors. Already in Bergmann's study, 55% said that doctors expected them to act independently [42]. In Burtchen's study, too, they complained about insufficient cooperation with doctors [33].

Success is another important factor in physiotherapists' job satisfaction. In a phenomenological study by Takeuchi, the success of physiotherapists is described primarily as a circular process that emerges during the course of their career and is developed on the basis of positive results in terms of patients, their career and reputation [43]. An employee's salary can also be seen as success at work: roughly one third of those surveyed for this study were dissatisfied with their salary and wanted better pay. This can lead to job dissatisfaction [44].

In order to deal with and compensate for the physical and psychosocial demands and strains, resources are needed to prevent mental stress reactions [35]. Physiotherapists employed in larger rehabilitation centres or hospitals often complain that they have too little scope and work under too much time pressure [8]. Since most of the subjects in the present study worked independently as practice proprietors or freelancers, the majority of them had more scope to arrange their working hours and breaks, and more influence on their own work. Varied work with different patients, the application of learned skills and expert knowledge and the feeling that the work being done is important and meaningful reinforce job satisfaction. Thus, nearly all of those questioned felt motivated and engaged, a feeling that was reinforced by good social relationships. A relaxed and collegial work climate makes a substantial contribution toward employees' health. If relationships between people at the workplace do not function, this leads to dissatisfaction [44,45]. Eighty per cent of the physiotherapists surveyed, however, described the atmosphere among colleagues at the workplace as pleasant and felt that they were part of a community. Professional interchange with colleagues about difficult cases or new techniques also helps in solving stressful problems and enhances one's self-esteem in respect of one's own professional competence.

Limitations

The response rate for this study was relatively low at 41%, as only 85 physiotherapists took part in the survey. Differing response behaviour may lead to selection bias. Physiotherapists who were fairly satisfied with their profession and therefore, with appropriate time management, had enough time to complete the questionnaire may have been the main participants in this study and may therefore have distorted the response behaviour positively. On the other hand, those who were very dissatisfied with their profession may also have taken the opportunity to express their discontent. These response behaviours may balance each other out and deliver a fairly accurate image of the reality. Since we only wrote to practices, and in the main independent physiotherapists participated in this study, the findings can hardly be transferred to employees in practices or hospitals.

Problems that were not addressed in our questionnaire but which, according to the results of the open question about other factors, have a major influence on the job satisfaction of physiotherapists, are statutory regulations due to the current catalogue of remedies as well as working with health insurers. These aspects should be included in further studies.

Conclusion

Despite the resource-related physical and psychosocial stress, there is a high rate of job satisfaction among physiotherapists. Limitations tend to be seen in statutory regulations and welfare benefits of the German healthcare system. In order to minimise the stress on physiotherapists, preventive measures are still required, especially in order to prevent awkward postures and infections. In addition, some changes in the regulations governing the healthcare system could ensure less bureaucracy and greater concentration on patients. Attention should be paid to sufficient protection for physiotherapists' resources so that this profession remains as satisfied as it is now.

Competing interests

The authors declare that they have no competing interests.

Authors' contributions

BB developed the questionnaire, curried out the survey, analyzed the data and wrote the first draft. CP supervised the survey and data analysis and gave substantial comments for the improvement of the first draft. AN performed data analysis of the routine data concerning accidents and occupational diseases and gave substantial comments for the improvement of the first draft. AS supervised the survey and data analysis and gave substantial comments for the improvement of the first draft. All authors read and agreed on the final form of the manuscript.

Author details

[1]University Medical Center Hamburg-Eppendorf (UKE), Institute for Health Services Research in Dermatology and Nursing (CVcare), Hamburg, Germany. [2]Institute for Statutory Accident Insurance and Prevention in the Health and Welfare Services (BGW), Department of Occupational Health Research, Hamburg, Germany. [3]University Medical Center Hamburg-Eppendorf, Institute for Health Service Research in Dermatology and Nursing, Martinistrasse 52, 20246 Hamburg, Germany.

References

1. Bash DS, Farber RS: **An examination of self-reported carpal tunnel syndrome symptoms in hand therapists, protective and corrective measures and job satisfaction.** *Work* 1999, 13:75–82.
2. Bork BE, Cook TM, Rosecrance JC, Engelhardt KA, Thomason ME, Wauford IJ, Worley RK: **Work-related musculoskeletal disorders among physical therapists.** *Phys Ther* 1996, **76**:827–835.
3. Campo M, Weiser S, Koenig KL, Nordin M: **Work-related musculoskeletal disorders in physical therapists: a prospective cohort study with 1-year follow-up.** *Phys Ther* 2008, **88**:608–619.
4. Cromie JE, Robertson VJ, Best MO: **Work-related musculoskeletal disorders and the culture of physical therapy.** *Phys Ther* 2002, **82**:459–472.
5. Grooten WJA, Wernstedt P, Campo M: **Work-related musculoskeletal disorders in female Swedish physical therapists with more than 15 years of job experience:Prevalence and associations with work exposures.** *Physiotherapy Theory and Practice* 2011, **27**:213–222.
6. Passier L, McPhail S: **Work related musculoskeletal disorders amongst therapists in physically demanding roles: qualitative analysis of risk factors and strategies for prevention.** *BMC Musculoskelet Disord* 2011, **12**:24.
7. Campo MA, Weiser S, Koenig KL: **Job strain in physical therapists.** *Phys Ther* 2009, **89**:946–956.
8. Gröbel S: **Psychosoziale Belastungen von PhysiotherapeutInnen. Querschnittsstudie zur Arbeitsbelastung mittels des Copenhagen Psychosocial Questionnaire.** *pt Zeitschrift für Physiotherapeuten* 2008, **60**(10):1068–1087.
9. Dulon M, Peters C, Wendeler D, Nienhaus A: **Trends in occupational airway diseases in german hairdressers: Frequency and causes.** *Am J Ind Med* 2011, **54**:486–493.
10. Nienhaus A, Kesavachandran C, Wendeler D, Haamann F, Dulon M: **Infectious diseases in healthcare workers - an analysis of the standardised data set of a German compensation board.** *J Occup Med Toxicol* 2012, **7**:8.

11. Nienhaus A, Schablon A, Preisser AM, Ringshausen FC, Diel R: **Tuberculosis in healthcare workers - a narrative review from a German perspective.** *J Occup Med Toxicol* 2014, **9**:9.
12. Deutscher Verband für Physiotherapie (ZVK) e.V: **Hier finden Sie Physiotherapiepraxen und freiberuflich tätige Physiotherapeuten in Ihrer Nähe.** https://www.physio-deutschland.de/patienten-interessierte/physiotherapeutensuche.html. 2014. 25-8-2014.
13. Kristensen TS, Hannerz H, Hogh A, Borg V: **The Copenhagen Psychosocial Questionnaire–a tool for the assessment and improvement of the psychosocial work environment.** *Scand J Work Environ Health* 2005, **31**:438–449.
14. Pejtersen JH, Kristensen TS, Borg V, Bjorner JB: **The second version of the Copenhagen Psychosocial Questionnaire.** *Scand J Public Health* 2010, **38**:8–24.
15. Nübling M, Stössel U, Michaelis M: **Messung von Führungsqualität und Belastungen am Arbeitsplatz: Die deutsche Standardversion des COPSOQ (Copenhagen Psychosocial Questionnaire).** In *Fehlzeiten-Report 2009*. Edited by Badura B, Schröder H, Klose J, Macco K. Berlin Heidelberg: Springer; 2010:253–261.
16. Nübling M, Stößel U, Hasselhorn HM, Michaelis M, Hofmann F: *Methoden zur Erfassung psychischer Belastungen - Erprobung eines Messinstrumentes (COPSOQ)*. Dortmund/Berlin/Dresden: Wirtschaftsverlag NW, Verlag für neue Wissenschaften; 2005.
17. Kersten M, Kozak A, Wendeler D, Paderow L, Nübling M, Nienhaus A: **Psychological stress and strain on employees in dialysis facilities: a cross-sectional study with the Copenhagen psychosocial questionnaire.** *J Occup Med Toxicol* 2014, **9**:4.
18. Kozak A, Kersten M, Schillmöller Z, Nienhaus A: **Psychosocial work-related predictors and consequences of personal burnout among staff working with people with intellectual disabilities.** *Res Dev Disabil* 2013, **34**:102–115.
19. Ilmarinen J: **The Work Ability Index (WAI).** *Occup Med (Lond)* 2007, **57**:160.
20. Cromie JE, Robertson VJ, Best MO: **Occupational health in physiotherapy: General health and reproductive outcomes.** *Aust J Physiother* 2002, **48**:287–294.
21. Nienhaus A, Costa JT: **Screening for tuberculosis and the use of a borderline zone for the interpretation of the interferon-gamma release assay (IGRA) in Portuguese healthcare workers.** *J Occup Med Toxicol* 2013, **8**:1.
22. Ringshausen FC, Schablon A, Nienhaus A: **Interferon-gamma release assays for the tuberculosis serial testing of health care workers: a systematic review.** *J Occup Med Toxicol* 2012, **7**:6.
23. Cromie JE, Robertson VJ, Best MO: **Work-related musculoskeletal disorders in physical therapists: prevalence, severity, risks, and responses.** *Phys Ther* 2000, **80**:336–351.
24. Jäger M, Luttmann A, Bolm-Audorff U, Schäfer K, Hartung E, Kuhn S, Paul R, Francks H-P: **Mainz-Dortmunder Dosismodell (MDD) zur Beurteilung der Belastung der LWS durch Heben oder Tragen schwerer Lasten oder durch Tätigkeiten in extremer Rumpfbeugehaltung bei Verdacht auf Berufskrankheit Nr. 2108 - Teil 1: Retrospektive Berlastungsermittlung für risikobehaftete Tätigkeitsfelder.** *Arbeitsmed Sozialmed Umweltmed* 1999, **34**:101–111.
25. Denton MA, Zeytinoglu IU, Davies S: **Working in clients' homes: the impact on the mental health and well-being of visiting home care workers.** *Home Health Care Serv Q* 2002, **21**:1–27.
26. Snodgrass SJ, Rivett DA, Chiarelli P, Bates AM, Rowe LJ: **Factors related to thumb pain in physiotherapists.** *Aust J Physiother* 2003, **49**:243–250.
27. McMahon M, Stiller K, Trott P: **The prevalence of thumb problems in Australian physiotherapists is high: an observational study.** *Aust J Physiother* 2006, **52**:287–292.
28. Girbig M, Deckert S, Kopkow C, Latza U, Dulon M, Nienhaus A, Groneberg D, Seidler A: **Work-related complaints and diseases of physical therapists - protocol for the establishment of a "Physical Therapist Cohort" (PTC) in Germany.** *J Occup Med Toxicol* 2013, **8**:34.
29. Campo M, Darragh AR: **Impact of work-related pain on physical therapists and occupational therapists.** *Phys Ther* 2010, **90**:905–920.
30. Harris LM, Cumming SR, Campbell AJ: **Stress and psychological well-being among allied health professionals.** *J Allied Health* 2006, **35**:198–207.
31. Santos MC, Barros L, Carolino E: **Occupational stress and coping resources in physiotherapists: a survey of physiotherapists in three general hospitals.** *Physiotherapy* 2010, **96**:303–310.
32. Pavlakis A, Raftopoulos V, Theodorou M: **Burnout syndrome in Cypriot physiotherapists: a national survey.** *BMC Health Serv Res* 2010, **10**:63.
33. Burtchen I: **Berufsbedingte Belastungen von Physiotherapeuten und ihre Bewältigung.** *Zeitschrift für Physiotherapeuten* 2006, **58**:2–5.
34. Speakman HG, Pleasant JM, Sutton GB: **The job satisfaction of physical therapists.** *Physiother Res Int* 1996, **1**:247–254.
35. Gröbel S: **Fühlen Sie sich heute erschöpft? Wenn Arbeitsanforderungen zur Belastung werden.** *pt Zeitschrift für Physiotherapeuten* 2008, **60**:1134–1137.
36. Randolph DS: **Predicting the effect of extrinsic and intrinsic job satisfaction factors on recruitment and retention of rehabilitation professionals.** *J Healthc Manag* 2005, **50**:49–60.
37. Neubauer I: **Arbeitszufriedenheit von Physiotherapeuten.** *physioscience* 2005, **1**:72–80.
38. Karasek RA: **Job demands, job decision latitude, and mental strain: Implications job redesign.** *Adm Sci Q* 1979, **24**:285–308.
39. Friedel H, Orfeld O: **Das Anforderungs-Kontroll Modell: Psychische Belastungen am Arbeitsplatz sind einfach zu ermitteln.** *Die BKK Zeitschrift für die betrieblichen Krankenkassen* 2002, **90**(2):50–54. Essen.
40. Peter R: **Berufliche Gratifikationskrisen und Gesundheit.** *Psychotherapeut* 2002, **47**:386–398.
41. Bundesministerium für Bildung und Forschung: **Richtlinie des Gemeinsamen Bundesausschusses über die Verordnung von Heilmitteln in der vertragsärztlichen Versorgung (Heilmittel-Richtlinie/HeilM-RL) in der Fassung vom 20. Januar 2011 /19. Mai 2011 in Kraft getreten am 1. Juli 2011.** *Bundesanzeiger* 2011, **4**:2247–2311.
42. Bergmann E, Menzel R, Bergmann KE, Bergmann RL: **Verbreitung von Übergewicht in der Bundesrepublik Deutschland.** In *Tätigkeitsbericht 1990 des Bundesgesundheitsamtes*, Volume 1990. Edited by Bundesgesundheitsamt. Verlag GmbH München: MMV Medizin; 1990:221–224.
43. Takeuchi R, O'Brien MM, Ormond KB, Brown SD, Maly MR: **"Moving Forward": Success from a Physiotherapist's Point of View.** *Physiother Can* 2008, **60**:19–29.
44. Eker L, Tuzun EH, Daskapan A, Surenkok O: **Predictors of job satisfaction among physiotherapists in Turkey.** *J Occup Health* 2004, **46**:500–505.
45. Barnes MR, Crutchfield CA: **Job satisfaction-dissatisfaction. A comparison of private practitioners and organizational physical therapists.** *Phys Ther* 1977, **57**:35–41.

Permissions

All chapters in this book were first published in JOMT, by BioMed Central; hereby published with permission under the Creative Commons Attribution License or equivalent. Every chapter published in this book has been scrutinized by our experts. Their significance has been extensively debated. The topics covered herein carry significant findings which will fuel the growth of the discipline. They may even be implemented as practical applications or may be referred to as a beginning point for another development.

The contributors of this book come from diverse backgrounds, making this book a truly international effort. This book will bring forth new frontiers with its revolutionizing research information and detailed analysis of the nascent developments around the world.

We would like to thank all the contributing authors for lending their expertise to make the book truly unique. They have played a crucial role in the development of this book. Without their invaluable contributions this book wouldn't have been possible. They have made vital efforts to compile up to date information on the varied aspects of this subject to make this book a valuable addition to the collection of many professionals and students.

This book was conceptualized with the vision of imparting up-to-date information and advanced data in this field. To ensure the same, a matchless editorial board was set up. Every individual on the board went through rigorous rounds of assessment to prove their worth. After which they invested a large part of their time researching and compiling the most relevant data for our readers.

The editorial board has been involved in producing this book since its inception. They have spent rigorous hours researching and exploring the diverse topics which have resulted in the successful publishing of this book. They have passed on their knowledge of decades through this book. To expedite this challenging task, the publisher supported the team at every step. A small team of assistant editors was also appointed to further simplify the editing procedure and attain best results for the readers.

Apart from the editorial board, the designing team has also invested a significant amount of their time in understanding the subject and creating the most relevant covers. They scrutinized every image to scout for the most suitable representation of the subject and create an appropriate cover for the book.

The publishing team has been an ardent support to the editorial, designing and production team. Their endless efforts to recruit the best for this project, has resulted in the accomplishment of this book. They are a veteran in the field of academics and their pool of knowledge is as vast as their experience in printing. Their expertise and guidance has proved useful at every step. Their uncompromising quality standards have made this book an exceptional effort. Their encouragement from time to time has been an inspiration for everyone.

The publisher and the editorial board hope that this book will prove to be a valuable piece of knowledge for researchers, students, practitioners and scholars across the globe.

List of Contributors

Paul T. J. Scheepers and Arné Oerlemans
Research Lab Molecular Epidemiology, Radboud Institute for Health Sciences, Radboudumc, 6500 HB Nijmegen, The Netherlands

Eline van Daalen
Research Lab Molecular Epidemiology, Radboud Institute for Health Sciences, Radboudumc, 6500 HB Nijmegen, The Netherlands
Present address: Ministry of Social Affairs and Employment, The Hague, The Netherlands

Robbert Cremers
Research Lab Molecular Epidemiology, Radboud Institute for Health Sciences, Radboudumc, 6500 HB Nijmegen, The Netherlands
Witteveen+Bos Consulting, The Hague, The Netherlands

Lucie Masen-Poos and Bonne Biesma
Department of Lung Diseases, Jeroen Bosch Hospital, 's-Hertogenbosch, The Netherlands

Frits G. B. G. J. van Rooy
Arbo Unie Expert Centre for Chemical Risk Management, Utrecht, The Netherlands

Hera Lichtenbeld
Oxility BV, Best, The Netherlands

Jorid B. Sørli, Ismo K. Koponen, Søren Thor Larsen, Peder Wolkoff and Asger W. Nørgaard
The National Research Centre for the Working Environment, Copenhagen, Denmark

Albert Nienhaus
Center of Excellence for Epidemiology and Health Services Research for Healthcare Professionals (CVcare), Institute for Health Service Research in Dermatology and Nursing, University Medical Center Hamburg-Eppendorf, Hamburg, Germany
Principles of Prevention and Rehabilitation Department (GPR), Institute for Statutory Accident Insurance and Prevention in the Health and Welfare Services (BGW), Hamburg, Germany

Paolo Chiodini
Medical Statistics Unit, Second University of Naples, Naples, Italy

Maria W G Nijhuis-van der Sanden
Radboud Institute for Health Sciences, IQ Healthcare, Radboud University Medical Center, Nijmegen, The Netherlands

Nathan Hutting and J Bart Staal
Radboud Institute for Health Sciences, IQ Healthcare, Radboud University Medical Center, Nijmegen, The Netherlands
Research Group Occupation and Health, HAN University of Applied Sciences, Nijmegen 6503 GL, The Netherlands

Josephine A Engels and Yvonne F Heerkens
Research Group Occupation and Health, HAN University of Applied Sciences, Nijmegen 6503 GL, The Netherlands

Marcial Velasco Garrido, Cordula Bittner, Volker Harth and Alexandra Marita Preisser
Institute for Occupational Medicine and Maritime Medicine (ZfAM), University Medical Center Hamburg-Eppendorf, Seewartenstrasse 10, 20459 Hamburg, Germany

Uwe Rose
Federal Institute of Occupational Safety and Health (FIOSH), Nöldnerstrasse 40-42, 10317 Berlin, Germany

Stefanie March
Institute of Social Medicine and Health Economics, Otto-von-Guericke-University of Magdeburg, Leipziger Str. 44, 39120 Magdeburg, Germany

Melanie Ebener and Jean-Baptist du Prel
Institute for Safety Engineering, University of Wuppertal, Gaußstr. 20, 42119 Wuppertal, Germany

Heather P. Lampel
Department of Dermatology, Duke University, Durham, North Carolina, USA

Susan Mwamungule, Henry Mwelwa Chimana and Geoffrey Kwenda
Department of Biomedical Sciences, School of Medicine, University of Zambia, Lusaka, Zambia

Sydney Malama
Health Promotions Unit, Institute of Economic and Social Research, University of Zambia, Lusaka, Zambia

Geoffrey Mainda and John Bwalya Muma
Department of Disease Control, School of Veterinary Medicine, University of Zambia, Lusaka, Zambia

Stefanie Schönrock, Anja Schablon and Claudia Peters
University Medical Center Hamburg-Eppendorf (UKE), Institute for Health Services Research in Dermatology and Nursing (CVcare), Martinistrasse 52, 20246 Hamburg, Germany

Albert Nienhaus
University Medical Center Hamburg-Eppendorf (UKE), Institute for Health Services Research in Dermatology and Nursing (CVcare), Martinistrasse 52, 20246 Hamburg, Germany
Department of Occupational Health Research, Institute for Statutory Accident Insurance and Prevention in the Health and Welfare Services (BGW), Hamburg, Germany

Abdulrahman Hamad Alrashed, Abdulrahman Abdulaziz Almana, Yazeed Ibrahim Altheiban, Mohammed Saud Aldosari, Nawaf Faleh Almudarra and Sulaiman Ali Alwabel
Department of Physiology, College of Medicine, King Saud University, Riyadh, Kingdom of Saudi Arabia

Sultan Ayoub Meo
Department of Physiology, College of Medicine, King Saud University, Riyadh, Kingdom of Saudi Arabia
Clinical Physiology, Department of Physiology (29), College of Medicine, King Khalid University Hospital, King Saud University, Riyadh 11461, Saudi Arabia

Tiina Föhr and Urho M. Kujala
Department of Health Sciences, University of Jyväskylä, FIN-40014 Jyväskylä, Finland

Asko Tolvanen
Methodology Centre for Human Sciences, Faculty of Social Sciences, University of Jyväskylä, FIN-40014 Jyväskylä, Finland

TeroMyllymäki and Raimo Lappalainen
Department of Psychology, University of Jyväskylä, FIN-40014 Jyväskylä, Finland

Elina Järvelä-Reijonen and Marjukka Kolehmainen
Institute of Public Health and Clinical Nutrition, University of Eastern Finland, Kuopio Campus, FIN-70211 Kuopio, Finland

Sanni Rantala, Riitta Korpela and Katri Peuhkuri
Medical Faculty, Pharmacology, Medical nutrition physiology, University of Helsinki, FIN-00014 Helsinki, Finland

Sampsa Puttonen
Finnish Institute of Occupational Health, Topeliuksenkatu 41 a A, FIN-00250 Helsinki, Finland
Institute of Behavioral Sciences, University of Helsinki, FIN-00014 Helsinki, Finland

Heikki Rusko
Department of Biology of Physical Activity, University of Jyväskylä, FIN-40014 Jyväskylä, Finland

Carlos Pérez-Diaz
Infectious Diseases Department, Clinica Marly, Bogotá, Colombia
Infectious Diseases Department, Hospital de la Samaritana, Bogotá, Colombia
Servicios y asesorías en infectología (SAI), Calle 50 # 13-62, 110231420, Bogotá, Colombia

Omar-Javier Calixto, Juan S. Bravo-Ojeda, Erika Uribe-Pardo, Yesid F. Mantilla-Florez, Fabian Benitez and Ada Duran
Servicios y asesorías en infectología (SAI), Calle 50 # 13-62, 110231420, Bogotá, Colombia

Álvaro A. Faccini-Martínez
Servicios y asesorías en infectología (SAI), Calle 50 # 13-62, 110231420, Bogotá, Colombia
School of Medicine, Universidad de la Sabana, Chia, Colombia

Carlos A. Botero-García
School of Medicine, Universidad Militar Nueva Granada, Bogotá, Colombia

Johana Osorio
School of Medicine, Fundación Universitaria Navarra, Neiva, Colombia

Terence Khai Wei Tay, Han Zhe Chan, Tunku Sara Tunku Ahmad, Kok Kheng Teh, Tze Hau Low and Nuraliza Ab Wahab
Department of Orthopaedic Surgery, Faculty of Medicine, University of Malaya, 50603 Kuala Lumpur, Malaysia

Anne Kristin Møller Fell
Department of Occupational and Environmental Medicine, Telemark Hospital, Ulefossveien 55, Skien 3710, Norway

Steffen Roth
Department of Occupational and Environmental Medicine, Telemark Hospital, Ulefossveien 55, Skien 3710, Norway
Department of Occupational and Environmental Medicine, University Hospital of North Norway, Tromsø, Norway

Peter Grešner, Radosław Świercz, Magdalena Beata Król, Ewa Twardowska, Jolanta Gromadzińska and Wojciech Wąsowicz
Department of Toxicology and Carcinogenesis, Nofer Institute of Occupational Medicine, 8, Sw. Teresy str., 91-348 Lodz, Poland

Katrin Bossmann, Sabine Bach, Conny Höflich, Anett Neumann, Wolfgang Straff and Katrin Süring
Environmental Medicine and Health Effects Assessment, Federal Environment Agency, Corrensplatz 1, 14195 Berlin, Germany

Kerttu Valtanen
Microbiological Risk Assessment, Federal Environment Agency, Corrensplatz 1, 14195 Berlin, Bossmann et al. Journal of Occupational Medicine and Toxicology Germany

Rita Heinze
Toxicology of drinking water, Federal Environment Agency, Heinrich-Heine-Str. 12, 08645 Bad Elster, Germany

Elia Noemi Gallegos Morales, Johannes Knierer, Anja Schablon and Jan Felix Kersten
Center of Excellence for Health Services Research in Nursing (CVcare), University Medical Center Hamburg-Eppendorf (UKE), Hamburg, Germany

Albert Nienhaus
Center of Excellence for Health Services Research in Nursing (CVcare), University Medical Center Hamburg-Eppendorf (UKE), Hamburg, Germany
Institute for Statutory Accident Insurance and Prevention in the Health and Welfare Services (BGW), Hamburg, Germany

Christian Eisenhawer, Michael K. Felten and Thomas Kraus
Institute of Occupational and Social Medicine, RWTH Aachen University, Pauwelsstraße 30, 52074 Aachen, Germany

Thomas Hager
Institute of Pathology, University Hospital of Essen, University of Duisburg-Essen, Hufelandstraße 55, 45147 Essen, Germany

Mikhail Gronostayskiy
Division of Thoracic Surgery, West German Lung Center, Ruhrlandklinik, University Hospital Essen, Tüschener Weg 40, 45239 Essen, Germany

Philipp Bruners
Department of Diagnostic Radiology, RWTH Aachen University, Pauwelsstraße 30, 52074 Aachen, Germany

Andrea Tannapfel
Department of Pathology, Ruhr-University Bochum, Bürkle de la Camp-Platz 1, 44789 Bochum, Germany

A. Romaniuk, M. Lyndin, V. Sikora
Department of pathology, Sumy State University, st. Privokzalnaya, 31, Sumy Postal code 40022, Ukraine

Y. Lyndina
Department of normal anatomy, Sumy State University, Sumy, Ukraine

S. Romaniuk
Cardiology department of Sumy regional hospital, Sumy, Ukraine

K. Sikora
Sumy Regional Clinical Perinatal Center, Sumy, Ukraine

Alexander Gerber, Doris Klingelhoefer, David A Groneberg and Matthias Bundschuh
Institute of Occupational, Social and Environmental Medicine, Goethe-University, Theodor-Stern-Kai 7, Haus 9b, Frankfurt am Main 60590, Germany

Monica Lamberti, Rossella Uccello, Maria Grazia Lourdes Monaco, Mariarosaria Muoio, Daniela Feola and Nicola Sannolo
Department of Experimental Medicine, Section of Hygiene, Occupational Medicine and Forensic, Medicine, Second University of Naples, Naples, Italy

Michael K Felten, Lars Knoll, Christian Schikowsky and Thomas Kraus
Institute of Occupational and Social Medicine, Medical Faculty, RWTH Aachen University, Aachen, Germany

Marco Das
Department of Diagnostic Radiology, Medical Faculty, RWTH Aachen University, Aachen, Germany
Department of Radiology, Maastricht University Medical Centre, Maastricht, Netherlands

Kurt G Hering
Department of Diagnostic Radiology, Knappschaftskrankenhaus, Dortmund, Germany

Alfred Böcking
Institute of Cytopathology, Heinrich Heine University, Düsseldorf, Germany
Institute of Pathology, Düren Hospital, Düren, Germany

Sintayehu Daba Wami, Daniel Haile Chercos, Awrajaw Dessie, Zemichael Gizaw, Atalay Getachew, Tesfaye Hambisa, Tadese Guadu, Dawit Getachew and Bikes Destaw
Department of Environmental and Occupational Health and Safety, Institute of Public Health, University of Gondar, Gondar, Ethiopia

Eileen M. Wanke David A. Groneberg
Institute of Occupational, Social and Environmental Medicine, Goethe-University Frankfurt Main, Theodor-Stern-Kai 7, 60590 Frankfurt am Main, Germany

Julia Schreiter and Burkhard Weisser
Department Sports Medicine and Training Science, Christian-Albrechts-Universität Kiel, Institute of Sports Science, Olshausenstrasse 74, 24098 Kiel, Germany

Martin Rüegger, Doreen Droste, Markus Hofmann, Marcel Jost and David Miedinger
Department of Occupational Medicine, Swiss National Insurance Fund Suva, Fluhmattstr. 1, CH 6002 Lucerne, Switzerland

Tiina Teisala, Sara Mutikainen, Mirva Rottensteiner and Urho M Kujala
Department of Health Sciences, University of Jyväskylä, Jyväskylä FIN-40014, Finland

Asko Tolvanen
Methodology Centre for Human Sciences, Faculty of Social Sciences, University of Jyväskylä, Jyväskylä FI-40014, Finland

Tuija Leskinen
Turku PET Centre, University of Turku, Kiinamyllynkatu 4-8, Turku FIN-20520, Finland

Jaakko Kaprio
Hjelt Institute, Department of Public Health, University of HelsinkiHelsinki FI-00014, Finland
Department of Mental Health and Substance Abuse Services, National Institute for Health and Welfare, Helsinki FI-00300, Finland
Institute for Molecular Medicine (FIMM), University of Helsinki, Helsinki FI-00014, Finland

Marjukka Kolehmainen
Institute of Public Health and Clinical Nutrition, Clinical Nutrition, University of Eastern Finland, Kuopio Campus, Joensuu FIN-70211, Finland

Heikki Rusko
Department of Biology of Physical Activity, University of Jyväskylä, Jyväskylä FIN-40014, Finland

Hamzeh Al Zabadi
Public Health Department, Faculty of Medicine and Health Sciences, An-Najah National University, West Bank, Nablus, Palestine
Master of Public Health Program, Faculty of Graduate studies, An-Najah National University, Nablus, Palestine

Yaser Nazzal
Master of Public Health Program, Faculty of Graduate studies, An-Najah National University, Nablus, Palestine

Christian Feldhaus
RWE Power AG, Essen, Germany

Birte Brattig, Anja Schablon and Claudia Peters
University Medical Center Hamburg-Eppendorf (UKE), Institute for Health Services Research in Dermatology and Nursing (CVcare), Hamburg, Germany

Albert Nienhaus
University Medical Center Hamburg-Eppendorf (UKE), Institute for Health Services Research in Dermatology and Nursing (CVcare), Hamburg, Germany
Institute for Statutory Accident Insurance and Prevention in the Health and Welfare Services (BGW), Department of Occupational Health Research, Hamburg, Germany
University Medical Center Hamburg-Eppendorf, Institute for Health Service Research in Dermatology and Nursing, Martinistrasse 52, 20246 Hamburg, Germany

Index